The Vocal Athlete

The Vocal Athlete

Wendy D. LeBorgne, PhD, CCC-SLP

Marci Daniels Rosenberg, BM, MS, CCC-SLP

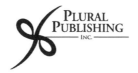

PLURAL PUBLISHING INC.

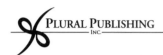

5521 Ruffin Road
San Diego, CA 92123

e-mail: info@pluralpublishing.com
Web site: http://www.pluralpublishing.com

Copyright © by Plural Publishing, Inc. 2014

Typeset in 10½ x 13 Garamond by Achorn International
Printed in the United States of America by McNaughton & Gunn, Inc.

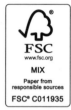

Illustration by Maury Aaseng. Copyright © 2013 Maury Aaseng. The authors give their thanks.

Library of Congress Cataloging-in-Publication Data

LeBorgne, Wendy DeLeo, author.
    The vocal athlete / Wendy D. LeBorgne, Marci Daniels Rosenberg.
        p. ; cm.
    Includes bibliographical references and index.
    ISBN 978-1-59756-458-8 (alk. paper)
    ISBN 1-59756-458-3 (alk. paper)
    I. Rosenberg, Marci Daniels, author.   II. Title.
    [DNLM: 1. Singing–physiology. 2. Voice Training. WV 501]
    QP306
    612.7'8—dc23
                                                2014005084

Contents

Preface

Meeting Industry Demands of the 21st-Century Vocal Athlete

Through our years of professional singing, training, and performance (resulting in an evolution to become voice pathologists and singing voice specialists), we have encountered a transition in the industry demands and injuries of the 21st-century vocal athlete. Today's commercial music industry demands versatility of vocal athletes who are now expected to be skilled in multiple styles of singing. Not only are these singers asked to perform vocal gymnastics on an eight-show per week schedule, these vocal athletes must also possess excellent acting skills and strong dancing ability to be competitive. These demands on the voice, body, and psyche necessitate a physically, vocally, and mentally fit singer who is agile and adaptable.

In a time when major opera companies are closing their doors, the commercial music industry boasts millions of viewers on a weekly basis through mainstream media outlets (e.g., "The Voice," "American Idol," "X-Factor"). Broadway shows grossed over 400 million dollars in 2012. And in the pop music market, in 2012 alone, physical albums, digital albums, and digital songs surpassed 1.65 billion units indicating a strong public desire and potentially lucrative business for commercial music singers. Yet, there are only two exclusively nonclassical vocal pedagogy training programs in the United States as of this writing. Therefore, these vocal athletes learn their craft by relying on god-given talent, they make their way by imitation, or they study with a voice teacher who may or may not have experience or training in the commercial music genre. Some of these choices may unfortunately lead to vocal problems if they cannot withstand demands of the profession. By no means do we suggest that classical voice pedagogy is not a valid and proven effective method of vocal training. However, even though running is part of a gymnastics floor routine, it would be unlikely that an Olympic gymnast would train exclusively with a running coach when he or she is required to perform backflips on a balance beam.

Similarly, this book was developed to aid singing teachers (of all genres), voice pathologists who work with singers, and the singers themselves in their understanding of the vocal mechanism, specific care of the body and instrument, and the science behind how we learn and how we can maximize performance for longevity in a commercial music market. Section I introduces the Structure and Function of the Voice as it applies to vocal athletes. Chapter 1 presents the mechanics, structure, and function of the singer's body, incorporating anatomy of body framework and the integration of movement and movement strategies for active performers. The next two chapters (Chapters 2 and 3) go beyond typical anatomy and physiology of the respiratory and laryngeal mechanisms. These chapters incorporate relevant research and functional utility of breath and sound production in the commercial music performer including topics on how dancers who sing use different breathing strategies and information on vocal fold vibration patterns in high demand voice users. Chapter 4 details the central command center (neurologic control) of the voice, from both a physical and emotional perspective. Included in Chapter 4 is information relevant to performance anxiety in vocal athletes. The final chapter (Chapter 5) in Section I sets up a basic understanding of vocal acoustics and resonance, and provides singers and teachers a user-friendly chapter on these often challenging topics using relevant singing illustrations.

As vocal health and fitness are paramount for amateur and elite vocal athletes for long-term careers, Section II—Vocal Health and Fitness, is devoted to providing a unique perspective on relevant topics for vocal athletes. Section II includes invited expert authors on the topics of: the impact of reflux on the singer (Chapter 7, Adam D. Rubin, MD, Cristina Jackson-Menaldi, PhD); what singers need to know when undergoing anesthesia (Chapter 8, Andrew Rosenberg, MD); and team members' roles on a multidisciplinary voice care team (Chapter 11, Leda Scearce, MM, MS). Chapter 6 details the how and why of phonotrauma on the vocal folds and provides insight into wound healing and injury prevention. The Life Cycle of the Voice (Chapter 9) provides an overview of the changes that happen to the singing voice throughout the lifespan with specific attention to the under 40 singers that populate the commercial music scene. Chapter 10 (Medicines, Myths, and Truths) confirms and dispels many of the common old wives' tales related to vocal health and hygiene, including tradition and alternative medical therapies.

The final section of this text (Section III—Vocal Pedagogy for the 21st Century Vocal Athlete) includes six unique chapters. These chapters span a review of both classical and belting pedagogy (Chapters 12 and 13) and the scientific studies on the how and why of belting in elite and student performers (Chapter 14). Currently, there is no book that incorporates this information into one text. The assumption that traditional classical pedagogy can support any style of singing is inconsistent with what singing science research is now showing about physiologic differences between classical and contemporary commercial music (CCM) styles of singing. Chapter 15 and Chapter 16 are based in how we learn and acquire new skills providing singing teachers (regardless of style) invaluable information on maximizing teaching and learner outcomes. The book concludes with an invited chapter on audio technology (Chapter 17, Matthew Edwards, BM, MM) and the understanding and use of current technology (e.g., microphones, sound boards, monitors) by every teacher and singer who sings in a commercial style.

We would be remiss without including functional exercises to develop and train the concepts discussed in this text. Therefore, over 60 exercises, from expert teachers all over the world, to accompany and parallel the concepts presented here are included in the sister workbook: *The Vocal Athlete: Application and Technique for the Hybrid Singer* by Rosenberg and LeBorgne, 2014.

Whether at the professional or novice level, or somewhere in between, there are limited resources for training commercial vocal styles relative to the number of singers who desire to sing. This book aims to provide scientifically based information without usurping the art of singing pedagogy to provide the 21st-century hybrid singer with a guide toward their goal of becoming a proficient and healthy CCM vocalist. This brings us back to the necessity for sound vocal instruction and technique to allow these singers to use their voices as safely as possible in order to promote vocal health in this group of singers who may already be at high-risk for encountering vocal problems.

This is now more important than ever, as musical theater and other CCM styles will continue to raise the bar for vocal performance demands. Composers will continue to be commissioned to write shows that will make money, especially during current economic strains when there is less willingness to finance works that aren't going to assure financial payoff. Therefore, singers will continue to be asked to "defy gravity" and generate more complex vocal acrobatics in order to stay employed. Ultimately, the CCM vocal athlete and teachers are charged with the task of providing voice students with a sound pedagogical technique that will (1) serve them well in their chosen vocal style, (2) allow the singer to cross over to varied vocal styles as demanded, and (3) promote vocal longevity and health.

hy•brid sing•er – (n). refers to the vocal athlete who is highly skilled performing in multiple vocal styles possessing a solid vocal technique that is responsive, adaptable, and agile in order to meet demands of current and ever-evolving vocal music industry genres.

Acknowledgments

This book would never have been possible without the support and mentorship of many people. My sincere appreciation to my first mentor in vocal pedagogy: Dr. Jeanette Ogg who sparked a lifelong love of voice science and pedagogy; my first mentor in voice therapy: Dr. Joseph Stemple who took me under his wing as a young clinician. Thank you to each and every vocal athlete with whom I have shared the stage or treated as a patient. You inspire an increased depth of understanding of the craft of musical theater and commercial music performance. To my physician and voice pathology colleagues at SOENTS, BBIVAR, the ENT Group, and ProVoice, thank you, Si, Steve, Jennifer K., Jennifer R., and Erin, you provide an ideal environment to learn and collaborate daily. Thanks to my mom, dad, and sister for your love. And finally, to Ed, Quinn, and Vaughn, this book would never have been possible without your constant hugs, love, and unwavering support.

—Dr. Wendy DeLeo LeBorgne

I have been fortunate to have had many mentors throughout the years beginning with some of my earliest voice teachers including Dr. Thom Houser, who inspired me to become a speech pathologist/singing voice specialist; Drs. Christy Ludlow and Ron Scherer were instrumental in my earlier development as a student of voice and speech science. Thank you to all of my colleagues at The University of Michigan, School of Music Theater and Dance, and the Departments of Speech Language Pathology and Otolaryngology, and specifically to Norman Hogikyan, Laryngologist. I have been so fortunate to be part of such an outstanding group of clinicians and professionals. I have truly treasured your collaboration and collegiality over the years. Most of all, thank you to all of my patients. You have taught me over the years how truly remarkable the voice is. I continue to learn daily from your lessons and am humbled to play a part in your voice rehabilitation. Finally, to my ever supportive husband Andrew and my beautiful daughters Lily and Charley. Without your constant support, love, and patience, this book could not have been written.

—Marci Daniels Rosenberg

We would sincerely like to thank Erin Donahue and Elizabeth Campbell for their time and critical proofreading of this book.

—Wendy DeLeo LeBorgne &
Marci Daniels Rosenberg

Contributors

Matthew Edwards, MM
Assistant Professor
Voice and Voice Pedagogy
Shenandoah University
Faculty
CCM Voice Pedagogy Institute
Winchester, Virginia
Chapter 17

Maria Cristina A. Jackson-Menaldi, PhD
Director
Lakeshore Professional Voice Center
Lakeshore Ear, Nose and Throat Center
Adjunct Full Professor
School of Medicine
Department of Otolaryngology
Wayne State University
St. Clair Shores, Michigan
Chapter 7

Wendy D. LeBorgne, PhD, CCC-SLP
Clinical Director
Voice Pathologist and Singing Voice
   Specialist
The Blaine Block Institute for Voice
   Analysis and Rehabilitation
Dayton, Ohio
ProVoice Center
Cincinnati, Ohio
Adjunct Assistant Professor
Musical Theatre-CCM/OMDA
Communication Sciences and Disorders,
   CAHS
Cincinnati, Ohio
*Chapters 1, 2, 3, 4, 5, 6, 9, 10, 12, 13, 14,
   15, 16*

Andrew Rosenberg, MD
University of Michigan
Ann Arbor, Michigan
Chapter 8

Marci Daniels Rosenberg, BM, MS, CCC-SLP
Speech-Language Pathologist
Voice and Singing Specialist
Vocal Health Center
Departments of Otolaryngology-
   Laryngology, Rhinology, and General
   Otolaryngology and Speech-Language
   Pathology
University of Michigan
Ann Arbor, Michigan
*Chapters 1, 2, 3, 4, 5, 6, 9, 10, 12, 13, 14,
   15, 16*

Adam D. Rubin, MD
Director
Lakeshore Professional Voice Center
Clinical Assistant Professor
Michigan State University
Adjunct Assistant Professor
University of Michigan
Department of Otolaryngology-Head and
   Neck Surgery
St. Clair Shores, Michigan
Chapter 7

Leda Scearce, MM, MS, CCC-SLP
Director
Performing Voice Programs and
   Development
Duke Voice Care Center
Division of Otolaryngology-Head and Neck
   Surgery
Duke Medical Center
Raleigh, North Carolina
Chapter 11

SECTION I

Structure and Function of the Voice

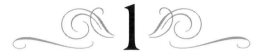

The Singer's Body: Alignment, Movement, and Intention

Introduction

Posture and alignment are among the foundational principles of good singing. Those who have had any sort of training as a singer have likely been taught about posture in some way or another. Singers are therefore aware that the vocal instrument extends beyond the throat. Often, the first impression of a performer is what the performer is conveying via his or her body and stance before we hear any sound. Vocal pedagogy emphasizes body alignment during singing, and most singers are aware of the important role that posture/alignment plays in optimal voice production and efficiency. Fortunately, voice and acting students have benefited from bodywork such as Alexander Technique™, Feldenkrais®, and pilates (to name a few) used to help establish and reinforce optimal musculoskeletal alignment and function at the most basic neuromuscular level.

Efficient use of the singer's body extends beyond good posture. In most styles of singing, including musical theater and opera, movement and/or dancing is incorporated into the performance. The task of the singer is to use the movement or dancing efficiently in order to serve the singing in a productive way, so that the two occur synergistically instead of existing as disparate entities working against one another. Often, the singer is also managing restricting costumes, moving set pieces, a raked stage, and pyrotechnics. Yet, voice lessons typically occur in a static environment with limited space to move. As a result, many singers learn to sing with good posture and alignment while standing somewhat still within the confines of the voice studio, but often are left to their own devices to navigate movement, choreography, and costumes when in a performance venue. This chapter discusses the basic anatomic and physiologic principles of posture and alignment. It also provides readers an overview to the many complementary and often essential methods used by many singers and actors to facilitate optimal voice production and performance when the desired alignment may be compromised. Relevant research findings on posture and alignment as it relates to the vocal athlete are reviewed.

Posture and Alignment

Consider what comes to mind when you think of your posture. Take a moment to stand erect and notice what you feel. What, in your mind, holds you upright? Do you balance on the balls of your feet, the heel, or on the center? Where do your ears lie relative to your shoulders? Is your chest collapsed, in a military stance, or neutral? How does your head feel balancing on your cervical spine? Are you actively holding your head up? Do you notice that you engage your neck strap muscles to assist in holding your head up? Now sing a short phrase of "Happy Birthday." Does your posture and/or muscular awareness change when singing is introduced? Physical awareness of the body during singing is important to maintain freedom and ease of both the voice and body. The singing student may not be aware of how the body is designed and put together, yet having a solid understanding the anatomy and physiology of the entire musculoskeletal system is an important part of learning good vocal technique and the impact that postural changes may have on vocal output.

Skeletal Structure

Put simply, the role of the skeleton is to provide the framework for the body and provide a place for origin or attachment of muscles. It is designed to efficiently distribute weight and work so that we can move freely without significant effort. When out of balance, the body system works less efficiently and voice production can be compromised. This section highlights some of the common locations for physical misalignment and concession of vocal technique as a result. Figure 1–1 shows a lateral view of the human skeleton. The figure was adapted for "What Every Singer Needs to Know About the Body"(Malde, 2009). Malde's book provides an extended resource for singers of all styles and is recommended for further reading regarding posture, alignment, and body mapping. The authors discuss in detail the six places of balance to facilitate optimal freedom of the body during singing. Imagine a vertical line traveling from head to the feet. The six places of balance, as described by Malde and colleagues (2009) include: (1) atlanto-occipital (A-O) joint, (2) arm structure, (3) thorax/lumbar spine, (4) hip joints, (5) knee joints, and (6) ankle joints. These areas all have dense sensory input to provide tactile feedback about how the body is moving.

The human head accounts for approximately 8% of the entire body mass and can average six to ten pounds. Adding a headpiece, wig, or mask will easily add a few more pounds for the cervical spine to support. The head is supported by the first cervical vertebra called the atlas, and this joins the bottom of the skull at the occiput via the atlanto-occipital joint (A-O joint), the first of the six places of balance. This is an important juncture because proper alignment of the head onto the cervical spine allows for freedom of movement of the head and neck without extraneous involvement of the neck strap muscles.

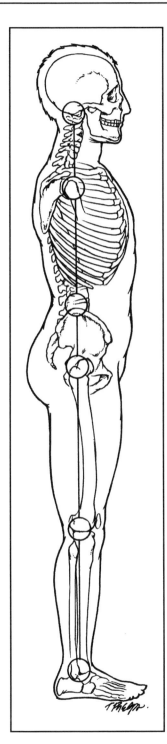

Figure 1–1. Places of balance skeleton, side view. By T. Phelps. Copyright 2008. Used with permission.

If a singer has extensive neck strap involvement during singing check to see if A-O alignment is off causing neck strap muscles to engage limiting freedom and range of motion both at rest and during singing.

When aligned, the A-O joint marks the middle of the skull. Figure 1–2 shows the head centrally aligned on the cervical spine. The cervical spine extends from the base of the skull down to the thoracic spine. The role of the cervical spine is to support the head. It contains seven vertebrae (C1–C7). The first two vertebrae (C1 and C2) allow for rotation of the neck (right and left), while C5–C7 allow for flexion (forward) and extension (backward). This portion of the spine houses and provides protection to the upper part of the spinal cord.

The thoracic spine refers to the upper and middle back. There are 12 vertebrae on the thoracic spine (T1–T12). Unlike the cervical spine, which is designed to be flexible, the thoracic spine trades flexibility for strength and stability in order to hold the body upright. The ribs are paired, with 12 ribs on each side. They are connected at each level of the thoracic vertebrae providing a protective cage for the lungs, heart, and other essential organs. The costal cartilage (Figure 1–3) connects the ribs to the sternum (breastbone). The sternocostal joints connect the cartilaginous portion of ribs two through six to the sternum. The expansion we are able to achieve with the ribs during inhalation is, in part related to the pliability of the costal cartilages. The costal cartilages will ossify (become more bone-like and less flexible) as we age. Thus rib cage expansion is decreased during the aging process. More detail about the

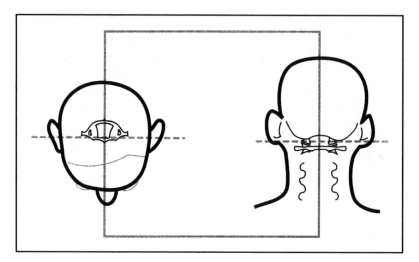

Figure 1–2. A-O joint location. By Conable. Copyright 2001. Used with permission.

skeletal and muscular structures of the ribs is discussed in the chapter on respiration.

The lumbar spine is commonly referred to as the lower back consisting of five vertebrae allowing for flexibility of this part of the spine. The vertebrae in the spinal column are connected with various ligaments and tendons, which further stabilize the spine and also prevent it from moving in a direction that is suboptimal or potentially injurious.

The pectoral girdle (or shoulder girdle), which includes the clavicle (collarbone) and scapula (shoulder blade) connects the arms to the axial (central) skeleton. The arms are not often thought of in terms of body alignment, but they play a crucial role in performance because the arms are involved in stability. Singers may use arm movement to add depth and communication to a performance by intentional movement and gesture, or the arms may hinder a performance by lying limply contributing nonintentional or distracting

movement. The pectoral girdle includes both the clavicle (collarbone) and the scapula (shoulder blade). These bony structures attach to the sternum via the sternoclavicular joint. The sternoclavicular joint extends out to the shoulder joint. At that point, the glenohumeral joint (shoulder joint) connects the pectoral girdle to the humerus (upper arm bone). The arm then extends to the elbow joint and finally wrist joints. These four joints allow for generous range of motion. Although one may not view the arms as having an impact on breathing, consider that the clavicle lies parallel to the floor and the clavicle and scapula are meant to suspend symmetrically over the spine and rib cage. Thus, aberrant posturing of the scapula, such as in a militaristic stance, can actually impede range of motion of the ribs during breathing (Malde, 2009).

The pelvic girdle which includes the following bony structures: sacrum, coccyx, ilium, ischium, and pubic bone, provides origins and attachments for muscles

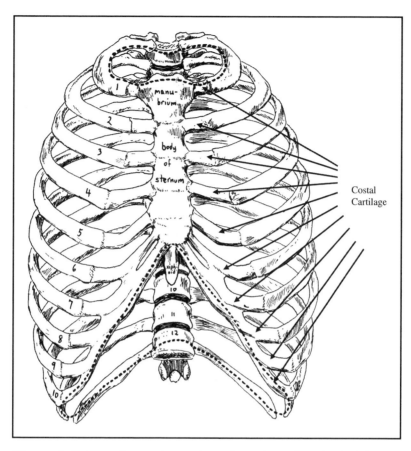

Figure 1–3. The ribs and costal cartilage (anterior view). Adapted from *The Body Moveable* (4th ed., p. 119), by D. Gorman, 2002, Ampersand Press.

that form the pelvic floor and lower abdomen. The pelvic girdle allows for the distribution of the weight of your upper body down to the femur, or thigh bone when standing. The head of the femur (thigh bone) articulates with the pelvic girdle at the acetabulum via a bulbous extension of the femur called the greater trochanter at the acetabulofemoral joint. This connection forms the hip joint and allows for rotation and movement of the upper portion of the leg and bending at the waist. It also serves as the connection from the lower limbs (legs) to the axial skeleton (spine). The leg consists of the femur (thigh bone), knee joint, the tibia (shin bone) and fibula (calf bone), the ankle joint, and the feet. A balanced stance below the knee requires that the points of balance above the knee be aligned. For further detail on anatomy discussed above, the reader is referred to "Atlas of Human Anatomy" (Netter, 1997) and "Clinically Oriented Anatomy" (Moore & Dalley, 2006).

> If a student is observed to have locked knees or rigid ankles, it may be advisable to evaluate alignment beginning from the top of the head and visually scanning down the body to assess where the posture breakdown occurs. If everything in the torso and upper body is appropriately aligned and balanced, the knees and ankles should also be balanced with evenly distributed weight.

Postural alignment of vocal athletes may be affected by costume design, set design, and physical character demands. One costume consideration that may significantly affect postural alignment and balance is the height and type of footwear worn by the performer. Vocal athletes often do not have much control over the type of shoe they wear. Therefore, it is advisable to do a significant amount of training and rehearsal in the type of shoe required to wear for performance in order to adjust alignment within those parameters, costume, character, and choreography demands. Heavy, bulky costumes, masks, and headpieces, may also require a period of physical adaptation for maximal performance.

In the realm of musical theater, choreography provides an added dimension to the physical demands placed on performers while engaging in high-level singing. Depending on the skill of the dancer and the intensity of the choreography and singing, compensation in alignment may result in a compromised vocal output. Triple threat performers must adapt to these physical demands and maintain core stability during singing and dancing to minimally alter physical alignment and posture. There is limited research on the impact of movement and dancing on voice because it is so difficult to measure.

Muscular Structures of the Neck

While the bony skeletal structures provide the framework for the human body, the muscles are responsible for positioning and movement. Efficient muscular balance is essential for optimal posture and voice production. The next segment reviews the primary muscles relevant for purposes of alignment and voice production (Moore & Dalley, 2006).

Extrinsic Laryngeal Muscles

Suprahyoid muscles—These muscles extend from the hyoid bone to the tongue base and play an important role in elevating the hyoid bone for swallowing and phonation. These muscles include the stylohyoid muscle, mylohyoid muscle, geniohyoid muscle, and digastric muscle. The latter three muscles also depress the mandible (lower jaw) when the hyoid bone is stabilized by the infrahyoid muscles. If the suprahyoid muscles become foreshortened or chronically tense, there is risk that the larynx will remain persistently high.

Infrahyoid muscles—These include the sternohyoid muscle, omohyoid muscle, sternothyroid muscle, and thyrohyoid muscle. These muscles each play a role in depressing (lowering) the hyoid bone and larynx for swallowing and phonation. Figures of these muscles can be viewed in Chapter 3 (phonation).

Constrictors—These include the superior, middle, and inferior constrictors that together form the sides and back wall of the pharynx (throat). These muscles narrow, or constrict the pharyngeal wall during swallowing and inadvertently can cause throat tightness during singing.

Deep Muscles of the Neck

Suboccipital muscles—These muscles extend and flex the head. Included in this group are the posterior, major, and minor rectus capitis muscles and the superior and inferior oblique capitis muscles. Trigger points of pain can occur in these muscles resulting from compensatory hyper flexion of the neck as when using binoculars or when wearing glasses that are not an accurate prescription. Supporting the head with the hand under the chin for long periods of time, as when sitting at a desk, can also foreshorten these muscles (Kostopoulos & Konstantine, 2001).

Anterior Neck Muscles—This group of muscles include the sternocleidomastoid muscle (SCM), levator scapulae muscle, trapezius muscle, and splenius capitis muscles. The SCM (see Chapter 3) extends the neck and allows for rotation of the head. Injury to this muscle can occur from a high-velocity movement such as whiplash, persistent forward neck posture, and inadequate support from a pillow. The levator scapulae muscle elevates scapula and the upper trapezius muscle stabilizes the scapula to help hold the shoulders up and back. Heavy shoulder bags or holding a phone between the shoulder and ear can created a prolonged stretch of the trapezius muscle (Kostopoulos & Konstantine, 2001). Splenius capitis muscle courses from the base of the skull to the seventh cervical vertebrae and the upper four thoracic vertebrae.

Jaw

The jaw is composed of the upper jaw (maxilla) and lower jaw (mandible). The mandible is a single, horseshoe-shaped bone that connects to the skull at the temporomandibular joint (TMJ). Figure 1–4 illustrates the temporomandibular joint. The TMJ is located directly in front of the ears. The primary muscles involved in closing the lower jaw are the masseter and the temporalis muscles. When the hyoid bone is stabilized by the infrahyoid muscles, the digastric muscles open the jaw, as do the geniohyoid and mylohyoid muscles. The lateral and medial pterygoid muscles allow the jaw to move from side to side.

The jaw muscles can contribute indirectly to laryngeal tension via the biomechanics of the suprahyoid muscles attaching to the hyoid bone inferiorly and the mandible and tongue superiorly (Cookman & Verdolini, 1999). The muscles of the jaw are innervated by cranial nerve V (trigeminal nerve) and the larynx is innervated by cranial nerve X (vagus nerve). Additionally, the possibility of neurological connections between the jaw and the larynx have been postulated at both the level of the brainstem and cortex (Luo, 1991; Travers, 1983; West, 1995).

Cookman and Verdolini investigated the relationship of mandibular activity and laryngeal function in 12 nonsingers. The authors looked at potential impact of jaw movement on vocal function, the relevance of jaw position or level of relaxation for impact on vocal function, and whether jaw opening impacts degree of vocal fold closure. All subjects repeated specific vocal tasks under various conditions altering jaw opening and level of bite pressure, and degree of vocal fold closure in the speaking range and in a higher range. Results of this study demonstrated the following: Increased jaw opening in the speaking range resulted in increased vocal fold closure, however jaw opening in the higher range yielded varied vocal fold closure results.

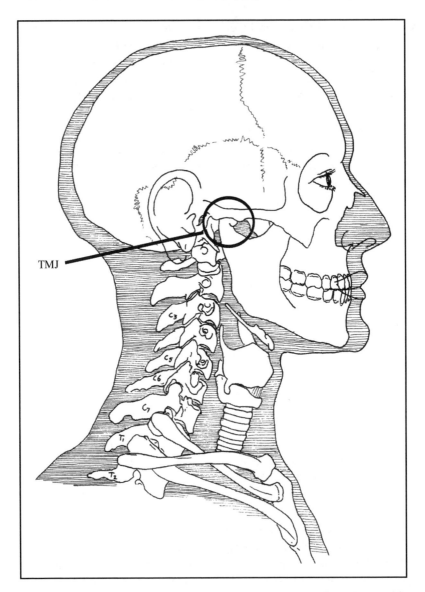

Figure 1–4. The temporomandibular joint. From *The Body Moveable* (4th ed., p. 152), by D. Gorman, 2002, Ampersand Press.

Biting gestures resulted in increased vocal fold closure in the speaking range for males regardless of the level of jaw opening. Additionally, females in this study demonstrated increased vocal fold closure at higher ranges when the jaw was in a relaxed, open state. The result that jaw opening increased vocal fold closure is contrary with both pedagogical and clinical thinking. The authors offer a biomechanical explanation for this contrary finding. They stated that perhaps the connection of the suprahyoid and submandibular muscular structures to the mandible allow for a compression and/or displacement of the larynx resulting in increased vocal fold closure. This study was completed on a small number of nonsingers and research findings are specific to this group. The results cannot necessarily be transferred to muscular patterns in a group of singers without further research into that specific population. Further research is required to confirm this finding over a larger subject pool of normal speakers and also in the singer population. Although done on a small group of subjects, this study is helpful to delineate the very complex biomechanical relationship between the larynx, jaw, and tongue.

Tongue

The tongue is considered the primary structure for articulation and therefore plays a vital role in speech and singing. Extending beyond what is visible in the mouth, singers are often surprised at how large the tongue is when anatomically diagramed. Biologically, the tongue's primary role is taste, chewing, and swallowing. It prepares and helps to move food posteriorly into the mouth to be swallowed. The tongue is divided into four regions: tip, blade, dorsum, and root. The tip is the anterior-most portion of the tongue, the blade is located behind the tip inferior to the alveolar ridge, and the dorsum is inferior to the soft palate. All of these structures are still visible within the oral cavity. The root of the tongue is the most posterior portion of the tongue (and is not visible in the oral cavity).

The muscles that comprise the tongue (glossus) are divided into extrinsic and in-trinsic muscles. There are four paired intrinsic muscles: (1) the superior longitudinal muscle which shortens the tongue and pulls the tip and lateral walls up—this muscle originates near the epiglottis and hyoid bone; (2) the inferior longitudinal muscle which makes up the undersurface of the tongue—it shortens the tongue and moves the tip and lateral sides of the tongue downward and also has fibers that connect to the styloglossus muscle; (3) the transverse muscle acts to flare the tongue like a fan and narrows and/or elongates the tongue; and (4) vertical muscle which flattens the tongue (Behrman, 2007). Figure 1–5 shows the intrinsic muscles of the tongue in both lateral and anterior frontal views.

The extrinsic muscles of the tongue are illustrated in Figure 1–6. These also include four paired muscle groups: (1) the genioglossus muscle is the largest and strongest of the extrinsic tongue muscles, and contraction of the posterior fibers protrudes the tongue forward. Conversely, contraction of the anterior fibers of the genioglossus muscle retracts the tongue. Contraction of both anterior and posterior fibers pulls the tongue down. The genioglossus muscle makes up the bulk of the tongue and attaches to the hyoid bone, (2) the styloglossus muscle is the antagonist to the genioglossus muscle and pulls the tongue up and forward during contraction. This muscle also pulls the side of the tongue upward, (3) the palatoglosus muscle serves both the tongue and soft palate elevating the tongue root. It also works with the styloglossus and genioglossus to create groove shape on the back of the tongue, and (4) the hyoglossus muscle originates at the hyoid bone and contraction of this muscle depresses and retracts the tongue. This muscle can also elevate the hyoid bone and larynx (Zemlin, 1998). Figure 1–7 shows a

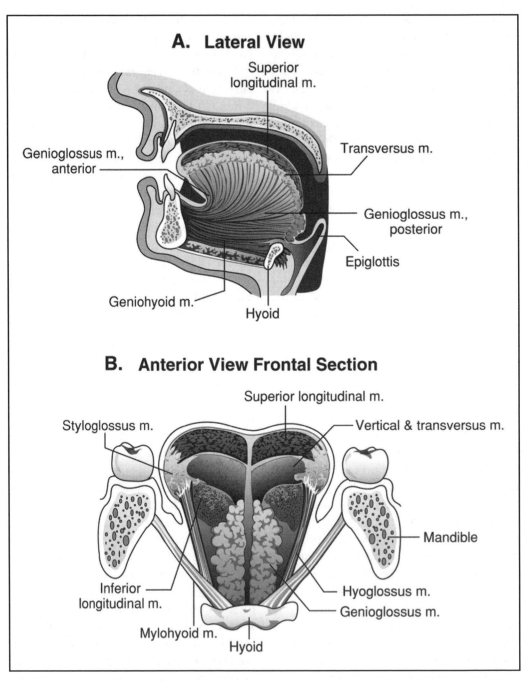

Figure 1–5. Complex intrinsic muscles of the tongue. From *Speech and Voice Science* (p. 266) by A. Behrman, 2013, Plural Publishing.

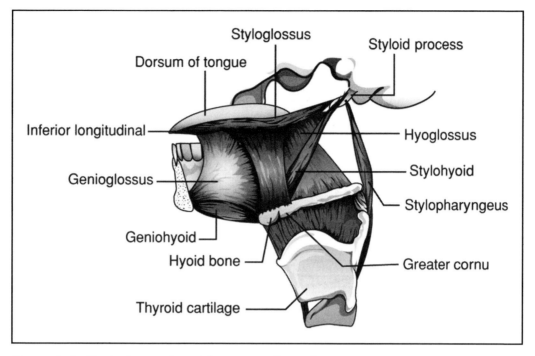

Figure 1–6. Extrinsic muscles of the tongue. From *Speech and Voice Science* (p. 266) by A. Behrman, 2013, Plural Publishing.

schematic representation of the functions of the muscles of the tongue.

Because the tongue is considered to be a soft compressible structure, movements in the anterior portion of the tongue can impact the tongue shape more posteriorly (Behrman, 2007). The fibers of the tongue muscles are to a degree interwoven with each other. As a result, varied parts of the tongue are used to articulate specific consonants. Changes in shape and tension of the tongue alter the resonating cavities resulting in different vowels.

Distorted vowels during singing and vocalizing can be an indication that there may be tongue tension present.

The importance in understanding the tongue and its relationship to the jaw and larynx cannot be underestimated for the vocal pedagogue, as the tongue and jaw are often implicated in technical problems. One common misconception associated with the tongue is that tongue and jaw movement are dependent on each other. Teachers often spend a significant amount of time fostering jaw/tongue independence, and this is well worth the time given the close biomechanical relationship between the tongue, jaw, and larynx.

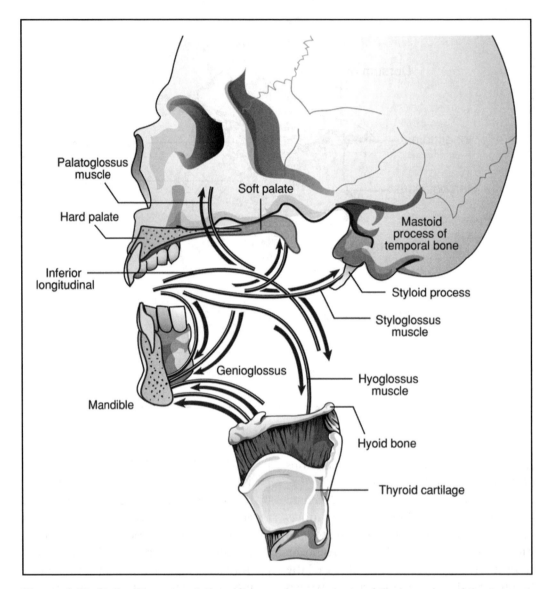

Figure 1–7. Stylized representation of general movements of the muscles of the tongue. From *Speech and Voice Science* (p. 265) by A. Behrman, 2013, Plural Publishing.

Assessing Posture and Alignment

Voice teachers and voice pathologists often address deviant posture and alignment when working with students or patients (respective to the profession). However, these professions typically do not receive formal training on how to complete a general physical assessment of posture and alignment. The research dedicated to the impact of posture and alignment on the singing voice is limited. Pertinent literature is reviewed below.

One of the seminal articles highlighting the importance of posture and head balance for singing was published in the early 1970s (Jones, 1972). In this paper, Jones discussed the utilization of Alexander Technique™ principles to increase awareness of releasing neck strap muscles during singing for a single female subject. A manual technique developed by Alexander was used in this study. It involved manually elongating the suboccipital muscles during singing to prevent them from foreshortening. The author used sound spectrograms during habitual neck position and again during manipulation. Jones reported improved resonance and sound quality perceptually and the singer reported improved tonal quality and increased ease of singing. The voice spectrograms demonstrated increased overtones during the manipulated tone production. Jones concluded, postural manipulation may be an effective teaching aid as it enhanced tonal quality, and increased student kinesthetic awareness of optimal head balance during singing. A limitation of this study was that the subject pool was limited to one, and results cannot be generalized to all singers. However, empirical pedagogical wisdom insinuates that optimizing head and neck balance may optimize voice production. More importantly, this article demonstrates that the value of posture and alignment in relation to optimal singing and voice production are not new concepts.

Sundberg, Leanderson, von Euler, and Knutsson (1991) examined the impact of body position and posture on subglottal pressure. These authors measured muscular activity of the intercostal muscles, diaphragm, and oblique muscles via surface electromyography (EMG) recordings on two baritone singers. The singers were asked to complete various vocal tasks including varying loudness, singing octave intervals, staccato, legato, and melismatic passages. They were asked to complete these tasks first upright, and then supine. Each singer began each task at nearly full lung volume and continued until lung volume was depleted. Results for these two subjects showed that they were able to compensate quickly and accurately for postural and lung volume changes, maintaining steady control over subglottal pressures during phonation. Each singer employed a unique breathing strategy, and this is consistent with other literature regarding the existence of more than one method of efficient respiration. Although these results cannot be generalized due to small number of subjects, they are consistent with what is seen and expect from performers in a variety of compromised postural circumstances (Sundberg, Leanderson, VonEuler, & Knutsson, 1991).

More recently, Schneider, Dennehy, and Saxon (1997) described the use of exercise physiology principles of overload, progressive muscular resistance, specificity, frequency, intensity, and endurance to promote optimal postural strength and balance. Within this paper, they delineate a series of exercises to strengthen the primary postural muscles of the neck, trunk, hamstrings, and soleus muscles. They recommended two to three times per week at a level of intensity suitable to impose increasing demands on the muscle. The training session included a warm-up followed by active muscle strengthening exercises ending with a cool down. This article was not presented as research, but as an exercise physiology primer as it related to strengthening postural muscles. The recommendations for exercises were based on previous studies on postural muscles, and the assumption was that application of the exercise physiology principles could be applied to optimize postural integrity and improve voice production (Schneider, 1997). This article represents one of the earlier articles emphasizing the importance of application of exercise physiology principles to voice, and this topic is discussed in greater detail in Chapter 15. Similar to Schneider and colleagues' article, Wilson Arboleda and Frederick (2008) wrote an educational article directed at speech pathologists working with voice patients regarding the importance of anatomy and physiology involving postural alignment.

These authors emphasize that there are several things to consider when assessing posture and alignment including both skeletal and muscular components. First, when thinking about muscular function, one must consider the agonist/antagonist relationship for body balance.

A second component to consider is muscular hyperfunction (excessive contraction) or muscular weakness. If a muscle

---

Think of a muscle (the agonist) as having a partnering muscle that works against it (the antagonist). Therefore, when the agonist is contracted, the antagonist is relaxed and vice versa (Smith, Weiss, & Lehmkuhl, 1996). The bicep/tricep pair is an example of an agonist/antagonist pair, and the action of relaxation of the antagonist upon contraction of the agonist is referred to as reciprocal inhibition (Powers & Howley, 2009). The concept of reciprocal inhibition is an important concept to keep in mind in terms of training vocal registers and is discussed in Chapter 15.

---

remains contracted for a long period of time, it can cause microtrauma, increasing the metabolic demands of the muscle, which, in turn reduces blood circulation to the area due to vasoconstriction. This results in stiffness and ischemia in the muscle that is chronically contracted and a concomitant weakness in the antagonist muscle that has been reactively stretched (Kostopoulos, 2001). It is important to maintain balance of tension and length of agonist/antagonist pairs avoiding a chronic stretch of the antagonist muscle, as the muscle can eventually succumb to a stretch weakness (DeDeyne, 2001; Dennehy, 1997).

Remediation of this type of problem involves not only relaxing and stretching the hyperfunctional agonist muscle, but also a restrengthening of the lengthened and weakened antagonist muscle (Gossman, 1982; McDonnell, 2005). Muscle physiology is discussed in greater detail in the chapter on exercise physiology.

Teachers and/or clinicians often rely on the history and complaints of the student or patient in order to determine aberrant posture and alignment in the absence of objective methods for measurement. Knowledge of history of physical injury, chronic pain, muscular soreness, and/or muscular fatigue is vital when assessing posture and alignment. Wilson Arboleda and Frederick (2008) highlight specific considerations when assessing posture and alignment as well as addressing common postural misalignments. These include shoulder rounding, neck thrusting, and upper crossed syndrome (combination of both; Figure 1–8).

Shoulder rounding has an appearance of shoulders that are both elevated, and rounded forward. This postural deviation is associated with hypercontraction of the chest and pectoral muscles with a resultant over stretching of the shoulder blade, or

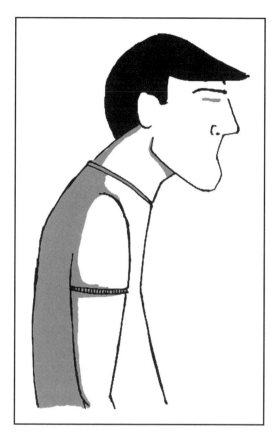

Figure 1–8. Upper crossed syndrome. From Wilson Arboleda and Frederick, 2008, used with permission.

restore the optimal length/tension balance between these agonist/antagonist muscles (Wilson Arboleda & Frederick, 2008).

Neck thrusting is another postural problem described by these authors. Characteristically, the appearance of the ears sitting anterior to the shoulders with the head extended results in stretched anterior neck muscles including the suprahyoid and infrahyoid muscles and a shortening of the suboccipital muscles. Recall from the section on anatomy and physiology that the suprahyoid and infrahyoid muscles are extrinsic laryngeal muscles responsible for stabilizing the larynx, and also allow for vertical movement of the larynx. This means that the muscles responsible for laryngeal lowering and elevation are at risk for sustaining a stretch weakness if the misalignment persists (McDonnell, 2005). An alteration in the position of the neck poses a risk of altering pharyngeal space reducing filer function during voice production (Heman-Ackah, 2005). If neck thrusting is observed, the student or patient would likely benefit from exercises to facilitate stretch of the suboccipital muscles, and exercises to strengthen the anterior neck muscles allowing for freedom of vertical movement of the larynx.

Therapeutic postural intervention utilizing physical therapy modalities demonstrated effectiveness in a single subject classical singer undergoing nine sessions of physical therapy over a four-month period (Staes et al., 2011). Physical therapy focused on treating both muscular and joint dysfunction. The subject was reported to have been compliant with the intervention plan. Post intervention measures of posture demonstrated normalized shoulder and head position and symmetrical positioning of the scapulae. Appropriate use of the cervical muscles to maintain cervical alignment rather than engaging sternocleidomastoid

scapular muscles. This in turn prevents the body from achieving proper alignment of the shoulders (Wilk, 2002). Consequently, shoulder rounding can lead to foreshortening of the rib cage and abdominal muscles because of the thoracic kyphosis (back rounding). This reduces range of motion of the rib cage during inhalation, impacting voice production. This is an excellent example of atypical tension length balance between an agonist/antagonist pair of muscles and its impact on surrounding muscular systems. Exercises designed to stretch the pectoral muscles while strengthening the scapular muscles may be necessary to muscles was also observed. Range of motion for the rib cage was also improved. The authors noted that the subject continued to have tight masseter muscles and reduced jaw opening after intervention. Post intervention measurements of voice demonstrated increased dynamic and pitch range as measured on a Voice Range Profile (VRP).

A basic knowledge and understanding of the primary muscles involved in posture and alignment is vital when training vocal athletes. Furthermore, understanding the relationship between agonist/antagonist muscle pairs and resultant problems from long-term misalignment and aberrant tension/length relationships between these muscle pairs is useful when determining appropriate exercises and stretches to benefit the student or patient. Knowledge of relevant musculoskeletal problems including history of injury is imperative for the voice teacher and/or voice pathologist to ensure proper referral of the student for further assessment by a physical therapist and/or physician when appropriate. Complaints of pain, dizziness, tingling, or other neurological symptoms warrant immediate referral to a physician.

Beyond Posture

There are a multitude of disciplines and methods that aim to maximize posture and alignment through a variety of physical training/body balance techniques. This portion of the chapter provides an overview of some of the most common training modalities. Additional references for the reader who seeks more detailed information are provided. Many of these methods were designed to learn in a hands-on

modality, and the authors encourage readers to seek out classes and workshops for further knowledge on these methods.

Feldenkrais Method®

Named after its creator, both a physicist and electrical engineer, Moshe Feldenkrais initially created his method to prevent being confined to a wheelchair after sustaining several injuries in his twenties playing soccer. Feldenkrais investigated the movement of the body with extensive focus on function with the overall goal being to maximize efficiency and minimize physical effort; an idea consistent with most vocal pedagogy styles. In order to achieve this, Feldenkrais postulated one must have heightened kinesthetic awareness to allow for increased sensory motor learning.

With his bodywork method, it is important to understand that even the smallest adjustment can lead to big changes. Sometimes in order to elicit these changes, Feldenkrais advocates speaking to our body in a language it understands. A teacher is not as likely to accomplish physical change by instructing a student to "relax her jaw" rather; he or she must use a more subtle language that speaks to the neurologic component of movement at a more micro level of functioning. This allows the learner to experience a more functional position at a subconscious level, which, in turn, theoretically results in freer movement.

The concept of slow and subtle movements are the salient features of Feldenkrais's kinesthetic lessons, designed to first break down and then rebuild and retrain physical barriers leading to tension. The Feldenkrais Method® has two primary components: awareness through movement (ATM) and functional integration (FI). FI

In short, we may say that the human brain is such as to make learning, or acquisition of new responses, a normal suitable activity. It is as if it were capable of functioning with any possible combination of nervous interconnections until individual experience forms the one that will be preferred and active. The actual pattern of doing is, therefore, personal and fortuitous. . . .

This great ability to form individual nervous paths and muscular patterns makes it possible for faulty functioning to be learned. The earlier the fault, occur, the more ingrained it appears, and is. Faulty behavior will appear in the executive motor mechanisms, which will seem later, when the nervous system has grown fitted to the undesirable motility, to be inherent in the person and unalterable. It will remain largely so unless the nervous paths producing the undesirable pattern of motility are undone and reshuffled into a better configuration—Feldenkrais.

ten, this neuromotor acquisition results in increased range of motion, reduced pain if applicable, and reduced tension.

Awareness through movement does not always involve one-to-one hands on interaction with a Feldenkrais practitioner. Rather, it may involve guided movement lessons where the practitioner leads a student or a class in a series of movements. The goal is to reorganize the nervous system to replace deviant movement patterns with more efficient and functional movement patterns. Many performers have acquired abnormal patterns of movement over their lifetime as a result of an injury or structural anomaly. Certainly, these can impact the freedom and functionality of voice output.

For further reading on Feldenkarais as it related to voice, the authors recommend "Singing with Your Whole Self: The Feldenkrais Method and Voice" (Nelson & Blades-Zeller, 2002).

Alexander Technique™

Frederick Matthias Alexander was a Shakespearean actor who suffered from recurrent hoarseness in the late 1800s. Doctors were unable to answer his repeated queries of why his hoarseness persisted despite Alexander's diligence to follow medical instruction of vocal rest. Alexander noted that as soon as he began to use his voice again, the hoarseness returned. He concluded that his hoarseness must be the result of something he himself was doing incorrectly. Subsequently, he began to examine his own physical behaviors that could be contributing to his vocal problems.

It was through his direct attention and observation paired with the realization that

involves working one to one with a certified Feldenkrais practitioner. It typically involves use of a treatment table and direct interaction between the student and the practitioner. The touch patterns are not invasive, and the student may or may not be consciously aware of intention of the touch or movement. However, conscious awareness is not imperative because the student may integrate the movement information at a neurologic level, resulting in establishment of a new habitual pattern of movement. Of-his own uncharacteristic habitual movements may have been contributing to his voice problems leading him to develop his method used commonly by actors today. Alexander Technique™ is about learning how *not* to do. Rather, it promotes replacing old dysfunctional habits with new ones. It emphasizes efficient, balanced muscle function not only when performing, but in daily activities such as brushing your hair and picking up a laundry basket. Jane Ruby Heirich (2005) in her book "Voice and The Alexander Technique™: Active Exploration for Speaking and Singing," summarizes the underlying concept of Alexander Technique™:

"Alexander found he had to re-educate his 'debauched kinesthesia' in order to understand what his sensory receptors were trying to report: for example, when sufficient muscular work was completed. His sense of what was comfortable, familiar, and 'right' changed; the unfamiliar eventually became comfortable" (Heirich, 2005).

One of the most useful ideas presented by Alexander is that the process is more important that the product. Meaning, the student should not spend all of his energy focusing on the desired goal, rather he should focus his energy on the journey undertaken to achieve the goal and how he is getting there. Ms. Heirich's book is designed as a workbook, leading the reader through an experience of different exercises and explorations of "nondoing" to free the body and the voice. Additional recommended reading includes *How to Learn the Alexander Technique* (Conable & Conable, 1995).

Body Mapping

Body mapping is a method used for both instrumentalists and singers. It is based on research supporting the notion that each anatomic structure has cortical representation in the brain and that each of us has varied conceptions, or misconceptions, as to how we are organized anatomically in the form of a somatotopic map (Nichols, 2009). The term body mapping was introduced by William Conable in the 1970s. Conable, a cello professor at Ohio State University, applied this principle to his cello students and found that maladaptive and dysfunctional movement patterns were sometimes due to a student's incorrect somatotopic map of their own muscles, joints, and bones structures resulting in movement patterns that were more reflective of this incorrect map resulting in dysfunctional movement patterns. He found that by correcting the student's internal map, their movement patterns improved. Because body mapping concepts may be new for some readers, consider the following as an idea of how body mapping works: take a moment and think about your arm. Where does your arm begin, what does it connect to? How many joints does it have? Now imagine that you are a young cello player, and your body map is organized so that your conception is that your arm begins at the shoulder joint, and your elbow is one inch higher than it actually is. Your movements, when playing, are based on this misconception, and therefore, the movement is suboptimal at the very least and could be dysfunctional, leading to potential injury. Solidification of this incorrect map results in ingrained aberrant movement pattern into your playing (or singing). Similar to Alexander's ideas of "debauched kinesthesia," Conable has referenced much of Alexander's work in his own writings and teachings. Conable worked with his students to correct their body map, giving them accurate representations of their own anatomy and associated movements by increasing conscious awareness. During body mapping training, the student is directed to be aware of his whole body and how other parts of their body are responding and functioning, as one set of movement patterns impact another.

Myofascial Release

Myofascial release is a technique used to address and treat the connective tissue that mediates the muscles and bones of the body. Fascial tissue is a three-dimensional web of tough connective tissue enveloping every structure in the body from head to toe. This connective tissue facilitates maintenance of skeletal structure and shape, keeping organs and viscera in place. Additionally, fascial tissue provides a degree of protection against mechanical impact upon the body and its internal structures. The fascia has an ability to adapt to changing biomechanical states. For example, it may alter help to reinforce ligaments adapting to demands of a specific type of repetitive athletic movement. Additionally, it adapts during wound repair. Unfortunately, the fascial tissue can also adapt in a way that is counterproductive. This can happen as a result of chronic, aberrant biomechanical behaviors (poor postural patterns), or even psychologically based body holding behaviors (Earls & Myers, 2010). Fascial tissue can become restricted resulting in binding of the structure(s) beneath it resulting in pain and dysfunction. Additionally, because the fascial web encompasses the entire body without distinct anatomic disruption, a restriction in one area can have a negative impact in a related area. Unfortunately, much of the imaging used to assess structural integrity such as CT scans, x-ray, and many other tests, do not show fascial tissue. Therefore, injury or dysfunction at this level is often not addressed. John Barnes, a physical therapist, popularized myofascial release in the physical therapy world, and he continues to teach workshops and seminars on his method. As described by Barnes, "Myofascial release is a three-dimensional application of sustained pressure and movement into the fascial system in order to eliminate fascial restrictions and facilitate the emergence of emotional patterns and belief systems that are no longer relevant or are impeding progress" (Barnes, 1990).

Rolfing

Ida Rolf was a PhD chemist who also studied homeopathic medicine while studying atom physics and the Swiss Technical University in Zurich. During the 1930s, she found she was unsatisfied with what were the standard medical treatments, and she sought knowledge in the areas of yoga, Alexander Technique™, osteopathic, and chiropractic medicine.

Over the years, Rolf began to compile a method she called structural integration, and she continued to develop this technique for the next several years. She authored a book on her method entitled *Rolfing: The Integration of Human Structures* (1977). Like the previously described methods, structural integration training is undertaken with a certified practitioner over several sessions (typically ten) with a cumulative effect during each subsequent session. The adjustments are small but

> "This is the gospel of Structural integration: When the body gets working appropriately, the force of gravity can flow through. Then spontaneously, the body heals itself." —Ida Rolph

> "Your body is your instrument for living. Your body is also your instrument for singing. Singing comes from the soul through the mind to the body." —Judith Carman

specific. Emphasis is not on muscles or massage. Rather, work is focused on releasing the fascia (the tissue surrounding the muscles). The intended result is a release and lengthening of the fascia with concomitant reorganization and optimization of alignment and posture.

Practitioners who do structural integration will differentiate Rolfing from myofascial release (MFR) in two primary ways: (1) Rolfing has a cumulative effect with each session building on the previous and (2) Rolfing focuses on the whole body and not just the area of pain or discomfort in order to maintain relief and benefit (Rolph, 1977).

Yoga

Originating from India, yoga is derived from a Sanskrit word meaning to focus ones attention, to attach, join, and bind. The intention of yoga is to achieve a spiritual and tranquil state striving toward optimal mental and physical health (mind-body balance). There are several types of yoga. One type commonly used in Western culture is Hatha Yoga, which incorporates asanas, or postures. The primary focus for Hatha yoga is meditation, exercise, and breathing (Iyengar, 1976). Hatha Yoga has gained popularity as a form of exercise and is used by singers, actors, and other performers. The strength and flexibility provided by yoga fosters core strength for posture and alignment. During the asanas, nasal breathing is used. Additionally, certain types of the yogic breath call for both abdominal and thoracic breathing with the abdomen expanding followed by the chest for inhalation and vice versa for exhalation. Imagery used for the yogic breath calls for visualization of the breath moving from the navel up through the throat during the inhalation and from the throat down to the navel during exhalation. This type of breath imagery is the contradictory of what is actually happening during the breathing cycle. That is not to say that singers cannot greatly benefit from yoga; however, singers should be aware of these breathing differences. Judith Carman, in "Yoga and Singing: Natural Partners" (2004) states that yoga and singing are both centered in the breath, but she also points out the differences between a full singer's breath and the full yogic breath that includes a clavicular component. She promotes the "Bee Breath," involving a resonant /hum/ with a hierarchical approach aiming to extend the breath and tone. Carman further discusses the benefits of yoga for mental focus, performance anxiety, and ability to connect emotion and meaning to performance by removing mental blocks and fears through guided meditation (Carman, 2004).

Pilates

Pilates was developed by Joseph Pilates over 80 years ago. Pilates training emphasizes strengthening the lower back, abdominal, and stabilizing muscles collectively referred to as "the core." A popular form of strength training for dancers, a primary goal of pilates, is to improve strength and balance, to establish long lean muscles, elongated spine, and prevent injury. Traditional pilates training includes use of a machine (reformer) to maximize results. The exercises prescribed by pilates are structured and do not vary. Today, a contemporary version of pilates does not require a machine or device, and the routines are broken down and varied from the original versions created by pilates. Resistance bands and stability balls allow for a wider practice of this method. Pilates training emphasis fluidity of movement, control, precision, and focus. Breathing during pilates exercises emphasizes forced exhalation to promote a subsequent full inhalation. The abdominals are pulled inward and upward emphasizing expansion of the lower lateral rib cage. Pilates and yoga often can complement one another as a paired fitness regimen; however, as with yoga, the singer is encouraged to note breathing differences. For further reading on pilates, readers are referred to *A Pilates Primer: A Combo Millennium Edition* (Pilates & Robbins, 2011), *Pilates Anatomy* (Izacowitz & Clippinger, 2011).

Chapter Summary

Vocal athletes and those who train them would likely agree that balanced posture and alignment are essential for optimal voice production regardless of genre. Performance demands are often not conducive to optimal posture and alignment, and these postural adjustments required by the directors, choreographers, costume designers, set designers, and character development differ drastically from the training environment most singers undergo. Because many voice teachers find value in bodywork, complementing vocal technique training, they will (and should) refer students to seek additional work in these areas when needed. Vocal athletes who are able to access some of the above complementary techniques

will likely reap the benefits of their investment. The similar target goal (optimal mind-body balance) of many of these techniques emphasize neuromuscular retraining, tapping kinesthetic feedback or reorganizing of structures rather than simply strengthening postural muscles. As with many training techniques, no one method is necessarily superior to another, and there are many more practices to achieve these goals than what was highlighted in this chapter. The reader is encouraged to seek out further readings as suggested in this chapter in addition to training workshops and hands-on seminars for further knowledge and skill acquisition.

References

Barnes, J. (1990). *Myofascial release: The search for excellence.* Paoli, PA: John F. Barnes, P.T. and Rehabilitation Services.

Behrman, A. (2007). *Speech and voice science.* San Diego, CA: Plural Publishing.

Carman, J. (2004). Yoga and singing: Natural partners. *Journal of Singing, 60*(5), 433–441.

Conable, B., & Conable, W. (1995) *How to learn Alexander Technique.* Columbus, OH: Andover Road Press.

Cookman, S., & Verdolini, K. (1999). Interrelation of mandibular laryngeal functions. *Journal of Voice, 13*(1), 11–24.

DeDeyne, P. (2001). Application of passive stretch and its implication for muscle fibers. *Physical Therapy, 81,* 819–827.

Dennehy, C., Saxon, K., & Schneider, C. (1997). Exercise physiology principles applied to voice performance: The improvement of postural alignment. *Journal of Voice, 11,* 332–333.

Gossman, M., & Sahrmann, S. (1982). Review of length-associated changes in muscle: Expiremental evidence and clinical applications. *Physical Therapy, 62,* 1799–1808.

Heirich, J. (2005). *Voice and the Alexander Technique* (2nd ed.). Berkeley, CA: Mornun Time Press.

Heman-Ackah, Y. (2005). Physiology of voice production: Consideration for the voice performer. *Journal of Singing, 62*, 173–176.

Isacowitz, R., & Clippinger, K. (2011). *Pilates anatomy.* Champaign, IL: Human Kinetics Publishers.

Iyengar, B. (1976). *Light on yoga.* New York, NY: Schoken Books.

Jones, F. (1972). Voice production as a function of head balance in singers. *The Journal of Psychology, 82*, 209–215.

Kostopoulos, D., & Konstantine, R. (2001). *The manuel of trigger point and myofascial release.* Thorofare, NJ: Slack Incorporated.

Luo, P., Wang, B., Peng, Z., & Li, J. (1991). Morphplogical characteristics and terminating patterns of masseteric neurons of the mesencephalic trigeminal nucleus in the rat: An intracellular horseradish peroxidase labeling study. *Journal of Comparative Neurology, 303*, 286–299.

Malde, M., Allen, M., & Zeller, K. (2009). *What every singer needs to know about the body.* San Diego, CA: Plural Publishing.

McDonnell, M., Sahrmann, S., & VanDillen, L. (2005). A specific exercise program and modification of postural alignment for treatment of cervicogenic headache: A case report. *Journal of Orthopedic Sports Physical Therapy, 35*, 3–15.

Moore, K., & Dalley, A. (2006). *Clinically Oriented Anatomy* (5th ed.). Philadelphia, PA: Lippincot Williams & Wilkins.

Nelson, S., & Blades-Zeller, E. (2002). *Singing with your whole self: The Feldenkrais Method for voice.* Lanham, MD: The Scarecrow Press, Inc.

Netter, F. H. (1997). *Atlas of human anatomy* (2nd ed.). East Hanover, NJ: Novartis.

Nichols, T. R. (2009). The scientific basis of body mapping. In M. Malde, M. Allen, & K-A. Zeller (Eds.), *What every singer needs to know about the body* (pp. 209–211). San Diego, CA: Plural Publishing.

Pilates, J., & Robbins, J. (2011). *A pilates primer: The combo millennium edition.* Ashland, OR: Presentation Dynamics LLC.

Powers, S., & Howley, E. (2009). *Exercise physiology: Theory and application to fitness and performance.* Boston, MA: McGraw Hill.

Rolph, I. (1977). *Rolfing: The integration of human structures.* Santa Monica, CA: Dennis Landman.

Schneider, C., Dennehy, C., & Saxon, K. (1997). Exercise physiology principles applied to vocal performance—the improvement of postural alignment. *Journal of Voice, 11*(3), 332–337.

Smith, L., Weiss, E., & Lehmkuhl, L. (1996). *Brunnstrom's clinical kinesiology.* Philadelphia, PA: F.A. Davis Company.

Staes, F. F., Jansen, L., Vilette, A., Coveliers, Y., Daniels, K., & Decoster, W. (2011). Physical therapy as a means to optimize posture and voice parameters in student classical singers: A case report. [Case reports]. *Journal of Voice, 25*(3), e91–101. doi: 10.1016/j.jvoice.2009.10.012

Sundberg, J., Leanderson, R., VonEuler, C., & Knutsson, E. (1991). Influence of body posture and lung volume on subglottal pressure control during singing. *Journal of Voice, 5*(4), 283–291.

Travers, J., & Norgren, R. (1983). Afferent projections to the oral motor nuclei in the rat. *Journal of Comparative Neurology, 220*, 280–298.

West, R., & Larson, C. (1995). Neurons of the anterior mesial cortex related to faciovocal activity in the awake monkey. *Journal of Neurophysiology, 75*, 1856–1869.

Wilk, K., Meister, K., & Andrews, J. (2002). Current concepts in the rehabilitation of the overhead athlete. *Americal Journal of Sports Medicine, 30*, 136–151.

Wilson Arboleda, B., & Frederick, A. L. (2008). Considerations for maintenance of postural alignment for voice production. *Journal of Voice, 22*(1), 90–99.

Zemlin, W. (1998). *Speech and Hearing Science Anatomy and Physiology* (4th ed.). Needham Heights, MA: Allyn and Bacon.

2

Respiratory Kinematics

Introduction

Breathing and breath support are the primary basis of power for all vocal athletes. Without an adequate power supply to support the vocal demands of performance, the voice cannot perform at an optimal level. Increased vocal output demands adequate and appropriate breath management. This chapter provides an overview of respiration for the singer encompassing a brief review of the "schools" of breathing techniques, anatomy, and physiology as it is warranted for teaching within the contemporary voice studio, and clinical research related to respiration in singers and actors. Training respiration in singers has a long history in the vocal pedagogy literature. This chapter is not meant to be an exhaustive exploration of respiratory pedagogy, but rather to provide the teacher with an understanding on the various schools of

breathing and resources for further study should they so choose. Similarly, the segment on anatomy and physiology provides the vocal pedagogue with tools to provide students with a proper understanding of the respiratory mechanism and the way it functions within the framework of the entire vocal mechanism. The final segment of this chapter provides the singing voice teacher with research supporting respiratory training in both singers and actors. The differences and similarities that exist in training respiration for both classical and contemporary commercial music (CCM) performers are discussed.

Historical Overview of Respiratory Pedagogy

The roots of modern day vocal pedagogy can be traced back to the first published pedagogical texts in 1723 by Pier Francesco Tosi. Tosi's text offers insight into specific training techniques and recommendations for singers. Literally, hundreds of texts have been written on training the classical voice since Tosi's initial publication. Elizabeth Blades-Zeller (1994) published an overview of current trends in training the classical voice within the United States providing a contemporary reflection of vocal training. This project interviewed 16 exemplary voice teachers from across the country on their pedagogical teachings and personal experiences. The plethora of literature on pedagogical methodology is vast and beyond the scope of this text for a comprehensive review. Therefore, examination of several well-known historical vocal pedagogy texts provides a basis for respiratory training techniques.

Much of what is reported, especially in the early literature, has a nonscientific basis. Rather, the writings provided detailed explanations of individual teachers regarding training techniques, which had produced some of the world's most highly regarded voices. Historical pedagogical references to training respiration, phonation, and articulation in Western classical singers to achieve optimal performance are based primarily in the Italian school of *bel canto* with some German and French influences (Blades-Zeller, 1994; Coffin, 1989; Miller, 1997). Two of the earliest published voice pedagogues, Pier Francesco Tosi and Giambasttisti Mancini deliver insight primarily into the training of the castrato voice. Although no castrati exist today, some of their suggested vocal techniques provide the basis for the training of the female voice. The roots of many of the 19th- and 20th-century voice teachers are traced back to the teachings of Manuel del Popolo Vincente Rodriguez Garcia (Garcia I), not

to be confused with Manuel Garcia II, the "father of modern otolaryngology." Garcia II took many of his pedagogical ideas and writing from his father, who was not only an excellent teacher, but also an excellent singer. In addition to an extensive performance career, many famous singers emerged from Garcia I's studio. His influential role on training the singing voice is observed throughout modern day literature on voice. Garcia I published *Exercises Pour La Voix* sometime between 1819 and 1822, which included 340 vocal exercises that reportedly could correct any vocal fault. His teachings advocated deep, slow, quiet breathing, which should always be employed by the singer prior to initiation of exercises or song, as not to engage in unnecessary laryngeal or respiratory tension.

Manuel Garcia II

Most of modern-day pedagogical voice exercises can be traced back to the writings of Garcia II, either by people who agreed with him and attempted to restate what he professed, or by people who disagreed with or misinterpreted his teachings and have developed pedagogical techniques in opposition. First and foremost, Garcia screened all singers that came to study with him. Minimum requirements were that of intelligence, good physical health, good vocal health, and an innate musical talent. Students, who did not possess musical ability, were advised not to pursue a professional singing career. A significant amount of time, 5 to 10 years, was spent training the voice prior to any performance. If voice teachers observed these strict, yet optimal guidelines today, many music schools would close due to the fact that they were not producing visible work in their singers. However, if one could take the time to train the vocal musculature for 5 years prior to introduction of song, one might be more prepared physically to handle the demands placed on the voice.

Proper respiration was considered the basis for all good singing technique, and those who lacked adequate respiratory control would never progress beyond a certain level of training. Garcia taught diaphragmatic breathing, requiring his students to maintain a noble posture with a raised chest (without stiffness or tension) and lowering of the diaphragm during inspiration. The inspiration was to be smooth and inaudible. Expiration was also to be a smooth controlled movement, with the focus on the diaphragm as the primary mediator of smooth exhalation.

Garcia warned that solely training breath for the beginning student may result in fatigue, but training the breath was the necessary basis for voice production of optimal quality. He wrote, "The breath, which holds the entire instrument under its subjection, exerts the greatest influence on the character of the performance and can make it calm or trembling, connected or detached, energetic or lifeless, expressive or devoid of expression" (Garcia, 1984, p. 35). With that statement, he leaves only four short exercises to train and strengthen the breath:

1. First one inhales slowly and during the space of several seconds as much breath as the chest can contain;
2. One exhales that air with the same slowness as with which it was inhaled;
3. One fills the lungs and keeps them filled for the longest time possible;
4. One exhales completely and leaves the chest empty as long as the physical

powers will conveniently allow (Garcia, 1984, p. 35).

Mathilde Marchesi

Mathilde Marchesi's teaching technique was also based on the Italian *bel canto* tradition, and she felt that one of the reasons for the significant decline in good singing technique was due to Wagner and the German school of singing. Specifically, Wagner's operas and the emergence of the German vocal pedagogical techniques resulted in a heavier vocal production that was more concerned with the text as opposed to the beauty of the vocal line (*bel canto*). As with Garcia, Marchesi believed that singers must possess an attractive appearance, have intact natural musical ability, and must study with her for a minimum of 2 years.

Marchesi believed respiration was to be diaphragmatic, and she did not believe in the use of corsets during singing. She cautioned against the use of corsets as they promoted lateral breathing by compressing the abdominal wall unnaturally. One of her techniques for teaching diaphragmatic breathing was to have the singer run up a staircase, then lie on the couch with a glass of water on their abdomen and force respiration, without a rippling in the glass of water. Another technique that she used to "strengthen the lungs" of a vocalist, involved blowing a feather while maintaining a distance of five to six steps away (Marchesi, 1901, 1967).

Lamperti

Unlike the Garcia family, the Lamperti family (Francesco [father] and Giovanni Battista

[son]) were not performers, but wrote and taught extensively on the art of singing. Franceso Lamperti was extremely disenchanted with the status of the singing voice and felt there had been a significant decline in the quality of the singer over time. Lamperti's text (1905) is based primarily on the study of respiration. He believed that if respiration was trained well, appropriate phonation and resonation would result. Singers were trained to inhale for 18 seconds in order that they might feel the *lutte vocale* (vocal struggle). The opposition of the inspiratory and expiratory muscles provides the basis for his training technique. In order for the singer to experience the correct *appoggio* (support of breath), one must first experience the struggle the muscles of respiration present at maximum inhalation. Once the singer has experienced this phenomenon, the feeling of "holding back the breath," by using active muscles of inspiration/expiration, can be attained. During any singing activity, the sensation of slight muscle tension should be felt in the respiratory muscles.

Shakespeare

One of Lamperti's pupils, William Shakespeare, wrote an excellent text based on the teachings of Lamperti. Shakespeare's text details information on respiration/breath management, phonation, resonation, registration, and faulty production. In Shakespeare's words, "singing must be regarded as the art of combining tune and speech in such a way that the notes are started in fullness, purity, and on the exact pitch intended" (Shakespeare, 1921, p. 7).

Shakespeare also believed that appropriate respiration and breath management was the basis for good sound production. At this point in history, the emergence of increased physiological understanding regarding the respiratory mechanism was beginning to evolve. Included in his text are figures of the muscles of respiration and their perceived actions. Several key points that Shakespeare emphasized in his teaching of respiration required a 10 to 20 second controlled exhalation. He also takes time in his discussion of breathing to report on the normal anatomy and physiology of respiration. Specifically, he notes abdominal expansion during inhalation as the diaphragm contracts, and he discusses lateral expansion of the rib cage. He professed that breath control was to be executed by the muscles of the thorax, not at the level of the larynx.

One of the most important issues related to breathing was that the audience should never see or hear the singer inspire. Clavicular breathing was never acceptable, especially on catch-breaths in the middle of a song. The shoulders were to remain free of tension as was the chest. Consistent with this line of thinking, once appropriate breathing patterns were learned, singers should never have to think about respiration during song. Shakespeare cautioned against being too full of breath, and the singer was always to have a breath reserve at the end of phrases. If there was no reserve of breath, automatically the throat would tighten to assist with breath control. The historical vocal pedagogues repeatedly report what is now known to be true today and have subsequently been able to prove with respiratory measures.

Vennard

William Vennard (1967) wrote one of the first complete texts on the science behind the singing voice. Unlike the previous voice pedagogues, Vennard did not include specific vocal exercises, but rather provided the singer with a basic discussion on acoustics. The fundamental physics of sound, sound waves, wave propagation, and clarification of terminology such as intensity, frequency, sonance, resonance, and timbre are included in the introductory chapters of his text. In his explanation of acoustics, Vennard discussed overtones, harmonics, and partials. He was far ahead of his time in his writings, and a basis for the present day study of vocal acoustics by voice scientists, voice pathologists, and modern day voice pedagogues has resulted.

Vennard's commentary on teaching breathing to singers included correct posture to support abdominal breathing as a necessity. The singer was advised to feel like a marionette puppet, with strings attached to the head, and sternum. Posture was not to be overemphasized, but rather gentle reminders of a raised chest and relaxed shoulders should be incorporated into each lesson. Vennard believed that no more than two lessons should be spent on breathing alone, but that correct habits should be reinforced during each lesson. If the singer was still exhibiting signs of clavicular breathing after a month of lessons, it could be assumed that the student was not practicing.

Vennard did not expect his students to memorize each muscle of inspiration and expiration, but a general anatomic understanding of the structure and function of muscles used for respiration was taught. He advised that teachers of singing should have an excellent knowledge of the anatomy and physiology of respiration, so they could correct the respiratory faults observed in their students. Clavicular breathing was considered by Vennard to be inefficient and was considered the "breath of exhaustion." The chest should remain raised during singing tasks, but should not

be solely involved in inspiration and expiration. Instead, the singer should practice abdominal/belly breathing. Vennard sums his breathing technique in three adverbs, "in, down, out" (Vennard, 1967, p. 29). Breath is taken "in" through the nose or mouth, breath goes "down" into the lungs and thorax, and causes them to expand "out."

Exercises Vennard used to promote abdominal breathing include: lying on the floor with a book on the abdomen and watching it rise during inhalation and fall during exhalation, or placing an object such as a book between the singer and a wall. As the singer inhales against the book, he or she should move away from the wall, and as exhalation occurs, the singer should move toward the wall. In addition to diaphragmatic breathing for song, Vennard explains the concept of muscular antagonism in terms of the specific muscles utilized during resting inspiration and expiration, and expiration for song. In conjunction with this concept, Vennard cites the cough reflex as an example that tone initiation should begin using a diaphragmatic attack.

In order for the singer to become aware of a diaphragmatic attack, Vennard suggests a panting exercise that results in a "bouncing epigastrium." Once this feat is mastered, the singer can hope to train breath control. Vennard considered breath control as the basis for increasing intensity of tone and maintaining air until the end of a musical phrase. When proper breath support is utilized, the singer should sense almost "holding the breath." In his own words, Vennard explains breath control:

The muscular antagonism which he must set up in order to maintain a stiff epigastrium against my pressure often enables him to sing a considerably longer phrase . . . Be sure that the "holding" is done by the diaphragm and by the intercostals, and *not by the larynx*. (Vennard, 1967, p. 34)

In order to train breath control, Vennard recommends that the singer inhale for five counts, hold the breath for ten counts, and then exhale slowly to five counts. It is the interpretation of these authors that when Vennard uses the term "holding," he is referring to the suspension of breath with an open glottis. Gradually, the length of the inhalation and exhalation should be increased. Once the singer has mastered the above technique, they should be able to take a quick inhalation and then exhale through slightly pursed lips for as long as possible. Maintaining an open throat, as in an /ɑ/ vowel during inhalation, the singer avoids tension within the larynx or pharynx prior to the initiation of phonation.

Contemporary Respiratory Pedagogical Training

Sullivan

Jan Sullivan wrote an article on belting, which included the following information on respiration for belting (1989). Postural alignment, specifically of the pelvic and pectoral girdles, is of paramount importance for proper respiration and breath support. Without appropriate pelvic alignment, one cannot expand the lower ribs, which in turn compromises diaphragmatic breathing. The pectoral girdle alignment helps to maintain noble posture and keep the head up. A raised head positioning allows for a raised larynx per Ms. Sullivan. Diaphragmatic breathing does not receive specific mention in her writings. However, she speaks of breathing in which "a more sideward, as well as forward, expansion of the upper abdomen (waist area) . . . helps in the retention or suspension of the open ribs as singing is taking place" (p. 48). Sullivan suggests that breathing for belting is slightly higher (anterior-posterior and lateral expansion is noted just below the rib cage) than that of classical opinion (lower abdominal expansion). Ms. Sullivan's discussion on breath support and attack are limited to a few sentences. She alludes to the *lutte vocale* (vocal struggle) when she addresses breath support. "One is retention of position of inhalation to keep ribs suspended outward instead of closing as if exhaling" (p. 49).

Coordinated tonal onset should be similar to staccato production or yelling. Ms. Sullivan suggests the term "accented legato" as the appropriate onset for belting. She defines "accented legato" as, "Quality of being smooth and connected yet each note has a muscular pulse from the support area of the upper abdomen-waist area as in staccato and/or yelling" (p. 45). If this technique is executed with the premise of staccato, minimal vocal fatigue should result. However, teaching staccato in the young or inexperienced singer often results in repeated hard glottal attacks. Also, Ms. Sullivan assumes that when people yell, they are doing so with proper abdominal breath support. Again, it is the opinion of the present authors, that not all yelling is correctly produced, and can result in vocal injury if it is repeatedly performed incorrectly.

Edwin

Singing teacher Robert Edwin (1998) provides another perspective to breathing for the belt voice. Edwin's recurring articles in the *NATS Journal* (The Bach to Rock

Connection) are based primarily in his experience with teaching. Advocating breath as the foundation for good singing technique, Edwin suggested training efficient breath management. He did not provide any explanation of what constitutes efficient breath management, nor did he provide insight as to whether breath management strategies used in training the classical singer are appropriate for the belter. One would assume that if belting is produced with intensity demands different from that of the classical singer, it may require a different breathing strategy.

Henderson

Within her chapter on performance technique in her book *How to Train Singers* (1991), Lara Henderson addressed the belting voice. Henderson advocated a solid basis for appropriate breath support based in the classical diaphragmatic breathing technique. Her text includes an entire chapter devoted to postural alignment and breathing technique. Similar to the classical pedagogues in her techniques, no significantly new information is offered in this text related to pedagogy training as it relates to breathing and breath management. However, Henderson is a strong believer in the Alexander Technique™ with respect to postural alignment.

Respiratory Pedagogical Summary

Historical and contemporary pedagogues tend to advocate that breath and breath support are key elements for optimal voice production in singers regardless of genre. However, the training modalities and implementation of training breath and breath management are highly variable from teacher to teacher. As science has attempted to quantify how singers breathe, there have become two general schools of teaching breathing; one is technical and relies heavily on the understanding of the anatomy and physiology of the respiratory mechanism and the second is based in imagery (Foulds-Elliott, Thorpe, Cala, & Davis, 2000; Pettersen, & Bjørkøy, 2007). Regardless of pedagogical choice, the basic understanding of the muscles of respiration and physiology is imperative for any singing teacher.

Anatomy and Physiology of the Respiratory Mechanism for the Singer

The respiratory system has traditionally been viewed as the base on which the voice is built. Therefore, it is imperative that those who teach singers have an excellent understanding of how the respiratory mechanism works. So often we hear phrases such as "sing from your diaphragm" or "breathe into your belly," which may set up inappropriate understanding of how the respiratory mechanism works. Through a better understanding of the respiratory mechanism, teachers will develop exercises for singers designed to maximize the training, efficiency, and coordination of these important muscles. As with any athlete, singers must train their muscles for strength, agility, flexibility, and stamina. Without an understanding of the respiratory musculature, teachers cannot not provide singers with the best training.

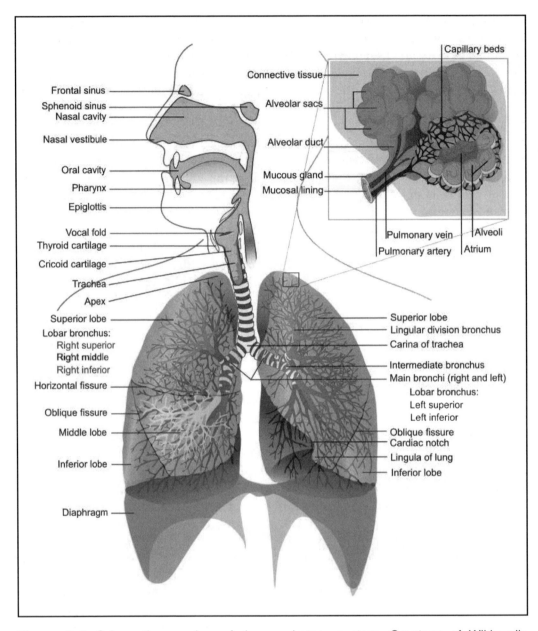

Figure 2–1. Schematic overview of the respiratory system. Courtesy of Wikimedia Commons.

Inspiration and Expiration for the Singer

There are several important components of the respiratory system vital for the preparatory inspiration prior to voice production. When you prepare to sing, you purposefully (actively) create a negative pressure in the lungs (either via diaphragm contraction or rib cage expansion), and air comes in through the mouth and/or nose, through the nasal, oral, and pharyngeal spaces, through the open vocal folds (glottis), through the trachea, bronchi, and into the lungs (Figure 2–1). At no point does air ever enter the diaphragm. Therefore, the term "diaphragmatic breathing" can be

quite confusing for many inexperienced singers.

Depending on how much breath is needed for a given phrase or intensity, varying amounts of abdominal and rib cage displacement are created resulting in varying levels of lung volumes. Inspiration always involves the activity of muscles. However, expiration (breathing out) has a passive component involving elastic recoil forces (think of a rubber band that has been overly stretched out). The more air you take into your lungs, the greater pressure you generate in the lungs, intercostals, and abdominal muscles. Therefore, if you "over-inflate" for the phrase that you need to sing, you have to work exceedingly hard to hold the air in (perhaps creating tension in other

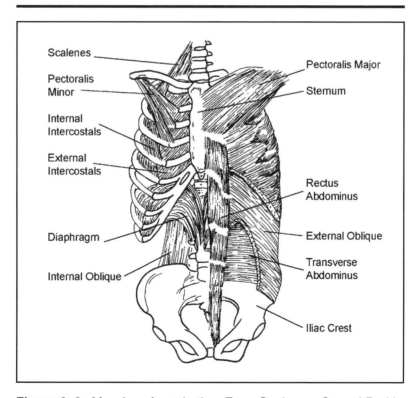

Figure 2–2. Muscles of respiration. From Sapienza, C., and Ruddy, B. H. (2013). *Voice Disorders* (2nd ed.). San Diego, CA: Plural Publishing. Used with permission.

TABLE 2–1. Accessory Inspiratory Muscles and Their Origins and Insertions and Major Expiratory Muscles and Their Origins and Insertions

Muscle	Function	Origin	Insertion
Levatores costartum	Accessory Inspiratory	Transverse processes of C7 to T12 vertebrae	Superior surfaces of the ribs immediately inferior to the preceding vertebrae
Serratus posterior superior	Accessory Inspiratory	The spinous processes of C7 through T3	The upper borders of the 2nd through 5th ribs
Sternocleido-mastoid	Accessory Inspiratory	Manubrium and medial portion of the clavicle	Mastoid process of the temporal bone
Scalenus	Accessory Inspiratory	C2–C7 vertebrae	The first and second ribs
Trapezius	Accessory Inspiratory	The spinous processes of the vertebrae C7–T12	At the shoulders, into the *lateral* third of the clavicle, and into the spine of the scapula
Pectoralis major	Accessory Inspiratory	The anterior surface of the clavicle; the anterior surface of the sternum, as low down as the attachment of the cartilage of the 6th or 7th rib	The crest of the greater tubercle of the humerus
Pectoralis minor	Accessory Inspiratory	3rd to 5th ribs, near their costal cartilages	The medial border and upper surface of the scapula
Serratus anterior	Accessory Inspiratory	The surface of the upper eight ribs	The entire anterior length of the medial border of the scapula
Subclavius	Accessory Inspiratory	Arises by a short, thick tendon from the first rib and its cartilage at their junction, in front of the costoclavicular ligament	The groove on the under surface of the clavicle

TABLE 2–1. *continued*

Muscle	Function	Origin	Insertion
Levator scapulae	Accessory Inspiratory	Arises by tendinous slips from the transverse processes of the atlas and axis and from the posterior tubercles of the transverse processes of the 3rd and 4th cervical vertebrae.	The vertebral border of the scapula
Rhomboideus major	Accessory Inspiratory	The spinous processes of T2 to T5	The medial border of the scapula
Rhomboideus minor	Accessory Inspiratory	The spinous processes of C7 and T1	The vertebral border near the point that it meets the spine of the scapula
Transversus thoracis	Accessory Inspiratory	The posterior surface of the body of the sternum, from the posterior surface of the xiphoid process, and from the sternal ends of the costal cartilages of the lower 3 or 4 true ribs	The lower borders and inner surfaces of the costal cartilages of ribs 2–6
Quadratus lumborum	Accessory Inspiratory	Arises by aponeurotic fibers from the iliolumbar ligament and the adjacent portion of the iliac crest	The lower border of the last rib for about half its length, and the apices of the transverse processes of the upper 4 lumbar vertebrae
Subcostal	Accessory Inspiratory	The inner surface of one rib	The inner surface of the 2nd or 3rd rib above, near its angle
Serratus posterior	Accessory Inspiratory	The spinous processes of T11 and T12 and L1–L3	The inferior borders of the lower 4 ribs, a little beyond their angles

continues

TABLE 2–1. *continued*

Muscle	Function	Origin	Insertion
Latissimus dorsi	Accessory Inspiratory	The spinous processes of T6–T12, iliac crest, and inferior 3 or 4 ribs	The humerus
Internal oblique abdominis	Expiratory	Inguinal ligament, Iliac crest, and the lumbodorsal fascia	Linea alba, xiphoid process, and the inferior ribs.
External oblique abdominis	Expiratory	Lower 8 ribs	Crista iliaca, ligamentum inguinale
Rectus abdominis	Expiratory	Pubis	Costal cartilage of ribs 5–7, xiphoid process of sternum

Source: Sapienza, C., & Ruddy, B. H. (2013). *Voice Disorders* (2nd ed.). San Diego, CA: Plural Publishing. Used with permission.

parts of the respiratory or laryngeal system; Iwarsson, Thomasson, & Sundberg 1998). Figure 2–2 shows a schematic of the muscles of inspiration and expiration, and shows the origins, insertions, and the muscle action. Table 2–1 lists the primary muscles of inspiration and expiration.

Primary Muscles of Inspiration

Diaphragm

The diaphragm is a dome-shaped muscle that separates the thoracic cavity from the abdominal cavity. The outermost portion of the diaphragm is muscular and the origins of these muscle fibers include the sternum (breastbone), ribs 7 through 12, and the lumbar vertebrae. The diaphragm muscle courses towards the middle of the body, inserting into the central tendon. Several important connections from the thorax course through the diaphragm to the lower body including the esophagus, aorta, and vena cava as well as several minor openings for nerves and blood vessels. Nerve supply to the diaphragm is provided by the phrenic nerve. During inspiration, the diaphragm contracts moving the abdominal cavity down and forward. This action increases rib cage expansion and results in negative pressure within the lungs.

External Intercostal Muscles

In addition to the diaphragm, the external intercostal muscles aid in inspiration. There are 11 pairs of external intercostal muscles (one set between each set of ribs). External intercostal muscles originate on the lower boarder of a rib and course downward to insert on the upper boarder of the rib below. When these muscles contract (toward the origin), they help to pull the rib cage up and out. These muscles are innervated by intercostal nerves (T1–T11).

Accessory Muscles of Inspiration

Other muscles that may play a role in inspiration include: sternocleidomastoid muscle and scalene muscle group (anterior, middle, and posterior). The sternocleidomastoid muscle (paired) originates from the sternum (breastbone) and clavicle (collarbone), and courses up to insert in the mastoid process (temporal bone of the skull). When this muscle contracts, it pulls the sternum and collarbone upward, and its action also involves turning the head. The scalene muscle group originates from cervical vertebrae two through seven and courses to insert into the first and second ribs. When the anterior and middle scalene muscles contract, they raise the first rib up and also aid in tilting the head to the same side as the contracted muscle. Contraction of the posterior scalene muscle helps to elevate the second rib and tilt the head to the same side.

Muscles of Expiration

Expiration is a passive event brought about by the elastic recoil forces of the previously stretched muscles (during inspiration) and lungs. However, during singing tasks, expiration often needs to be controlled by the active muscles of respiration including: internal intercostal muscles, rectus abdominus muscle, external oblique muscle, internal oblique muscle, and transverse abdominus muscle. These muscles are commonly referred to as the abdominal muscles. By using these muscles to help control expiratory flow, singers are able to manage long sung phrases. Coordination of proper expiratory airflow is often the basis of what vocal teachers consider

appropriate breath support. Challenges for vocal athletes arise when abdominal muscle strength and control is suboptimal for performance demands. If the expiratory musculature is compromised, laryngeal muscle compensation is often utilized to maintain adequate sound production.

Internal Intercostal Muscle

The internal intercostal muscles originate, course, and insert in the opposite direction from the external intercostal muscles discussed above. These 11 paired muscles originate from the top of a rib and course upward, inserting into the bottom of the rib above it. When the internal intercostal muscles contract, they act to draw the ribs down and inward, decreasing rib cage size.

Rectus Abdominus Muscle

This muscle, when highly toned with little excess body fat, is the "six-pack" of the abdominals. It originates from the pubic bone (in the pelvic girdle) and courses upward to insert into the bottom of the sternum and the costal cartilages of ribs five, six, and seven. Besides its active function in controlling respiration, this muscle is important for maintaining posture.

External Oblique Muscle

Originating from ribs 5 through 12, the external oblique muscles, course down and forward to attach to the iliac crest (pelvic girdle). When it contracts, this muscle pulls the chest down and helps to compress the abdominal cavity.

Internal Oblique Muscle

The internal oblique muscles originate from the pelvic girdle (iliac crest) and course upward and toward midline of the body, ultimately inserting into a tendon called the linea alba. Often considered the antagonist to the diaphragm, contraction of the internal oblique muscles results in compression of the abdomen.

Transverse Abdominus Muscle

The deepest of the abdominal muscles, the transverse abdominus muscle lies deep to the internal oblique. The origin of this fan-shaped muscle includes part of the pelvic girdle, the thoracic spine, and some of the lower ribs. Subsequently, it fans out and courses toward the center of the body. As with the other abdominal muscles, transverse abdominus muscles act to help compress abdominal contents.

Respiratory Kinematics for Vocal Athletes—What the Research Tells Us

Isolation of the respiratory system alone as it relates to the singing voice is essentially impossible. All components of voice must work together for optimal voice production in vocal athletes. Posture influences respiration, and the singer's body as it pertains to alignment and posture is discussed in detail in the following chapter. In general terms, gravity imparts a large inhalatory force for a body in an upright position, but, it imparts an exhalatory force in a supine (lying down on your back) position. (Thus, one of the reasons singers learning to breathe are often asked to lay on the floor is because it provides a natural positioning to promote appropriate breathing.) Singers of commercial music are rarely standing still singing; rather their bodies tend to be in constant motion through moving, jumping, and dancing all potentially changing both the postural influences on the respiratory system and the pressures and volumes of the lungs due to aerobic demands of the performance. This section of the text provides the singer with some understanding of the physiologic work completed on various vocal and physical athletes as it pertains to breathing.

Respiratory Kinematics of the Classical Singer

The most substantial research on respiratory kinematics in singers has been completed on classically trained vocalists. Although this text is aimed at the non-classical artist, there are very few studies specifically devoted to respiration in non-classical singers (Hoit, Jenks, Watson, & Cleveland, 1996). Unfortunately, one cannot generalize the research findings of one group across genres, but the information gained from previous classical studies may provide a basis for considering physiologic training discussion in commercial music singers.

Research on How Singers Breathe

Research regarding breathing and the singing voice has focused on several areas: (1) breathing strategies singers use at rest, speech, and song (i.e., rib cage and abdominal movements), (2) implications of muscles involved in breathing for singing, (3) influence of training on the way singers breathe, (4) role of emotion in breathing patterns of singers, and (5) considerations for respiratory muscle strength training in athletes (Carroll, Sataloff, Heuer, Spiegel, Radionoff, & Cohn,1996; Collyer, Kenny, & Archer, 2009; Foulds-Elliott, Thorpe, Cala, & Davis, 2000; Griffin, Woo, Colton, Casper, & Brewer, 1995; Hoit, Jenks, Watson, & Cleveland,1996; Illi, Held, Frank, & Spengler, 2012; Leanderson, Sundberg, & von Euler, 1987; Paulus, Flagan, Simmons, Gillis, Kotturi, Thom, . . . Swain, 2012; Petitt, 1994; Pettersen, 2005, 2006; Pettersen & Bjørkøy, 2007; Pettersen, Bjørkøy, Torp, & Westgaard, 2005; Pettersen & Eggebo, 2010; Pettersen & Westgaard, 2004, 2005; Rolf, Sundberg, & von Euler, 1987; Rothernberg, Miller, Molitor, & Leffingwell, 1987; Stathopoulos & Sapienza, 1993; Sundberg, Leanderson, von Euler, & Knutsson, 1991; Thomasson & Sundberg, 2001; Thorpe, Cala, Chapman, & Davis, 2001; Watson & Hixon, 1985; Watson, Hixon, Stathopoulos & Sullivan, 1990; Watson, Williams, & James, 2012).

Seminal work in respiratory kinematics (motion of the body during breathing) reveals that classically trained singers use a large amount of their total vital capacity when singing. More specifically, when the respiratory kinematics of singers' breathing strategies are compared between speech and song, singers take in a higher volume of breath and end their phrases with a lower volume, regardless of gender. Researchers also found that as there was increased rib cage volume, there was decreased abdominal volume and that the excursion of both rib cage and abdominal movement was greater during singing than in speech (Watson et al., 1990). Classical singers have also been shown to manipulate breath pressure in order to maintain subglottic pressure regardless of posture (Sundberg et al., 1991). Studies have confirmed that elite singers do not all use the same breathing strategies to produce voice during performance and that singers tend to have a distinct individual respiratory pattern. Generally speaking, endomorph body types tend to be abdominally based in their patterns, and ectomorph body types tend to be rib-cage based (Collyer et al., 2009). When trained singers were asked to alter their breathing patterns when given verbal direction, it was found that although they were able to functionally change their muscle patterns at the onset, but they unconsciously gravitated back to their typical breathing patterns (Collyer et al., 2009). However, they did indicate that even singers with strongly engrained breathing patterns were able to alter what they did with verbal cues.

The muscles of respiration have long been a source of controversy regarding involvement of specific muscle groups during song. In recent years, there has been much attention to the involvement and action of a variety of abdominal and strap muscles and their role in voice production. Findings indicate that some of the strap muscles of the neck, which are often associated with clavicular or inappropriate breathing patterns may actually be active during some parts of inhalation and sound production. It is important that the reader not equate active or engaged muscle activity with hyperfunction. Readers are encouraged to delve into the literature related to the specific muscles that may be of interest during singing provided in the references at the end of this chapter.

Breathing and Emotion

Breathing is often emotionally based, and breathing patterns change as a result of and a response to emotional stimulus. Audiences pay for an emotional connection to the singer. Therefore, singers are required to covey sentiment without allowing emotion to negatively impact their respiration during singing. Sundberg, Elliot, Gramming and Nord (1993) reported, breathing patterns during neutral speech were noted to be low and smooth whereas during emotive speech there was a significant increase in respiratory variation. When singers were asked to perform an aria under two different conditions: typical practice room and as if they were singing for an audience, researchers found that when the singers imagined they were "performing," they used their breath differently based on their emotional stimulus (Foulds-Elliot et al., 2000).

Respiratory Strength Training

Strength training of muscles is a component of any athlete's workout routine (in conjunction with flexibility, agility, stamina, and task-specific training). Vocal athletes generally do not think about building muscle strength in the muscles for breathing, but studies related to inspiratory and expiratory muscle strength training indicate that these muscles can indeed improve in actual strength and resultant function. For the singer, this may mean that improved respiratory muscle strength would change the effort level needed to produce voice. However, there are no specific studies on professional singers at this time, and further research on this subset of individuals is warranted.

The present research specifically related to breathing for commercial music singers is sparse. Hoit and colleagues (1996) looked at the breathing patterns of country music singers during speech and song. Findings indicated that the breathing patterns of country singers during speech were similar to nonsingers. Interestingly, during country music singing, the

performers used similar breathing strategies to speaking. This is in contrast to the findings of classical singers who use different breath strategies for speech and song. The researchers indicated that the speech/song breathing patterns may be similar because country music singers in this study generally did not have significant vocal training with respect to respiration. Also, much of country music is speech-based in its performance, and therefore, the singers may employ similar breath strategies between speech and song.

Chapter Summary

Breath and breathing strategies are paramount for optimal vocal performance regardless of genre. Understanding of the mechanisms of breathing for speech and song in the commercial music singer is warranted to facilitate efficient performance. The research supporting the understanding of breathing indicates there is much variability in the way professional singers breathe and their breathing strategies. Of specific interest is the fact that the majority of music theater performers and many pop performers are often actively engaged in dancing when singing, and this impacts their breathing dynamics. Although the level of physical activity on breathing technique notably distinguishes respiratory behaviors and patterns of certain music theater performers from that of other vocal performers, it is perhaps the most difficult to examine their respiratory kinematics given the dynamic nature of these types of performances. Yet, training and modifications of technique can be beneficial in developing breathing strategies that are most effective for a given performer and performance demands.

References

Blades-Zeller, E. (1994). Vocal pedagogy in the United States: Interviews with exemplary teachers of applied voice. *Journal of Research in Singing, 17*(2), 1-87.

Carroll, L., Sataloff, R., Heuer, R., Spiegel, J., Radionoff, S., & Cohn, J. (1996). Respiratory and glottal efficiency measures in normal classically trained singers. *Journal of Voice, 10*(2), 139-145.

Coffin, B. (1989). *Historical vocal pedagogy classics.* Metuchen, NJ: The Scarecrow Press.

Collyer, S., Kenny, D., & Archer, M. (2009). The effect of abdominal kinematic directives on respiratory behavior in female classical singing. *Logopedics Phoniatrics Vocology, 34*, 100-110.

Edwin, R. (1998). Belting 101. Parts 1 and 2. *Journal of Singing, 55*(1 & 2), 53-55, 61-62.

Foulds-Elliott, S., Thorpe, C., Cala, S., & Davis, P. (2000). Respiratory function in operatic singing: Effects of emotional connection. *Logopedics Phoniatrics Vocology, 25*, 151-168.

Garcia, M. (1984). *A complete treatise on the art of singing: Part One*, D. V. Paschke (Trans. & ed.). New York, NY: Da Capo Press. (Original work published 1841).

Griffin, B., Woo, P., Colton, R., Casper, J., & Brewer, D. (1995). Physiological characteristics of the supported singing voice. A preliminary study. *Journal of Voice, 9*(1), 45-56.

Henderson, L. (1991). *How to train singers.* West Nyack, NY: Parker Publishing.

Hoit, J., Jenks, C., Watson, P., & Cleveland, T. (1996). Respiratory function during speaking and singing in professional country singers. *Journal of Voice, 10*(1), 39-49.

Illi, S., Held, U., Frank, I., & Spengler, C. (2012). Effect of respiratory muscle training on exercise performance in healthy individuals: A systematic review and meta-analysis. *Sports Medicine, 42*(8), 707-724.

Iwarsson, J., Thomasson, M., & Sundberg, J. (1998). Effects of lung volume on the glottal source. *Journal of Voice, 12*(4), 424-433.

Lamperti, G. (1905). *The technics of Bel Canto*, T. Baker (Trans.). New York, NY: G. Shirmer.

Leanderson, R., Sundberg, J., & von Euler, C. (1987). Breathing muscle activity and subglottal pressure dynamics in singing and speech. *Journal of Voice, 1*(3), 258-261.

Marchesi, M. (1901). *Ten singing lessons.* New York, NY: Harper & Brothers.

Marchesi, M. (1967). *Vocal method* (2nd ed.). Milwaukee, WI: G. Schirmer.

Miller, R. (1997). *National schools of singing.* Lanham, MD: The Scarecrow Press.

Paulus, M., Flagan, T., Simmons, A., Gillis, K., Kotturi, S., Thom, N., . . . Swain, J. (2012). Subjecting elite athletes to inspiratory breathing load reveals behavioral and neural signatures of optimal performers in extreme environments. *PLoS ONE, 7*(1), e29394.

Petitt, M. (1994). Quiet breathing and breathing for singing: Anatomic and physiologic parameters. *Journal of Research in Singing, 18*(1), 21-39.

Pettersen, V. (2005). Muscular patterns and activation levels of auxiliary breathing muscles and thorax movement in classical singing. *Folia Phoniatrica, 57*(5-6), 255-277.

Pettersen, V. (2006). Preliminary findings on the classical singer's use of the pectoralis major muscle. *Folia Phoniatrica, 58*(6), 427-439.

Pettersen, V., & Bjørkøy, K. (2007). Consequences from emotional stimulus on breathing for singing. *Journal of Voice, 23*(3), 295-303.

Pettersen, V., Bjørkøy, K., Torp, H., & Westgaard, R. (2005). Neck and shoulder muscle activity and thorax movement in singing and speaking tasks with variation in vocal loudness and pitch. *Journal of Voice, 19*(4), 623-634.

Pettersen, V., & Eggebo, T. (2010). The movement of the diaphragm monitored by ultrasound imaging: Preliminary findings of diaphragm movements in classical singing. *Logopedics Phoniatrics Vocology, 35,* 105–112.

Pettersen, V., & Westgaard, R. (2004). The association between upper trapezius activity and thorax movement in classical singing. *Journal of Voice, 18*(4), 500–512.

Pettersen, V., & Westgaard, R. (2005). The activity patterns of neck muscles in professional classical singing. *Journal of Voice, 19*(2), 238–251.

Rolf, L., Sundberg, J., & von Euler, C. (1987). Role of diaphragmatic activity during singing: A study of transdiaphragmatic pressures. *Journal of Applied Physiology, 162*(1), 259–270.

Rothernberg, M., Miller, D., Molitor, R., & Leffingwell, D. (1987). The control of air flow during loud soprano singing. *Journal of Voice, 1*(3), 262–268.

Shakespeare, W. (1921). *The art of singing.* Bryn Mawr, PA: Oliver Ditson.

Stathopoulos, E., & Sapienza, C. (1993). Respiratory and laryngeal function of women and men during vocal intensity variation. *Journal of Speech and Hearing Research, 36*(1), 64–75.

Sullivan, J. (1989). How to teach the belt/pop voice. *Journal of Research in Singing and Applied Vocal Pedagogy, 13*(1), 41–56.

Sundberg, J., Elliot, N., Gramming, P., & Nord, L. (1993). Short-term variation of subglottal pressure for expressive purposes in singing and stage speech: A preliminary investigation. *Journal of Voice, 7*(3), 227–234.

Sundberg, J., Leanderson, R., von Euler, C., & Knutsson, E. (1991). Influence of body posture and lung volume on subglottal pressure control during singing. *Journal of Voice, 59*(4), 283–291.

Thomasson, M., & Sundberg, J. (2001). Consistency of inhalatory breathing patterns in professional operatic singers. *Journal of Voice, 15*(3), 373–383.

Thorpe, C. W., Cala, S., Chapman, J., & Davis, P. (2001). Patterns of breath support in projection of the singing voice. *Journal of Voice,* 15(1), 86–104.

Vennard, W. (1967). *Singing: The mechanism and the technic.* New York, NY: Carl Fischer.

Watson, P., & Hixon, T. (1985). Respiratory kinematics in classical (opera) singers. *JSHR, 28,* 104–122.

Watson, P., Hixon, T., Stathopoulos, E., & Sullivan, D. (1990). Respiratory kinematics in female classical singers. *Journal of Voice, 4*(2), 120–128.

Watson, A., Williams, C., & James, B. (2012). Activity patterns in latissimus dorsi and sternocleidomastoid in classical singers. *Journal of Voice, 26*(3), e95–e105.

3

Laryngeal Anatomy, Physiology, and Function During Singing

Introduction

The function of the human larynx as a means of vocal expression provides one of the distinguishing features separating human beings from other living animals. The capacity to generate and shape sound into verbal communication allows us to interact in a way that is unique to the human race. The ability to sing a lullaby to a child, or perform a song for an audience adds to the marvel of the many functions of the human larynx, even though verbal communication and singing are merely a secondary function of this highly versatile structure. This chapter provides an overview of the anatomy and physiology of the larynx. An overview of vocal fold vibration and laryngeal control of pitch and loudness is also discussed.

Role of the Larynx

The human larynx's primary role is noncommunicative. It is that of airway protection. The larynx houses the vocal folds, which serve to: (1) delineate the entrance to the upper respiratory system acting as a protective valve to prevent undesired objects, food, or liquid from entering into the airway, and (2) act as a functional valve allowing for buildup of air pressure below the closed vocal folds in order to volitionally and forcefully expectorate, or cough out an undesired object if it inadvertently has entered the airway. Its functionality continues helping in a valsalva maneuver, which allows for bearing down for lifting of heavy objects, defecation, or child bearing.

The highly evolved and refined functions of the human larynx, which include communicative and artistic functions, are secondary roles that are not integral to airway protection and breathing. The ability to produce sound in distress is not unique to humans; however, the ability to express emotions, and shape sounds into different languages or song distinguishes the human voice from many other animals.

As a sound generator, the larynx is incredibly flexible, capable of producing a wide array of frequencies and qualities. The following section describes the anatomy and physiology of the larynx including its structural framework and neighboring attachments. It emphasizes the adjustable nature of the larynx for control of frequency (pitch) and intensity (loudness). Readers desiring a more in-depth review are referred to several excellent articles and texts referenced in this chapter and listed in the bibliography (Armstrong & Netterville, 1995; Behrman, 2007; Moore, 2006; Netter, 1997; Titze, 1994; Zemlin, 1998).

Basic Laryngeal Anatomy and Physiology

The anatomy of the larynx is best thought of in terms of cartilages, joints, ligaments, membranes, intrinsic laryngeal muscles (which have both their origin and attachment within the framework of the larynx), and extrinsic laryngeal muscles (where either the origin or the attachment is outside the framework of the larynx), with a network of nerves and blood supply to the muscles.

There are two cartilages called the thyroid cartilage and cricoid cartilage and one bone, thee hyoid bone, which compose the primary external framework of the larynx. Within this cartilaginous housing are the vocal folds. There are 13 intrinsic laryngeal muscles (six paired and one unpaired)

and secondary cartilages (epiglottis, arytenoid cartilages, cuneiform cartilages, and corniculate cartilages). External to the laryngeal framework are the nine paired extrinsic muscles and ligaments. The role of the extrinsic muscles is to raise (laryngeal elevators) or lower (laryngeal depressors) the larynx in the neck. The larynx is situated directly under the base of the tongue extending down to the superior portion of the trachea. Relative to the cervical spine, the larynx extends down the 3rd, 4th, and 5th cervical vertebrae. Figure 3–1 illustrates the position of the larynx relative to the head and neck. On average, the structural framework of the larynx in men is 44 mm in length and 43 mm in diameter, whereas women on average measure 36 mm and 41 mm (Behrman, 2007). Surrounding the larynx posteriorly and laterally is the pharynx, referred to in lay terms as the back of the throat. The pharynx is composed of three parts: nasopharynx (back of the nose to just above the palate), oropharynx (palate to base of tongue), and laryngopharynx (base of tongue to vocal folds/upper esophageal inlet).

Framework of the Larynx

The larynx is a floating structure attached to the tongue above and the trachea below, allowing it to move several centimeters upward and downward. This flexibility (elevation and lowering) is necessary for a timely, protective response during laryngeal reflexes such as airway protection during a swallow. The thyroid cartilage, cricoid cartilage, and the hyoid bone compose the external laryngeal framework.

The Hyoid Bone

The hyoid bone is a horseshoe-shaped bone that is the only bone not attached to

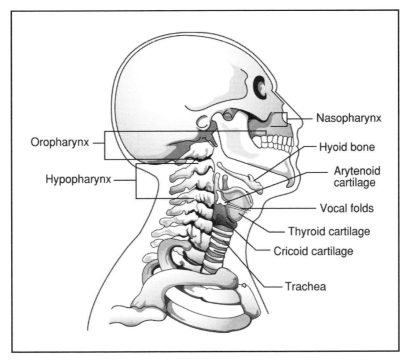

Figure 3–1. Laryngeal cartilaginous structures in anatomic relationship. Adapted from *The Larynx: A Multidisciplinary Approach* (2nd ed., p. 34) by M. P. Fried, 1996, Mosby.

another bone in the body (tongue above and cartilage below). The hyoid bone suspends the larynx, and muscular pull or push on this bone results in elevation or depression of the entire laryngeal mechanism. The hyoid bone suspends the larynx superiorly and attaches to the superior process of the thyroid cartilage via the thyrohyoid ligaments and membrane. The superior aspect of the hyoid bone attaches to the base of the tongue via the glossoepiglottic ligaments. Because many of the tongue muscles have attachments to the hyoid bone (digastric, mylohyoid, geniohyoid, hyoglossus), it is not uncommon for singers who have tongue tension, consequentially to have resulting laryngeal tension due to hyoid muscle attachments.

The Thyroid Cartilage

Inferior to, or underneath the hyoid bone is the thyroid cartilage, which is the largest cartilage of the laryngeal framework. The thyroid cartilage consists of two laminae, which join anteriorly (toward the front of the body) forming the prominence commonly referred to as the Adam's apple. The thyroid cartilage does not join completely in the back. The superior portion of the thyroid cartilage connects to the hyoid bone and the inferior portion connects to the cricoid cartilage via muscular and ligament attachments. Specifically the thyrohyoid muscle attaches to the hyoid bone above, and the cricothyroid muscle attaches to the cricoid cartilage below. The muscles and their impact on laryngeal function are discussed below.

The Cricoid Cartilage

The cricoid cartilage is the third primary structure of the laryngeal framework. It sits inferior to the thyroid cartilage, and it completely encircles the upper-most portion of the airway/trachea. The shape of the cricoid cartilage is often described as a signet ring. This cartilage serves as a base for the larynx and in addition to the cricothyroid muscle; the cricoid cartilage also provides muscular attachments for the posterior cricoarytenoid muscles and the lateral cricoarytenoid muscles.

The Arytenoid Cartilages

Housed within the laryngeal vestibule are the arytenoid cartilages. These are paired, pyramidal shaped cartilages, which sit on top of the posterior portion of the cricoid. At the base of these pyramids are the muscular process posteriorly, and the vocal process anteriorly. The top part of the arytenoid pyramidal structure is called the apex.

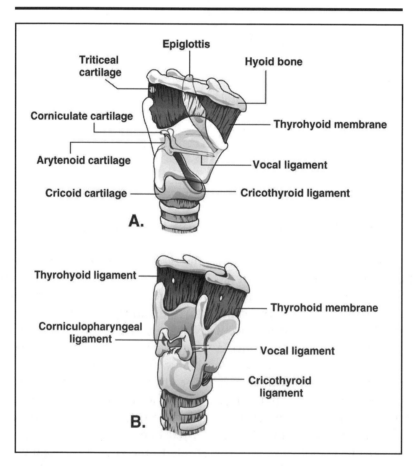

Figure 3–2. Lateral view (*left*) and sagittal section (*right*) of laryngeal ligaments. Adapted from *Atlas of Human Anatomy* (p. 78), 2001, Springhouse, PA: Springhouse Corporation.

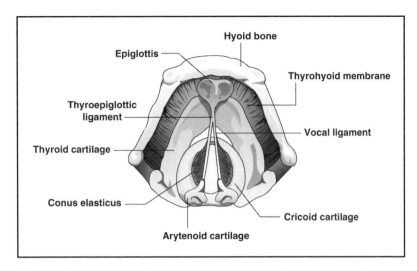

Figure 3–3. Laryngeal ligaments as viewed from above. Adapted from *The Larynx: A Multidisciplinary Approach* (2nd ed., p. 38), by M. P. Fried, 1996, Mosby.

These projections are important because they serve as origin and insertion points for many of the muscular portions of the vocal folds. The thyroarytenoid muscle attaches the vocal process of the arytenoid cartilages to the thyroid cartilage. Additional intrinsic muscles of the larynx that originate or attach to the arytenoid cartilages include: transverse arytenoid muscles, posterior cricoarytenoid muscles, lateral cricoarytenoid muscles, and oblique arytenoid muscles. The vocal process and muscular process allow for the vocal folds to be positioned in order to abduct (open) and adduct (close) the vocal folds. Figures 3–2 and 3–3 demonstrate various views of the laryngeal ligaments and cartilages.

Joints of the Larynx

The larynx has several types of joints to allow for movement. The primary joints are the cricothyroid joints and cricoarytenoid joints. Each provides a different type of movement within the larynx.

The Cricothyroid Joints

The cricothyroid joints are formed at the juncture of the inferior horn of the inner surface of thyroid cartilage to the lateral portion of the exterior surface for the cricoid cartilage bilaterally. These joints govern the relative angle of the thyroid cartilage to the cricoid cartilage. The relationship and structure of the thyroid and cricoid cartilages allows for versatility in range of motion largely due to the two types of movements these joints allow, including a rotary movement (tipping movement) and a sliding movement (posterior to anterior). The cricothyroid joints are supported by the cricothyroid ligaments, which stabilize the position of the thyroid cartilage unless the cricothyroid muscle is contracted. The role of the

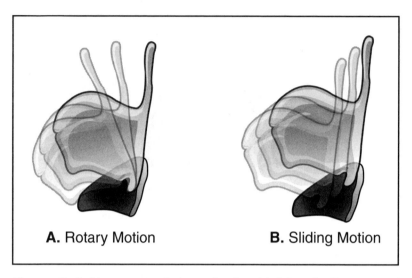

A. Rotary Motion   **B.** Sliding Motion

Figure 3–4. Movement of the cricothyroid joint **A.** Rotary and **B.** Sliding. From *Speech and Voice Science, 2E* (Figure 5–19, 1st ed., p. 134) by A. Behrman, 2013, Plural Publishing.

cricothyroid muscle is further described below. Figure 3-4 shows the role of the cricothyroid joint (rotary and sliding movement) and impact on the angle of the thyroid cartilage relative to the cricoid cartilage.

The Cricoarytenoid Joints

The cricoarytenoid joints are multiaxial joints formed at the articular facets of the arytenoid cartilages and cricoid cartilages. These joints are stabilized by the cricoarytenoid ligaments. The cricoarytenoid joints allow the arytenoids to both rock and glide, allowing for versatility in their movements such as rotation in medial-lateral or anterior-posterior directions (Figure 3–5). The intrinsic laryngeal muscles attaching to the muscular process of the arytenoid cartilage are the lateral cricoarytenoid muscle (LCA) and the posterior cricoarytenoid muscle (PCA) further described in the segment on muscles below. Movement of

the cricoarytenoid joint is directly related to the contraction of these two muscles relative to each other, as they are agonist/ antagonist pairs. For example, contraction of the LCA will move the tip of the medial edge of the muscular process of the arytenoid cartilage toward the midline, resulting in adduction of the vocal folds. Conversely, contraction of the PCA will move the muscular process of the arytenoid cartilage away from the midline resulting in abduction of the vocal folds. The range of motion afforded by both the cricothyroid and cricoarytenoid joints allows for a flexibility that enables singers to quickly adjust vocal positioning folds during various vocal tasks.

Muscles of the Larynx

Muscles are a specialized group of cells within the body that contract when stimulated by a nerve impulse. When at rest, skel-

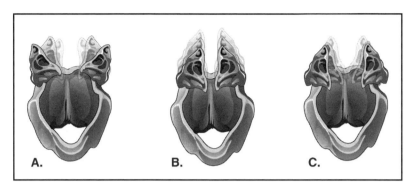

Figure 3–5. Movement of bilateral cricoarytenoid joint: **A.** primary, **B.** small amount of sliding, **C.** minor rotation). From *Anatomical and Physiological Bases of Speech* (p. 150), by D. R. Dickson and W. Maue-Dickson. Copyright 1982 Elsevier. Reprinted with permission from Elsevier.

etal muscles are generally long and lean. When contracted, they become foreshortened and increase in bulk. Muscles are capable of foreshortening up to half their resting length; however, more typically they function within 10% to 20% of their resting length (Behrman, 2007; Lieber, 2010).

Many muscles in the body have a partner muscle performing an opposite action. These partners are referred to as agonist/antagonist pairs. A commonly thought of example agonist/antagonist pairs would be the bicep and tricep muscles of the arm. When the bicep is contracted, the tricep is not acting in its primary role and vice versa. Both muscles need to be functioning and toned for the arm to be fully functional, but they are not both acting as agonists simultaneously. The cricothyroid muscle (CT) and thyroarytenoid muscle (TA), described below, are an agonist/antagonist pair, and the interaction and coordination of these two muscles play an important role in regulating pitch, intensity, and quality of the sound source.

Extrinsic Laryngeal Muscles

The muscles in the larynx can be thought of in terms of their relationship and connection to the laryngeal framework. The extrinsic muscles surround the outer portion of the cartilaginous framework and have various attachments to the tongue, jaw, clavicle, sternum, and hyoid bone. These muscles serve to stabilize the larynx, and

> Agonist: Muscle that causes motion to achieve a movement.
> Antagonist: A muscle that can move the joint opposite to the movement produced by the agonist.
> Synergist: A subcategory of an agonist muscle that helps another muscle accomplish a movement.
> Stabilizer: A muscle that contracts with no significant movement to maintain a posture or fixate a joint.

also allow for the adjustment of the vertical position (up and down movement).

Infrahyoid Muscles

Extrinsic muscles attaching at the hyoid bone or inferior to the hyoid bone are referred to as infrahyoid muscles. These include the sternohyoid muscle, sternothyroid muscle, thyrohyoid muscle, and omohyoid muscle. The sternohyoid muscle originates on the sternum (breastbone) and the clavicle (collarbone). It courses upward and attaches into the hyoid bone. When the sternohyoid muscle contracts, it pulls the hyoid bone down and depresses the larynx. The sternothyroid muscle begins at the sternum and attaches into the oblique line of the thyroid cartilage. Similar to the sternohyoid, when the sternothyroid muscle contracts, it acts to pull the thyroid cartilage downward. The thyrohyoid muscle originates at the oblique line of the thyroid cartilage and attaches to the inferior boarder of the hyoid bone. When the thyrohyoid muscle contracts, it decreases the space between the thyroid cartilage and the hyoid bone. Finally, the omohyoid muscle (*omo* means shoulder) actually originates on the scapula (shoulder blade), courses through a fascial loop on the clavicle, and attaches to the hyoid bone. Contraction of the omohyoid results in stabilization and depression of the hyoid bone. The nerves that are responsible

---

There are 12 pairs of cranial nerves, which come directly off of the brainstem and 31 pairs of spinal nerves that correspond to the segments of the spinal cord (cervical , thoracic, lumbar, and sacral). See Chapter 4 for a more detailed description of motor and sensory nerves.

---

for innervating the infrahyoid muscles include cervical nerves C1–C3.

Table 3–1 and Figures 3–6A and 3–6B delineate these muscles and their attachments.

Suprahyoid Muscles

Muscles attaching superior to the hyoid bone are called suprahyoid muscles. These muscles allow for movement or stabilization of the hyoid bone. The suprahyoid muscles include: mylohyoid muscle, digastric muscle (anterior and posterior bellies), stylohyoid muscle, and geniohyoid muscle. The mylohyoid muscle originates from the mandible and attaches to the hyoid bone. Contraction of this muscle either elevates the hyoid bone or depresses the mandible depending on which of the two bony structures is stable. Motor innervation to the mylohyoid muscle is provided by cranial nerve V (trigeminal nerve).

The digastric muscle is composed of two parts: the anterior belly and the posterior belly, which are connected by a tendon in the middle. The anterior belly originates on the inner surface of the mandible and courses toward the hyoid bone inserting into the intermediate tendon. The posterior belly of the digastric originates at the intermediate tendon and courses to insert on the mastoid process of the temporal bone (skull). Together, contraction of both the anterior and posterior bellies of the digastric serves to elevate the hyoid and also move it anteriorly. Interestingly, the anterior belly of the digastric has nerve innervation via cranial nerve V (trigeminal nerve), while the posterior belly is innervated by cranial nerve VII (facial nerve).

The geniohyoid (*genio* means chin) moves both the tongue and the hyoid anteriorly and widens the pharynx during swallowing. The origin of the geniohyoid muscle arises from near midline of the in-

TABLE 3–1. Extrinsic Laryngeal Muscles

Muscle	Attachments	Function
Suprahyoid Muscles		
Stylohyoid	Temperal bone (styloid process) to hyoid	Raises hyoid bone posteriorly
Mylohyoid	Mandible to hyoid	Raises hyoid bone anteriorly
Digastric	Two bellies, anterior and posterior:	
Anterior	Mandible to hyoid	Raises hyoid bone anteriorly
Posterior	Temporal bone (mastoid process) to hyoid	Raises hyoid bone posteriorly
Geniohyoid	Mandible to hyoid	Raises hyoid bone anteriorly
Infrahyoid Muscles		
Thyrohyoid	Thyroid to hyoid	Brings thyroid cartilage and hyoid bone closer
Sternothyroid	Sternum to thyroid	Lowers thyroid cartilage
Sternohyoid	Sternum to hyoid	Lowers hyoid bone
Omohyoid	Scapula to hyoid	Lowers hyoid bone

Source: Adapted from *Clinical Voice Pathology: Theory and Management* (3rd ed., p. 34). By J. C. Stemple, L. E. Glaze, and B. G. Klaben, 2000, Plural Publishing.

side of the mandible and courses directly back to attach into the body of the hyoid bone. Cervical nerve 1 (CN1) provides motor innervation to this muscle.

The stylohyoid serves to both retract and elevate the hyoid bone. Originating from the styloid process (on the temporal bone of the skull), this muscle courses down and forward inserting onto the hyoid bone. The stylohyoid muscle parallels the digastric muscle. Motor function to this muscle comes from cranial nerve VII (facial nerve).

See Figures 3-6A and 3-6B, which show the muscles from the front, and Figure 3-7 which depicts possible muscular action of the neck strap muscles (A) and tongue and suprahyoid muscles (B) on laryngeal position.

Intrinsic Laryngeal Muscles

The intrinsic muscles of the larynx are encased within the laryngeal framework of the

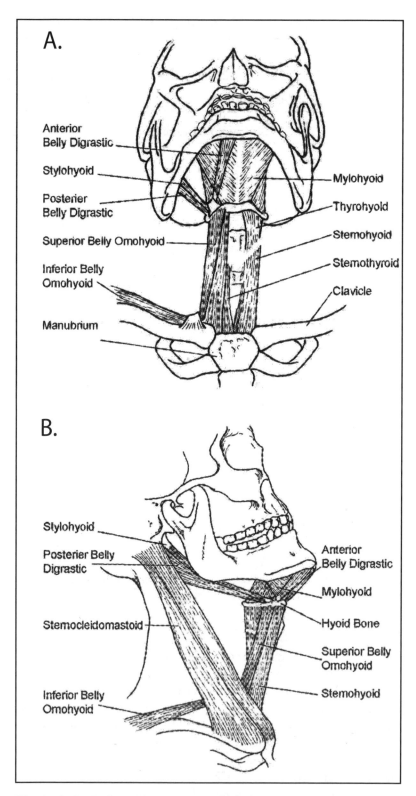

Figure 3–6. A. Anterior view of suprahyoid and infrahyoid muscles **B**. Lateral view of extrinsic muscles. From *Voice Disorders, 2e*, by C. Sapienza and B. Hoffman Ruddy. Copyright 2013, Plural Publishing. Reprinted with permission.

thyroid and cricoid cartilages. The primary functions of these muscles are to: (1) abduct or open for breathing, and (2) adduct, or close for airway protection or phonation, (3) tense to increase length, or (4) relax to shorten length. The adductors serve to move the vocal folds medially. They include the thyroarytenoid muscle, lateral cricoarytenoid muscle, and interarytenoids muscle. The posterior cricoarytenoid muscle is the only intrinsic muscle that serves to abduct the vocal folds. The cricothyroid muscle serves as the tensor resulting in lengthening of the vocal folds while the thyroarytenoid muscle serves as a tensor, relaxer, or adductor depending on other muscle action.

Adductors: Thyroarytenoid, Lateral Cricoarytenoid, Interarytenoids

The thyroarytenoid (TA) originates at the interior surface of the thyroid cartilage just below the thyroid notch (Adam's apple). The place of origin is referred to as the anterior commissure, and from this point, the TA extends posteriorly along the thyroid cartilage bilaterally. The TA terminates at the muscular process of the arytenoid cartilages. This muscle comprises the bulk of the vocal folds and can be further thought of in two parts: the thyrovocalis and thyromuscularis. Contraction of the TA shortens and increases the bulk of the vocal folds functionally lowering pitch. Motor innervation to the TA is provided by cranial nerve X (vagus), specifically by the recurrent laryngeal branch. The microanatomy of the TA muscle is further described below.

The lateral cricoarytenoid (LCA) muscle originates on the superior border of the cricoid cartilage and extends into the muscular process of the arytenoid cartilages bilaterally. A primary adductor of the vocal folds, contraction of the LCA positions the

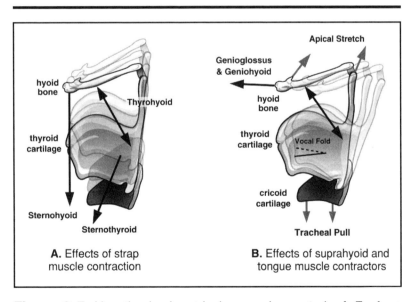

Figure 3–7. Hypothesized extrinsic muscle control of F_0 from contraction of the **A.** strap muscles, and **B.** suprahyoid and tongue muscles. From "Laryngeal and Extra Laryngeal Mechanisms of F_0 Control" by Honda in F. Bell-Berti and L. J. Raphael (Eds.), 1985, *Producing Speech: Contemporary Issues* (p. 223). New York, NY: American Institute of Physics Press. Reprinted with permission.

It is important to note the relationship between movement of the tongue, larynx, and supraglottic structures via these connections, as tension and imbalance in these structures can possibly impact physiology during singing. For example, the larynx is fixed inferiorly to the trachea; however, it is completely suspended superiorly via the above-mentioned infrahyoid and suprahyoid muscles making the larynx in essence a passive vessel amid a sea of competing musculature. It is this relationship of the larynx to these extrinsic muscles and their connections to the surrounding structures of the upper torso, cervical spine, tongue, and jaw that can make the larynx and vocal tract vulnerable to physical imbalance and muscular tension. As with most styles of singing, attention to balance and coordination of these muscles is important to facilitate free, adaptable, and responsive sound, allowing a hybrid singer to sing in multiple styles.

arytenoid cartilages medially, approximating the vocal processes of the arytenoids via movement of the cricoarytenoid joint. This allows for closure of the glottis by approximating the vocal processes of the arytenoids. This muscle is also innervated by the recurrent branch of the laryngeal nerve (branch of CNX).

The interarytenoids (IA) are composed of two muscles. The transverse muscle is unpaired and essentially connects the lateral portion of the arytenoid cartilage to the contralateral arytenoid cartilage. The oblique muscle is a paired muscle. It runs diagonally from the base of the muscular process of one arytenoid cartilage traveling up toward the apex of the other arytenoid cartilage. The arrangement of the interarytenoids allows them to aid the LCA in adducting the vocal folds for phonation and airway protection. Motor innervation of the IA is also the recurrent laryngeal nerve (RLN), branch of CNX.

Abductor: Posterior Cricoarytenoid

The posterior cricoarytenoid (PCA) is the only abductor. It is a paired muscle that runs from the posterior aspect of the cricoid cartilage upward to the muscular process of the arytenoid cartilage on the same side. When the PCA contracts, it rotates the vocal process away from the midline, thus opening, or abducting the vocal folds. This muscle is the agonist muscle to the LCA, as it imposes the opposite movement when contracted without opposition from LCA muscle. The motor innervation of the PCA comes from a branch of the recurrent laryngeal nerve (CNX).

Tensor: Cricothyroid

The cricothyroid (CT) is the primary tensor muscle of the vocal fold. It is a paired muscle that courses from the anterior portion of the cricoid cartilage and connects vertically to the inferior border of the thyroid cartilage and posteriorly to the lower portion of the thyroid cartilage. Contraction of the CT narrows the space between the superior border of the cricoid and the inferior border of the thyroid anteriorly. As described earlier, this narrowing tilts the thyroid cartilage downward, lengthening and tensing the vocal folds via the cricothyroid joint. The motor function to the CT is provided by the external branch of the superior laryngeal nerve (SLN), which is also a branch of CNX.

Relaxer: Thyroarytenoid

The thyroarytenoid, discussed in detail above, acts as an adductor, relaxer, and tenser depending on the surrounding muscle activity. Figure 3-8 shows intrinsic laryngeal musculature from various views, and Figure 3-9 shows schematic representation of their primary actions. Table 3-2 lists the actions of the intrinsic muscles of the larynx.

Review of Nerve Supply to the Intrinsic Muscles

In order for any muscle to contract or relax (motor function), it has to have a signal to do so from the brain, in the form of nerve conduction. The larynx receives its motor innervation from the vagus nerve CNX. Specifically two branches: the recurrent laryngeal nerve (RLN) innervates all of the

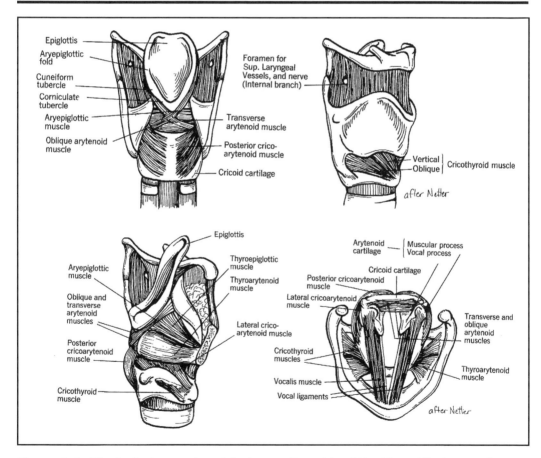

Figure 3–8. The intrinsic muscles of the larynx. From *Vocal Health and Pedagogy: Science and Assessment, Second Edition,* by R. Sataloff. Copyright 2006. Plural Publishing. Reprinted with permission.

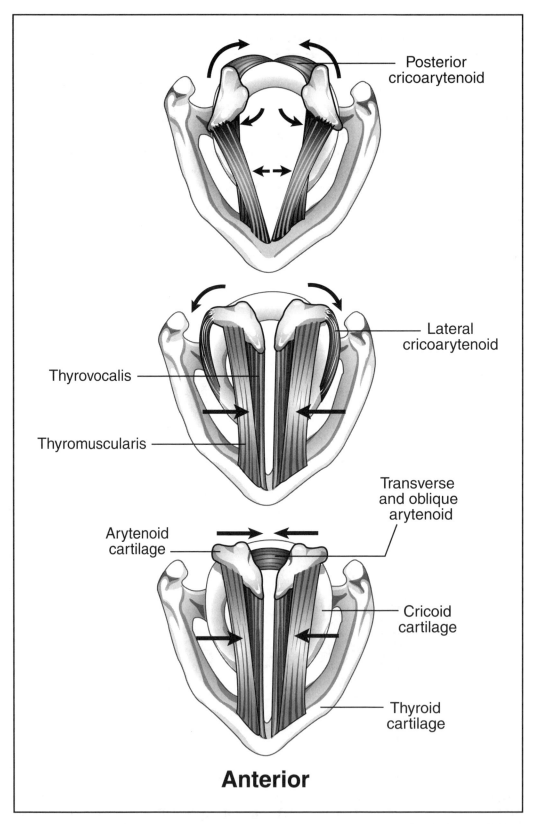

Figure 3–9. Superior view of general activity of intrinsic laryngeal muscles. From *Speech and Voice Science, Second Edition* by A. Behrman. Copyright 2013. Plural Publishing. Reprinted with permission.

TABLE 3–2. Intrinsic Laryngeal Muscle Functions

Parameters	
Function	Adduction or abduction of the vocal folds
Length	Shortening or lengthening the true vocal folds
Thickness	Thickening or thinning of the body of the vocal folds
Edge	Sharpening or rounding the free edge of the vocal folds
Tension	Increasing or decreasing stiffness of the vocal folds

Muscle Actions					
	CT	**TA**	**LCA**	**IA**	**PCA**
Function	Tensor	Adductor	Adductor	Adductor	Abductor
Length	Longer	Shorter	Shorter	—	NA
Thickness	Thinner	Thicker	Thicker	—	NA
Edge	Sharper	Rounder	Rounder	—	—
Tension	Stiffer	Stiffer	—	—	—

Source: Adapted from *Clinical Voice Pathology: Theory and Management* (3rd ed., p. 41). By J. C. Stemple, L. E. Glaze, and B. G. Klaben, 2000, Plural Publishing.
CT = cricothyroid; *TA* = thyroarytenoid; *LCA* = lateral cricoarytenoid; *IA* = interarytenoid; *PCA* = posterior cricoarytenoid; *NA* = not applicable.

intrinsic laryngeal muscles except for the CT. The cricothyroid receives its innervation from the external branch of the superior laryngeal nerve (SLN). The separate innervation of the TA and CT allows for independent motor control of these muscles. In addition to motor function, the sensory function of the larynx is also provided by the vagus nerve. Specifically, the internal branch of the superior laryngeal nerve provides sensory function for the larynx above the vocal folds, and the recurrent laryngeal nerve provides sensory function below the vocal folds. Both motor and sensory function are vital for controlling the many variables of singing such as modulating pitch and register changes independently.

Microstructure of the Vocal Folds

The anatomic laryngeal structures and their functions have been discussed previously; however, further discussion of the vocal folds is warranted to understand their complex behavior during phonation. The microanatomy of the vocal folds can be thought of as a system of layers (Fujimara, 1981; Gray, 2000; Gray, Hirano, & Sato, 1993; Hirano, 1974, 1977). Each vocal fold layer is composed of different biomechanical attributes, histology, and cellular make-up, allowing for a unique matrix vital for human voice production. The outermost layer

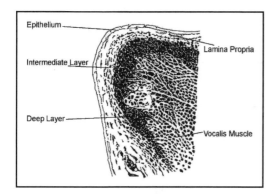

Figure 3–10. Histologic layers, as seen from a cross-section of the vocal fold mid-portion. From *Voice Disorders, Second Edition,* p. 33, by C. Sapienza and B. Hoffman Ruddy, 2013, Plural Publishing. Used with permission.

chemical and mechanical assault (Bartlett & Thibeault, 2011). Additionally, the epithelial cells help facilitate hydration of the vocal folds, which is critical for efficient vibratory function (Gray, 2000). The epithelium overlays the superficial, intermediate, and deep layers of the vocal folds, collectively called the lamina propria (LP). Figure 3–10 shows a photomicrographic slice of the adult male vocal fold in a cross section. Figure 3–11 shows a schematic representation of the same layers of the vocal fold, including fiber density and organization of each layer.

The biomechanical attributes of the LP and its overlying epithelium play a predominant role in vibration of the vocal folds. The noncellular materials found within the three layers of the lamina propria are referred to as the extracellular matrix (ECM). The ECM is composed of fibrous proteins such as collagen and elastic in addition to interstitial fluids, and these are described below. When vocal fold injury occurs, the manner in which the ECM is remodeled during wound healing is vital because the

of the vocal folds is the epithelium. The epithelium is covered by a veil of mucous. These mucous secretions emerge from glands, which sit below the vocal folds and within the laryngeal vestibule and are important for efficient vocal fold vibration (Behrman, 2007). This mucoserous coating serves as a protective blanket against both

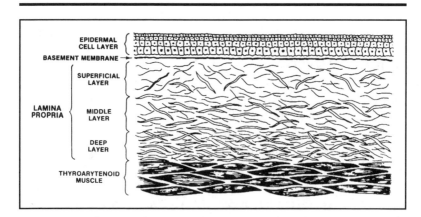

Figure 3–11. Structure of the basement membrane zone of the vocal folds. From "Basement Membrane Zone Injury in Vocal Folds," by S. D. Gray, 1991, in *Vocal Fold Physiology* by J. Gauffin and B. Hammarberg (Eds.), Singular Publishing. Reprinted with permission.

ECM makeup has direct impact on the biomechanical properties of the vocal fold tissue (Bartlett & Thibeault, 2011). The process of wound healing is discussed further in Chapter 6.

The epithelium is approximately 0.05 to 0.10 mm in thickness and has ridges on the surface (Titze, 1994). Other properties within the vocal fold mucosa, which compose the ECM, are interstitial fluids, such as hyaluronic acid, which are in-between the elastin and collagen fibers. The interstitial fluid is important because it is thought to provide shock absorption during vocal fold vibration (Bartlett & Thibeault, 2011). It has been postulated that this layer is well-designed to withstand the consistent frictional forces and sheering stresses incurred by the vocal folds during the impact of phonation. This is because the nonmuscular layers of the vocal folds are organized with variations in the width creating areas of reinforcement at the points of greatest contact (Hirano, 1977; Hirano, Kurita, & Nakashima, 1981). Histological studies of the vocal folds have demonstrated a thickening of the mucosal tissue in areas of the fold where collisional forces are greatest (Titze, 1994). Just under the epithelium is the basement membrane zone, which connects to the lamina propria via anchoring fibers. In some instances, when there is injury to the vocal folds (i.e., vocal fold nodules), the anchoring fibers detach from the lamina propria (Titze & Verdolini Abbot, 2012).

The superficial layer of the LP is also referred to as Reinke's Space. It is approximately 0.05 mm in thickness and is composed of loosely organized, but highly pliable elastin fibers. Elastin is a fibrous protein, which allows for flexibility and viscoelastic properties of the vocal folds allowing them to elongate and then return to their neutral state (Bartlett & Thibeault, 2011; Hirano, Kurita, & Nakashima, 1981).

The fibers are not organized in a parallel fashion along the free edge of the vocal fold. In fact, the fibers are somewhat randomly arranged within a gelatinous consistency. The density of fibers in the outer layer is very low relative to the intermediate and deep layers of the vocal fold allowing for pliability of the mucosal tissue of the vocal fold. This pliability is necessary to allow for changes in length of the vocal fold during phonation. Under the superficial layer

The more dense the collagen fiber, the less elastic the tissue is, making it more resistant to changes in length. Therefore, the vocal folds are the most pliable on the superficial layer and become increasingly more resistant to changes in length within the intermediate and deeper layers of the LP. These five layers have been referred to differently in terms of biomechanical schemes. Hirano described a two-layer body-cover scheme. The body refers to the muscle and the deep layer of the LP, and cover refers to the intermediate, superficial, and epithelium (Gray, 2000; Gray et al., 1993; Hirano, 1974, 1977; Hirano et al., 1981). In a three-layer scheme, the mucosa consists of the epithelium and superficial layer of LP, the transition consists of the intermediate and deep layers of the LP, also referred to as the vocal ligament and the third layer is the body, or TA muscle. Regardless of the two-layer or three-layer approach, the interaction of the cover and the body of the vocal folds are critical for fine control singing and registration, and this is discussed in greater detail.

is the intermediate layer of the LP. It is approximately 1 to 2 mm in thickness and is populated predominantly with elastin fibers in comparison with the superficial layer. In this layer, the elastin fibers are more organized and are interwoven lying in a parallel orientation along the free edge of the vocal fold.

The deepest layer of the LP is 1 to 2 mm in thickness and is the most densely populated layer. Collagen fibers and a fibrous protein lying in an organized, parallel fashion along the edge of the vocal fold within this layer help to provide strength to the vocal folds. There is some overlap of the connective fibers of the intermediate and deep layers of the LP. The thyroarytenoid muscle sits next to the deep layer of the LP, with the muscle fibers running in an anterior to posterior direction. This anterior-posterior coursing of the fibers lies in the same orientation as the elastin and collagen fibers of the intermediate and deep layers of the LP. In summary, the layers increase in density and stiffness as they move away from the mucosal edge of the vocal fold moving deeper toward the thyroarytenoid (TA) muscle.

Vocal Fold Vibration

There have been several theories describing voice production. The myoelastic aerodynamic theory is the most widely accepted theory. Although the theory sounds daunting, broken down it means myo (muscle), elastic (stretch), aero (air), dynamic (constantly changing), or in simple terms, with changing muscle stretch/contraction and changing airflow movement, the vocal folds vibrate. It was initially described by a German anatomist named Johannes Muller and was later expanded in greater detail by Van den Berg in 1958. This theory described by Muller was based on experiments using excised larynges creating vocal fold vibration by sending a stream of air from below excised vocal folds, while altering the longitudinal tension by imposing an outside force upon them.

Two events were confirmed based on this experiment. First, when the vocal folds were brought together toward the midline, they vibrated in the presence of an air stream coming from below (subglottal pressure). Second, when the tension of the vocal folds was increased, they vibrated at a faster rate (Van den Berg, 1958). To further understand these basic physiologic principles, an understanding of the Bernoulli effect is required.

Simply stated, the Bernoulli effect is the occurrence of a drop in pressure created when a liquid or gas increases in velocity as it passes through an area of constriction (Borden, 1994; Titze, 1994). This principle can be demonstrated by holding two pieces of paper facing each other in front of the lips and blowing a stream of air through the center of the two papers. This will cause the papers to approximate toward each other via the suction effect of the Bernoulli principle. Now consider how this principle plays a role in vocal fold vibration. It is important to note that the opening and closing of the vocal folds during vibration must be distinguished from the abduction and adduction of the vocal folds for breathing and phonation respectively. The arytenoid cartilages maintain closure during vocal fold vibration; they do not open and close with each vibration.

There are several things occurring biomechanically that allow for vocal fold vibration. Recall the myo-elastic aerodynamic theory of phonation. The aerodynamic component refers to the Bernoulli effect, which aids in pulling the mucosal cover of the vocal folds together to perpetuate vocal fold vibration. The myo-elastic component refers to the adduction (coming together) of the vocal folds via neuromuscular muscle (myo)contraction of the adductory muscle of the larynx, and the elastic component refers to the biomechanical properties of the layers of the vocal folds allowing for both displacement and recoil of vocal fold tissue during vocal fold vibration. The displacement occurs via actions of external forces including both aerodynamic and muscular forces. The recoil, or return to a neutral state occurs when these forces cease. For example, when the CT is active, the vocal folds will elongate. This elongation is permitted to occur because of both the stretching properties of the TA muscle and the elastic properties of the epithelium and lamina propria. When the vocal folds are elongated via contraction of the CT, the vocal folds become increasingly tense and taught, resulting in a faster vibration rate. When CT contraction stops, the muscular and nonmuscular layers of the vocal fold return or recoil back to their resting state when unopposed by other external forces.

Therefore, vocal fold vibration is reliant on: (1) neuromuscular control to adduct or approximate the vocal folds, (2) biomechanical attributes of displacement and recoil allowed for by the elastic properties of the vocal fold layers, and (3) driving force of air pressure, to facilitate aerodynamic activities of subglottal pressure and Bernoulli effect to help perpetuate vocal fold vibration. All of these must occur in order to initiate and maintain vocal fold vibration. A disturbance of any of these actions results in suboptimal phonatory efficiency and vocal output. For example, if you have any type of vocal fold pathology (nodules, polyp, cyst, etc.), it is the disruption of vocal fold vibration and alteration of vocal fold closure that in part creates the resulting hoarseness.

One Vibratory Cycle

One episode of opening and closing is referred to as one cycle of vibration. The listener perceived pitch is determined by the number of cycles occurring within one second and is referred to as the fundamental frequency (F_0). For example, if a singer sings an A4, the vocal folds have open and closed 440 times/second. If a louder (more intense) sound is produced, the amplitude of vibration (excursion of the vocal folds from midline and back) is increased because subglottal pressure must increase. The relative involvement of both body and cover are dynamic and changing as the singer changes frequency, intensity, and timbre. The degree of activation of TA versus CT and ratio of cover versus body may be important considerations in terms of vocal register (i.e., chest voice, head voice, mix).

Looking more specifically at the interaction of the three events discussed above, let us break down one cycle of vocal fold vibration: The vocal folds are approximated via contraction of the adductory muscles of the larynx (TC, LCA, IA). As exhalation occurs, the driving force of air pressure from the lungs is met with resistance against the now adducted vocal folds. As the subglottal air pressure just below the closed vocal folds increases, the elastic properties of the vocal folds eventually succumb to the pressure, resulting in a displacement of the nonmuscular layer of the vocal folds laterally, away from the midline. When this opening occurs, the vocal folds open first at the underside, or inferior margin, followed by the upper border, which lags behind. Essentially, the inferior and superior margins of the nonmuscular layers of the

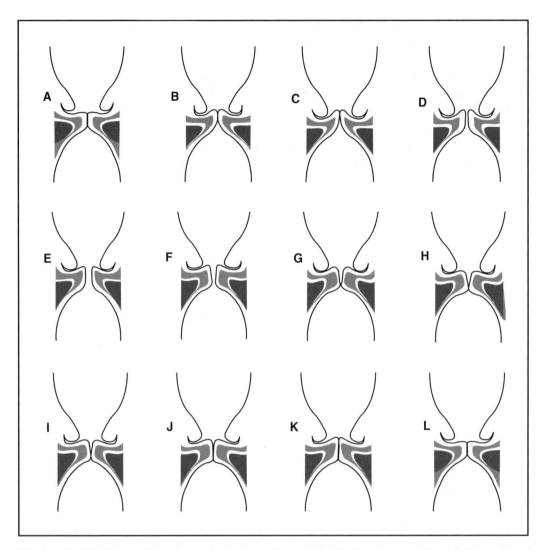

Figure 3–12. Schematic of coronal view of vocal fold vibratory motion. Schematic of coronal section of the vocal folds. From *Speech and Voice Science, Second Edition* by A. Behrman. Copyright 2013 by Plural Publishing. Reprinted with permission.

vocal folds are moving in opposite directions with the inferior margin achieving its full lateral excursion while the superior margin is still opening. Consequently, the inferior margin has begun approximating again while the superior margin is at its widest excursion. In essence, the inferior margin is always leading the superior margin of the vocal fold. This vibration pattern is referred to as the amplitude of vibration. When the inferior margin of the vocal fold is opening, the superior margin is closed, forming the apex of a triangle, with the inferior margin serving as the wider base.

At this snapshot during vocal fold vibration, the glottis is in a convergent shape (Behrman, 2007; Titze, 1994). Figure 3–12 depicts a schematic representation of one

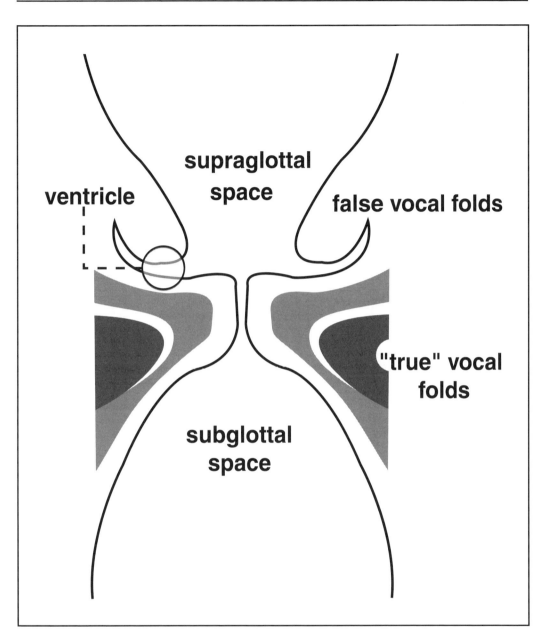

Figure 3–13. Schematic of coronal section of vocal folds. From *Speech and Voice Science, Second Edition* by A. Behrman. Copyright 2013 by Plural Publishing. Reprinted with permission.

full cycle of vocal fold vibration in a coronal (frontal) view. Figure 3–13 is a schematic representation of a coronal section (frontal) of the vocal folds. Figure 3–14 shows the same representation of one cycle of vocal fold vibration viewing the vocal folds from above. This glottal configuration is crucial because it allows for a buildup of subglottal air pressure generating a robust lateral movement of the cover of the vocal

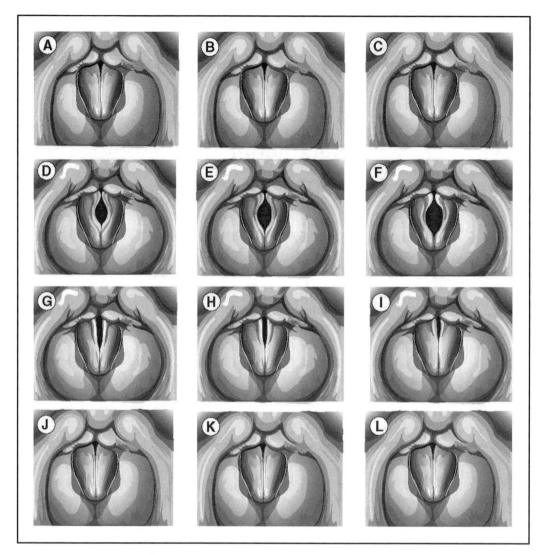

Figure 3–14. Schematic of superior view of vocal fold vibratory motion. From *Speech and Voice Science, Second Edition* by A. Behrman. Copyright 2013 by Plural Publishing. Reprinted with permission.

fold once it succumbs to the buildup of air pressure beneath. When both inferior and superior margins of the vocal fold are open, airflow is now passing through the glottis, and there is a drop in pressure across the level of the vocal folds. The vocal folds are now initiating closure of the glottis beginning with the inferior margin partly due to buildup of restorative forces. The geometry of the glottis is now in the opposite configuration with the triangle now inverted into a divergent shape. It is at this point in the vibratory cycle that the Bernoulli effect occurs as the transglottal

> It is helpful to note that total energy existing in the larynx can be classified as either potential energy (stored energy/pressure), or kinetic energy (motion). Because we know that the total sum of energy must always be the same, if one increases, the other must decrease. In other words, when the air molecules pass through the glottis and a faster rate (to maintain the same speed), kinetic energy (motion) has increased.

air pressure, or the air pressure across the glottis drops and the inferior margin is then pulled closed. This drop in pressure within the glottis deserves further explanation.

Laws of physics mandate that the rate of airflow traveling from the lungs through the larynx, vocal tract, and ultimately out of the mouth must be constant. Meaning, the air molecules must be traveling at the same speed at every point during this journey no matter how narrow the space becomes at any given point. This becomes particularly important when the air molecules reach the glottis. At this point, the same number of molecules must pass through the glottis at the same rate as the more open spaces above and below the glottis in order to avoid a bottleneck. Therefore, at the greatest narrowing, the rate of movement of the air molecules must speed up, resulting in a drop in pressure at the same point.

Supraglottic Influence on Vibration

Once above the glottis, the space is no longer as narrow, resulting in reduced kinetic

energy and increased potential energy and the air slows down (Baken, 2006). With the vocal folds adducted, there is a resultant agitation or excitation of the air molecules just above the glottis. This burst of agitated air molecules travels above the glottis into the vocal tract where it is shaped into sound.

When the air passes through the vocal folds (becomes supraglottic), another important component to vocal fold vibration occurs. This is the occurrence of self-sustained vocal fold vibration via the shaping of the vocal tract. Ingo Titze has described in detail the mechanics behind self-sustained vocal fold vibration, which are vital for efficient voicing. Self-sustained vocal fold vibration can be achieved by introducing a narrowing at any supraglottic point (e.g., ventricular folds, pharynx, and lips) along the vocal tract, creating a semi-occluded vocal tract. An increase in acoustic pressure at the point of narrowing creates a backpressure or redirection of some of the acoustic output back down toward the vocal folds. As a result, the backpressure facilitates a small amount of abduction during phonation. This improves vocal economy because the backpressure helps to neutralize or "un-press" the vocal folds allowing them to generate more efficient aerodynamic power. Voice pedagogues and speech pathologists often

> Students who have difficulty with intonation may have issues related to this delicate coordination of TA and CT activation balanced with subglottal air pressure rather than solely an issue of ear training.

use many variations of a semi-occluded vocal tract exercises (i.e., lip trills, hums) to facilitate efficient voice production. The impact and considerations on singing and control of registration are discussed further in Chapter 14 (Titze, 1994; Titze & Verdolini Abbot, 2012).

Intrinsic and Extrinsic Muscle Involvement in Pitch Regulation

Titze, Luschei, and Hirano (1989) reported that isolated activation of the TA could either raise or lower F_0 depending on pitch and volume. Increased TA activation at a low F_0 and intensity resulted in a raise in F_0, whereas increased TA activation at a high pitch and a louder intensity resulted in a decrease in F_0. Another study investigated the activity of the CT muscle during descending glides. When the frequency glide started in a high range, the relaxation of the CT was the primary controller of the fall in pitch. However, when the glide began in the mid-range of the voice, the CT was less active, and the neck strap muscles played a more prominent role during the descending glide (Erikson, Baer, & Harris, 1983).

The role of extrinsic laryngeal muscles in control of pitch is particularly interesting for singers as engagement of the neck muscles is typically viewed pedagogically as "poor technique" (see Figures 3–6A and 3–6B). Studies on less experienced classical singers have demonstrated laryngeal elevation when producing higher pitches, whereas, experienced classical singers maintained a more neutral laryngeal position (Shipp & Izdebski, 1975). This finding is consistent with traditional classical singing, when laryngeal posture is typically maintained in a stable, neutral to low position during singing to maintain an optimal resonating environment. However, it would not necessarily apply to all CCM vocal styles where the laryngeal range of motion is increased (mimicking the movement of speech patterns) and not typically maintained in a stable lowered position (Titze, 2007).

Vocal Intensity

Singing loudly and belting (which requires increased vocal intensity) are often required elements for the successful commercial music singer. Understanding the mechanisms of how increased vocal intensity is achieved

To get a sense of how the effects of duration, speed, and degree of vocal fold closure effect sound production, perform this simple variation on a clapping exercise: (1) move your hands 6 inches apart and instead of clapping in perfect closed hands-open hands rhythm, press your hands closed for two seconds and only open for one (duration); (2) move your hands 6 inches apart and clap as hard fast as you can (effects of speed/velocity); and (3) move your hands 6 inches apart and clap them as hard as you can, but only allow your fingers to touch during the clap, not your whole hand (degree of closure). Note the changes in the sound of the clap produced with each exercise. Note the feelings on your hand with each exercise and imaging the vocal fold translation of this clapping exercise.

becomes imperative for those who teach and sing these vocal styles. There are three aspects of vocal fold behavior during phonation that should be considered for adequate control of vocal intensity: duration of vocal fold closure, the speed of vocal fold closure, and the degree of vocal fold closure (Behrman, 2007). The duration refers to how long the vocal folds remain closed during the closed phase of the vibratory cycle. The longer the closed phase of vibration, the greater the buildup of subglottal air pressure beneath the vocal folds is required to overcome the impedance to blow them apart again, resulting in increased energy is transmitted outward through the glottis. The faster the speed (velocity) at which the vocal folds close abruptly results in excitation and energy transmitted to the air molecules directly above the glottis (Gauffin & Sundberg, 1989). Finally, the degree of closure or medial compression is important for intensity control. A complete closure of the glottis reduces loss of air through the glottis and allows for better buildup of subglottal air pressure.

Phonatory Onset

Initiation of sound (glottal onset) can be achieved in a variety of ways because of the pliable and responsive nature of the vocal folds. The three primary styles of glottal onset are: simultaneous (coup de glotte), breathy, and glottal. Koike (1967) described the characteristics of each of these types of phonation onset. The simultaneous onset is the well-coordinated and gentle approximation of the vocal folds. The onset of airflow occurs simultaneously with the onset of vocal fold vibration. The degree of medial compression of the vocal folds is relatively gentle. The involvement of the LCA, CT, IA, and TA initiate their movements in a gradual manner prior to voicing. This type of glottal onset also has onset of vibration occurring in concert with onset of airflow. The adductor muscles become active prior to initiation of voicing and the medial compression of the vocal folds is stronger relative to simultaneous and breathy phonatory onset. Modern high-speed laryngeal imaging has allowed us to now see that vibration/excitation of laryngeal tissue occurs before phonation starts (as the vocal folds are approximating), and airflow is happening in the coup-de-glotte onset (Ahmad, Yan, & Bless, 2012; Freeman, Woo, Saxman, & Murry, 2012).

The breathy onset involves initiation of airflow prior to initiation of the vocal folds adducting fully. The adductors gradually increase before voicing, and the vocal folds are closely approximated, but not fully adducted (Koike, 1967). The breathy onset is not typically used in classical style or musical theater styles but may be appropriate for certain jazz or pop vocal styles.

In contrast with either simultaneous or breathy onsets, during hard glottal attacks, the vocal folds were noted to be closed prior to the onset of phonation and subsequently blown apart, in a much more violent fashion (than the coup de glotte), which has been observed under high-speed imaging (Ahmad et al., 2012; Freeman et al., 2012). The hard glottal attack is not considered as efficient as simultaneous onset, and it has been associated with vocal fold pathology due to the extended medial compression of the vocal folds as compared with simultaneous or breathy onset (Koike, 1967). Glottal attacks are discouraged in a pathologic voice and are often a target behavior for elimination in speech and song. Several contemporary commercial music styles, such as musical theater, pop, jazz, and R & B, use glottal onsets as a stylistic choice. This is stylistically appropriate and may be used judiciously by a thoughtful and vocally healthy singer.

Vibrato

Vibrato is defined as "a quasi-periodic modulation of the fundamental frequency" (Sundberg, 1982). Both a modulation of the frequency and amplitude of the fundamental frequency are characteristic of vibrato. A consistent, even, vocal vibrato is a highly valued attribute in the classical singer (Mason & Zemlin, 1976; M. McLane, 1985; Miller, 1966). Aesthetically pleasing rates and the extent of classical singing vocal vibrato have changed in vocal music across time and genre of literature. Vibrato, or lack of noticeable vibrato, is one acoustic feature reported in the literature differentiating belting from classical singing (Estill, 1988; Miles & Hollien, 1990; Schutte & Miller, 1993; Sundberg, Gramming, & Lovetri, 1993).

Although rate of vibrato (measured in hertz, Hz) and extent of vibrato (measured in decibels (dB) may vary from singer to singer, there is an acceptable range of "normal" that has been defined among classical singers (Dejonckere, Hirano, & Sundberg, 1995; Horii, 1989; Rothman & Arroyo, 1987; Shipp, Leanderson, & Sundberg, 1980; Titze, 1994). Performance styles of early music suggested a decreased rate of vocal vibrato (2.0–6.9 Hz) as compared with present day standards (4.5–6.5 Hz; Hakes, Doherty, & Shipp, 1990; Titze, 1994). During the first half of the 20th century, faster vibrato rates (6–7 Hz) were considered aesthetically pleasing. Yet, Titze reported that

one of the great operatic tenors by current standards, Luciano Pavarotti, maintained a vibrato rate approximately 5.5 Hz.

The literature reports classical singers maintain vibrato in as much as 95% of every song (Mason & Zemlin, 1976). Robison, Bounous, and Bailey (1994) found that baritones with the most aesthetically pleasing voices maintained vibrato in their tones more than 80% of the time. Further confirming the importance of vibrato as a perceptual marker of good classical singing, a study by Ekholm, Papagiannis, and Chagnon (1998) found that the degree of vocal beauty in the classical singing voice was highly correlated with singers who possessed a consistent and even vibrato.

There is minimal research on the use and type of vibrato used in commercial music. Of the available literature on belting, Robison et al. (1994) reported the most aesthetically pleasing belter possessed vibrato in more than 50% of their song. However, the Robison study only employed teachers and connoisseurs of the classical voice. Therefore, it is not surprising that classical music lovers would rate a belt voice with a consistent vibrato as the most aesthetically pleasing. Robison et al. (1994) did not directly report vibrato rates of belters but suggested that they have a "moderately faster and narrower" vibrato in comparison with the classically trained baritones within the study. The average rate of vibrato of the baritones in the Robison et al. study was reported to be 5.3 to 5.4 Hz. The rate of acceptable vibrato reported in the classical voice ranges from 4.5 to 6.5 Hz (Dejonckere et al., 1995; Horii, 1989; Rothman & Arroyo, 1987; Seashore, 1932; Shipp et al., 1980; Titze, 1994).

LeBorgne (2001) examined the role of vibrato in the belt voice looking at differences between delay of onset of vibrato between elite and average belters across six vowels. Profile plots revealed a trend that appeared to show elite belters may have a shorter delay of onset of vibrato than average belters. Because this study was focused on the belt voice, an overview of some of the findings from this study is further described below.

Delay of Onset of Vibrato

LeBorgne (2001) found no statistically significant difference in the delay of onset of vibrato between elite and average belters. However, based on the results, there appeared to be a trend that the elite belters presented with less of a delay of the vibrato than the average belters. Specifically, the less the delay of vibrato, the more aesthetically pleasing the voice was perceived. There were observed differences in the delay of onset of vibrato between the vowels. Perhaps it is a stylistic choice of the singer that in those particular words a delay of vibrato is warranted. One of the reasons singers are hired in the professional arena is because of their uniqueness. As such, each singer may choose to use vibrato in a different way within the particular songs they perform.

Vibrato Rate

Analysis of vibrato in the LeBorgne (2001) study on belters was obtained for the entire vowel, as well as three distinct portions of the vowel (head, middle, and tail). Findings indicate no significant differences between groups with respect to the overall vibrato rate or amplitude (extent) of the vibrato. Interestingly, findings also revealed that the overall average rates of vibrato in the elite belters were comparable with the reported rates of vibrato in classical singers.

Vibrato Amplitude

With respect to amplitude (extent) variation of the vibrato, the reports in the literature suggest very small changes (2–3 dB) in classical singing (Horrii, 1989). The relatively small variance of amplitude reported in the classical literature indicates it is not thought to have a significant effect on the perception of overall intensity. Findings from the LeBorgne study suggested that increased amplitude variation of the vibrato found in belters may implicate amplitude of vibrato as a source of increased intensity for belters. Furthermore, belters may have greater amplitude (extent) of vibrato than reported in the classical literature for singers.

One possible explanation regarding the influence of vibrato on intensity relates to the amplitude variation of the vibrato. The amplitude variation is typically reported to be quite small (2–3 dB). However, several authors indicate that the influence of the amplitude variation results in an increase and decrease in overall intensity, because as the frequency of vibrato rhythmically varies around the fundamental, it causes fluctuations in the harmonics (Dejonckere et al., 1995; Horii, 1989; Schutte & Miller, 1993). The slight shifting of harmonics influences the amount of interaction with the formants for the sustained vowels. As the harmonics align more closely with the formants for a given vowel, the overall intensity of that vowel will increase. It is also this variation in harmonics and formant interaction that may influence the perceived ring in the voice. To further support this theory, Titze et al. (1999) found that at a maximum intensity point in a *messa di voce*, where the sound pressure level (SPL) was essentially constant, there appeared to be an increase in the amount of vocal vibrato that may have contributed to the perceived loudness. Titze writes, "The combination of this vibrato increase and higher spectral content is likely to add to the perception of increased loudness" (p. 2938).

Magnitude of Vibrato

Elite belters were found to have a greater magnitude of change within the rate of vibrato suggesting that the elite belters may have been perceived as having a different rate of vibrato than the average belters. Also, the magnitude of the extent of vibrato produced by the elite belters was significantly different across certain vowels. These subtleties may be the nuances that differentiate the elite and average belters. Choosing to alter the vibrato may influence the color of words or phrases in order to convey various emotions (LeBorgne, 2001).

The author surmised that belters maintain vibrato rates similar to classical singers. However, differences in the magnitude of the rate and amplitude of vibrato appear not only to be greater in belters, but also significantly different between elite and average belters. Vibrato rates also appear to be influenced by the vowel performed. LeBorgne (2001) concluded that further investigation into the use of vibrato in belting is warranted.

Chapter Summary

This chapter has provided an overview of anatomy and physiology of the laryngeal structures, discussion of microanatomy of the vocal folds, as well as an introduction to vocal fold vibration. It is important to have a clear understanding of the role of the vocal folds during phonation as CCM pedagogy continues to move toward a functional approach to vocal training. Additionally, as pedagogues, we must keep in mind that individual singers may execute a specific vocal task differently and still be physiologically appropriate as we each have normal anatomic variability. Part of guiding the student through vocal training and development is helping them find their most efficient path for voice production, understanding that there will be some differences across singers because of anatomic and physiologic variability.

References

Ahmad, K., Yan, Y., & Bless, D. (2012). Vocal fold vibratory characteristics in Northern female speakers from high-speed digital imaging. *Journal of Voice, 26*(2), 239–253.

Armstrong, W., & Netterville, J. (1995). Anatomy of the larynx, trachea, and bronchi [Review]. *Otolaryngologic Clinics of North America, 28*(4), 685–699.

Baken, R. (2006). An overview of laryngeal function for voice production. In R. Sataloff (Ed.), *Vocal health and pedagogy: Science and assessment*. San Diego, CA: Plural Publishing.

Bartlett, R., & Thibeault, S. (2011). *Bioengineering the vocal fold: A review of mesenchymal stem cell applications*. Rijeka, Croatia: InTech.

Behrman, A. (2007). *Speech and voice science*. San Diego, CA: Plural Publishing.

Borden, H. R. (1994). *Speech science primer: Physiology, acoustics and perception of speech* (4th ed.). Baltimore, MD: Williams & Wilkins.

Dejonckere, P., Hirano, M., & Sundberg, J. (1995). *Vibrato*. San Diego, CA: Singular Publishing.

Ekholm, E., Papagiannis, G., & Chagnon, F. (1998). Relating objective measurements to expert evaluation of voice quality in Western classical singing: Critical perceptual parameters. *Journal of Voice, 12*(2), 182–196.

Erikson, D., Baer, T., & Harris, K. (1983). *The role of the strap muscles in pitch lowering*. San Diego, CA: College-Hill Press.

Estill, J. (1988). Belting and classic voice quality: Some physiological differences. *Medical Problems of Performing Artists*, 37–43.

Freeman, E., Woo, P., Saxman, J., & Murry, T. (2012). A comparison of sung and spoken phonation onset gestures using high speed digital imaging. *Journal of Voice, 26*(2), 226–238.

Fujimara. (1981). Body-cover theory of the vocal fold and its phonetic implications. In K. Stevens & M. Hirano (Eds.), *Vocal fold physiology*, 271–281.

Gauffin, J., & Sundberg, J. (1989). Spectral correlates of glottal voice source waveform characteristics. *Journal of Speech and Hearing Research, 32*, 556–565.

Gray, S. D. (2000). Cellular physiology of the vocal folds. *Otolaryngologic Clinics of North America, 33*(4), 679–698.

Gray, S., Hirano, M., & Sato, K. (1993). Molecular and cellular struture of vocal fold tissue. In I. Titze (Ed.), *Vocal fold physiology: Frontiers in basic science*. San Diego, CA: Singular Publishing.

Hakes, J., Doherty, T., & Shipp, T. (1990). Trillo rates exhibited by professional early music singers. *Journal of Voice, 4*(4), 305–308.

Hirano, M. (1974). Morphological structure of the vocal cord as a vibrator and its variation. *Folia Phoniatric, 26*, 89–94.

Hirano, M. (1977). *Structure and vibratory behavior of the vocal folds: Current results, emerging problems, and new instrumentation*. Tokyo: Tokyo University Press.

Hirano, M., Kurita, S., & Nakashima, T. (1981). *The structure of the vocal folds*. San Diego, CA: University of Tokyo Press.

Horii, Y. (1989). Acoustic analysis of vocal vibrato: A theoretical interpretation of data. *Journal of Voice, 3*(1), 36–43.

Koike, Y. (1967). Experimental studies on vocal attack. *Otorhinolaryngology Clinics Kyoto, 60*, 663–688.

LeBorgne, W. (2001). *Defining the belt voice: Perceptual judgements and objective measures* (PhD dissertation). University of Cincinnati, ProQuest, UMI Dissertations Publishing.

Lieber, R. (2010). *Skeletal muscle structure, function, and plasticity: The physiological basis of rehabilitation* (3rd ed.). Baltimore, MD: Lippincott, Williams & Wilkins.

Mason, R., & Zemlin, W. (1976). The phenomenon of vocal vibrato. *The NATS Bulletin, 22*(3), 12–17, 37.

McLane, M. (1985). Artistic vibrato and tremolo: A survey of the literature. *Journal of Research in Singing, 8*(2), 21–43.

Miles, B., & Hollien, H. (1990). Whither belting? *Journal of Voice, 4*(1), 64–70.

Miller, R. (1966). Vibrato in relation to the vocal legato. *The NATS Bulletin, 22*(3), 10–11, 21.

Moore, K. & Dalley. A. (2006). *Clinically oriented anatomy* (5th ed.). Philadelphia, PA: Lippincot Williams & Wilkins.

Netter, F. H. (1997). *Atlas of human anatomy* (2nd ed.). East Hanover, NJ: Novartis.

Robison, C., Bounous, B., & Bailey, R. (1994). Vocal beauty: A study proposing its acoustical definition and relevant causes in classical baritones and female belt singers. *The NATS Journal*, 19–30.

Rothman, H., & Arroyo, A. (1987). Acoustic variability in vibrato and its perceptual signifigance. *Journal of Voice, 1*(2), 123–141.

Schutte, H., & Miller, D. (1993). Belting and pop, nonclassical approaches to the female middle voice: Some preliminary considerations. *Journal of Voice, 7*(2), 142–150.

Seashore, C. (1932). *Psychology of the vibrato in voice and instrument.* Iowa City, IA: University Press.

Shipp, T., & Izdebski, K. (1975). Vocal frequency and vertical larynx positioning by singers and non singers. *Journal of* the *Acoustical Society of America, 58*(5), 1104-1106.

Shipp, T., Leanderson, R., & Sundberg, J. (1980). Some acoustic characteristics of vocal vibrato. *Journal of Research in Singing, 4*(1), 18-25.

Sundberg, J. (1982). Effects of the vibrato and the 'singing formant' on pitch. *Journal of Research in Singing, 5*(2), 3-17.

Sundberg, J., Gramming, P., & Lovetri, J. (1993). Comparisons of pharynx, source, formant, and pressure characteristics in operatic and musical theatre singing. *Journal of Voice, 7*(4), 301-310.

Titze, I. (1994). *Principles of voice production*. Englewood Cliffs, NJ: Prentice Hall.

Titze, I. (2007). Belting and high larynx position. *Journal of Singing, 63*(5), 557-558.

Titze, I., Long, R., Shirley, G., Stathopoulos, E., Ramig, L., Carroll, L., & Riley, W. (1999). Messa di voce: An investigation of the symmetry of crescendo and decrescendo in a singing exercise. *Journal of the Acoustical Society of America, 105*(5), 2933-2940.

Titze, I., Luschei, E., & Hirano, M. (1989). The role of the thyroarytenoid muscle in regulation of fundamental frequency. *Journal of Voice, 3*, 213-224.

Titze, I., & Verdolini Abbot, K. (2012). *Vocology: The science and practice of voice habilitation*. Salt Lake City, UT: The National Center for Voice and Speech.

Van den Berg, J. (1958). Myoelastic-aerodynamic theory of voice production. *Journal of Speech and Hearing Research, 1*, 227-244.

Zemlin, W. (1998). *Speech and hearing science anatomy and physiology* (4th ed.). Needham Heights, MA: Allyn and Bacon.

4

Neurologic Control of Voice Production

Voice, speech, and song production are nothing short of an amazing electrical circuit, the complexities of which are increasingly understood because of advancements in neuroscience and neuroimaging. Human vocal production for singing requires a complex series of events to occur with respect to motor planning (brain), typical motor pathways (to the muscles of respiration, laryngeal musculature, and articulatory musculature), appropriately timed execution of muscle contractions (for pitch and rhythmic accuracy), the ability to sequence (so that one can sing an entire phrase accurately), and a sensory feedback loop (perception of performance) (Jürgens, 2009; Zatorre, Chen, & Penhune, 2007). These events typically take place without conscious forethought in most singers. This chapter provides a general understanding of the neurological pathways for voice production in relevant terms for singers to

know, if nothing more than for an appreciation of all of the "behind the scenes" action that is occurring during optimal vocal performance. Additionally, two important components of elite voice performances that are often overlooked in chapters related to neurological vocal production are covered: (1) emotional component of vocal production and (2) impact of performance anxiety/stage fright.

Working from the Top Down: From the Singer's Brain to the Singer's Body

A basic understanding of normal human neuroanatomy and physiology is necessary for vocal pedagogues and performers. Many professional artists have likely never been introduced to the motor and sensory

TABLE 4–1. Overview of Structure and Function of CNS, PNS, and ANS

	Structure	Function
Central Nervous System (CNS)	Brain, brainstem, cerebellum, and spinal cord	Master control center
Peripheral Nervous System (PNS)	31 pair spinal nerves/ 12 pair cranial nerves	Connects brain to muscles/ organs and sends sensory information back to brain
Autonomic Nervous System (ANS)	Interfaces with PNS & CNS	Flight or fight system

pathways required to produce physical movement, respiration, vocal production, or coordinated articulatory movements. Yet, every day in performance, billions of neural pathways are learned (motor-learning) and executed (through synaptic connections), resulting in dramatic performance for both the artist and audience to encounter an auditory and often visceral experience (Pa & Hickok, 2008; Pantev, Engelien, Candia, & Elbert, 2001). In simplest terms, the motor and sensory control of voice production starts in the brain and goes to the muscles to be activated for a given task. Sound is produced because muscle action occurs, and sound vibrations/sensory feedback returns to the ear, which tells the brain how successful the body/voice was in the vocal attempt.

Prior to a comprehensive understanding of vocal production from start to finish, a breakdown of the three major divisions of neural function are necessary. Table 4–1 provides a general overview of the three systems (central nervous system, peripheral nervous system, and autonomic nervous system), their primary components, and general function.

Central Nervous System

Cerebral Cortex

The human brain (Figure 4-1), brainstem, cerebellum, and spinal cord make up the central nervous system (CNS). The largest part of the human brain, the cerebrum, is divided into two hemispheres (right and left) and four lobes (frontal lobe, parietal lobe, temporal lobe, and occipital lobe; Figure 4-2). The two hemispheres of the brain are connected by a bundle of nerves called the *corpus callosum*. The corpus callosum acts to transfer important information from the right side of the brain to the left side of the brain and vice versa. Although both hemispheres of the brain are utilized during speech and song, most individuals have a dominant side of the brain (either left or right). All the connections in the CNS are considered upper motor neurons (UMN). A neuron is a cell type that transmits motor or sensory information to and from the brain to the muscles/organs and back.

Table 4-2 indicates the general structure and function of the cerebral lobes and hemispheres.

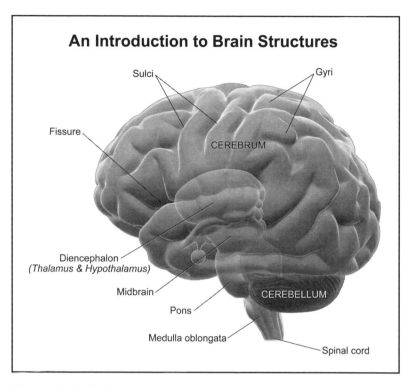

An Introduction to Brain Structures

Sulci

Gyri

Fissure

CEREBRUM

Diencephalon
(Thalamus & Hypothalamus)

Midbrain

Pons

CEREBELLUM

Medulla oblongata

Spinal cord

Figure 4–1. Surface features of the brain. Courtesy of Wikimedia Commons.

Although the brain may appear to be made up of random ridges (gyri), grooves (sulci), and valleys (fissures), through neuroimaging techniques, brain mapping for specific motor and sensory functions have been identified to unique parts of the brain.

Brainstem

The brainstem is located at the posterior (back) portion of the brain and acts as the connector between the brain and the spinal cord. All of the motor (*corticospinal tract*) and sensory paths (*posterior column-medial lemniscus pathway* and *spinothalamic tract*) go through the brainstem to get from the brain to the body and return information from the body back to the brain. The brainstem is composed of three main parts: medulla oblongata, midbrain, and pons (Figure 4–3). In addition to providing a pathway, the brainstem helps to regulate heart rate, quiet respiration, and sleep/wake cycles. Within the midbrain portion of the brainstem are several very important elements suspected to play a role in speaking, singing and musical performance (*periaqueductal gray (PAG)* and *reticular formation*) (Jürgens, 2009; Ozdemir, Norton, & Schlaug, 2006). Additionally, cranial nerves (Figure 4–4) III to XII come off of the brainstem, including all of the nerves responsible for voice

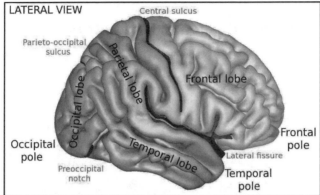

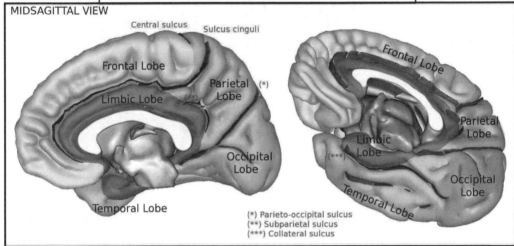

Figure 4–2. Brain lobes, main sulci, and boundaries. Courtesy of Wikimedia Commons.

(X-vagus) and articulation (V-trigeminal, VII-facial, IX-glossopharyngeal, X-vagus, XI-spinal accessory, XII-hypoglossal).

Cerebellum

The cerebellum (hindbrain) sits behind the cerebral cortex and coordinates fine motor control and equilibrium (balance). Like the cerebrum, it is divided into two hemispheres and has many gyri (*folia*). Processing input from the cerebral cortex, brainstem, and sensory neurons, the cerebellum (Figure 4–5) initiates volitional muscle contraction, coordinates fine motor movement, and provides awareness for where the body is in space. For performers, normal cerebellar function is vital for execution of physical, vocal, and instrumental musical skill.

Basal Ganglia

The basal ganglia (Figure 4–6) is a part of the forebrain and has been implicated in the aspect of timing and sequencing as

TABLE 4–2. Central Nervous System

Structure	Function
Right Hemisphere	overview processing, random processing, intuitive, artistic/hands-on, often considered "musical" side
Left Hemisphere	linear processing, sequential processing, logical, symbols/mathematic formulas
Frontal Lobe	memory, emotion, motor planning, decision making, personality, concentration
Parietal Lobe	sensation, body awareness (proprioception), goal-directed voluntary movements
Temporal Lobe	hearing, long-term memory, one of the fear centers, categorization of objects, intellect
Occipital Lobe	vision, interpretation of images

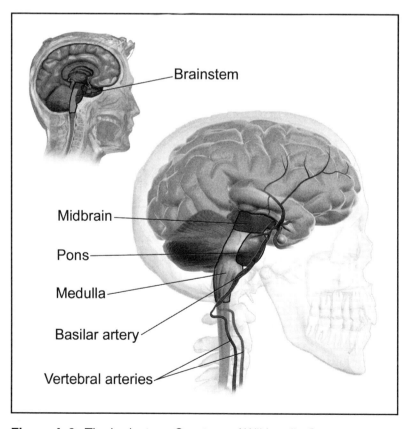

Figure 4–3. The brainstem. Courtesy of Wikimedia Commons.

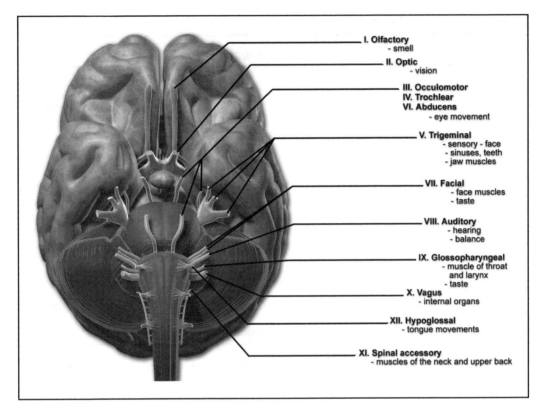

Figure 4–4. The human cranial nerves and their areas of innervations. Courtesy of Wikimedia Commons.

it pertains to musical performance. Disruption or injury to the basal ganglia often results in coordinated movement deficits.

Peripheral Nervous System

Once the motor and sensory nerves leave the spinal cord, they become part of the peripheral nervous system (PNS; Figure 4-7) and are considered lower motor neurons (LMN). The cranial nerves (12 pairs) and spinal nerves (31 pairs) compose the PNS. The cranial nerves can either be solely motor nerves, solely sensory, or mixed (motor and sensory). The spinal nerves consist of the eight cervical nerve pairs, twelve thoracic nerve pairs, five lumbar nerve pairs, five sacral nerve pairs, and one coccygeal nerve pair, and are all mixed nerves (motor and sensory). When the nerve leaves the spinal cord, it terminates at the neuromuscular junction (NMJ). The NMJ (Figure 4-8) is the place where chemicals (*acetylcholine* and *noradrenaline*) are released resulting in muscle fiber contraction. Once the muscle fiber contracts, a feedback (sensory) loop is sent back to the brain. These feedback loops help to determine sensations such as stretch and pain.

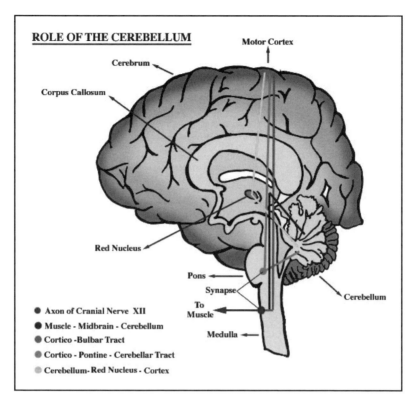

Figure 4–5. Role of the cerebellum. Courtesy of Dr. Patrick McCaffrey of CSU, Chico.

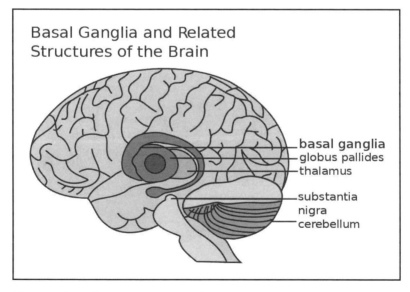

Figure 4–6. Basal ganglia and related structures of the brain. *Source*: John Henkel/ Wikimedia Commons /public domain.

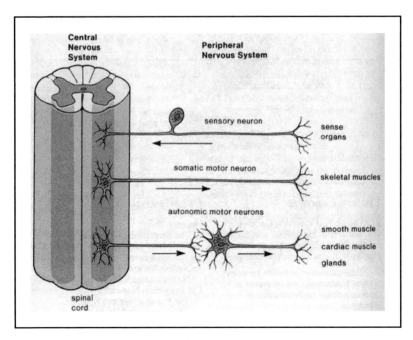

Figure 4–7. Communication between the brain and the spinal nerves that leave the cord. *Source*: Review of the Universe, Neurons and Nerves, Spinal Cord on website, universe-review.ca.

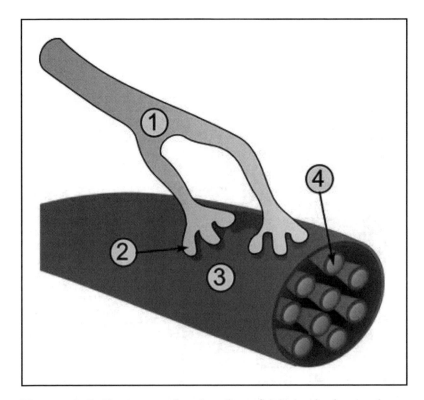

Figure 4–8. Neuromuscular junction (global view). 1. Axon. 2. Synaptical junction 3. Muscle fiber. 4. Myofibrils. Courtesy of Wikimedia Commons.

Autonomic Nervous System

The autonomic nervous system (ANS) is actually a division of the PNS, but is often considered separately. Best known as the "fight or flight" system, the ANS controls smooth (visceral) muscles and regulates functions such as heart rate, blood pressure, blood flow, digestion, perspiration, salivation, breathing rate, urination, and sexual arousal. Generally, the ANS does not fall under conscious control, but for elite performers, learning to manage visceral responses becomes a vital aspect of daily performing. Music performance anxiety (MPA) affects the lives of most performers at some point in their career, and vocal artists can be severely affected by the results of ANS response: dry mouth, rapid heart rate, increased respiratory rate, sweaty palms, and shaky knees. Further discussion of MPA is found in the section below.

Summary of Neuromotor and Neurosensory Pathways for Voice Production

Before taking the initial breath to initiate a sung phrase, millions of electrical connections are happening to accurately execute

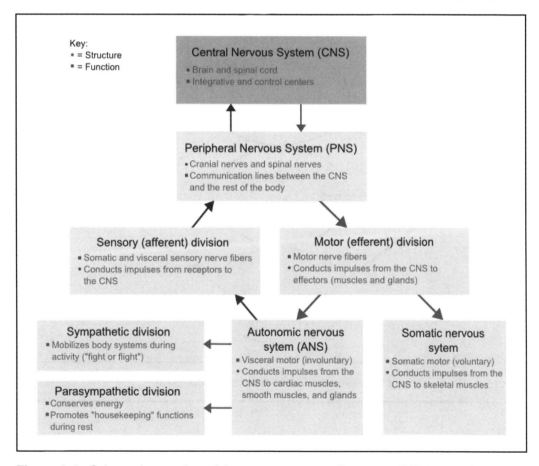

Figure 4–9. Schematic overview of the nervous system. Courtesy of Wikimedia Commons.

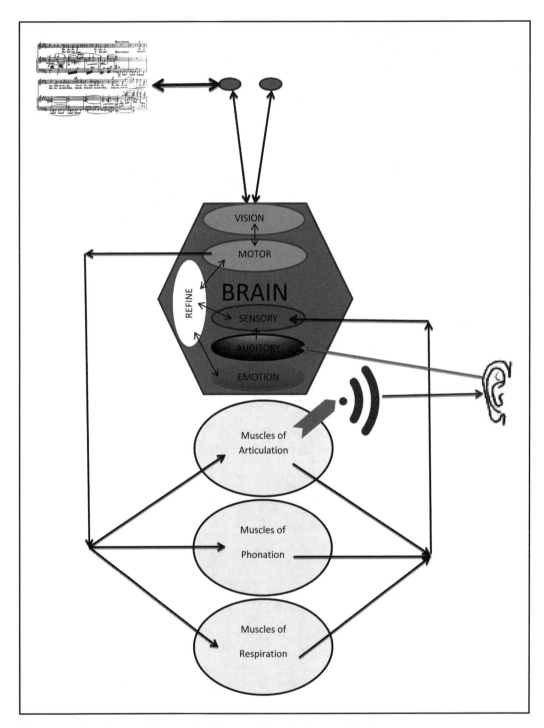

Figure 4–10. Schematic neurologic overview of voice production.

a musical utterance (never mind the dancing stage combat/puppetry that is going along with it). The circuitry to execute and coordinate motor activities is a complex system of signals sent out from the brain (CNS) to the muscles and organs of the body (PNS and ANS) which relays information back to the brain about how accurately the task was executed (Figure 4-9). The schematic (Figure 4-10) is a representation of what occurs from the brain, to the muscles, and back during vocal performance as it pertains to respiration, phonation, and articulation. In addition, the brain continues to monitor for postural control during movement, visual input (reading a score/script), and the emotional component of performance.

There are several seminal articles written on the neural control of voice in humans for both speech and song (Belin, Zatorre, Lafaille, Ahad, & Pike, 2000; Brown, Martinez, Hodges, Fox, & Parsons, 2004; Brown, Martinez, & Parsons, 2006; Chartrand & Belin, 2006; Chen, Penhune, & Zatorre, 2008; Kleber, Veit, Birbaumer, Gruzelier, & Lotze, 2010; Jürgens, 2002; 2009; Zarate & Zatorre, 2005; 2008; Zatorre, Belin, & Penhune, 2002). Within the genre of opera singers specifically, there has been research that documents the areas of the brain and feedback loops that are utilized based on number of years of experience (Kleber et al., 2010. The ability for the singer to listen to the sound produced, interpret what they hear, and make adjustments accordingly has also been mapped to specific parts of the brain and specific brain pathways (Chartrand & Belin, 2006; Jones & Keough, 2008; Kriegstein & Giraud, 2004; Murbe, Pabst, Hofmann, & Sundberg, 2004; Schulz, Varga, Jeffires, Ludlow, & Braun, 2005). There is also evidence to suggest that because of the way in which one learns music, there is a physiological difference in the brain of the musician and nonmusician. Specifically, preliminary evidence of keyboard players suggests areas of the brain that are bigger in keyboard musicians compared to nonmusicians, including the motor area, the listening (auditory) area, and the part of the brain that is responsible for integrating the visual-spatial information (Gaser & Schlaug, 2003). Performers require repetitive, accurate, muscle conditioning (e.g., voice lessons and daily practice) resulting in accurate motor learning with minimal conscious control (see the motor learning chapter for detailed information).

Musical Performance Anxiety and Emotional Aspects of Singing

Unlike instrumentalists, whose performance is dependent on accurate playing of an external musical instrument, the singer's instrument is uniquely intact and subject to the emotional confines of the brain and body in which it is housed. Severe musical performance anxiety (MPA) can be career threatening for all musicians, but perhaps the vocal athlete is most severely impacted (Spahn, Echternach, Zander, Voltmer, & Richter, 2010). The majority of literature on MPA is dedicated to instrumentalists, but the basis of its definition, performance effects, and treatment options can be considered for vocal athletes (Anderson, 2011; Brantigan, Brantigan, & Joseph, 1982; Brugués, 2011a, 2011b; Chanel, 1992; Drinkwater & Klopper, 2010; Fehm & Schmidt, 2006; Fredrikson & Gunnarsson, 1992; Gates, Saegert, Wilson, Johnson, Shepherd, & Hearne, 1985; Kenny, Davis, & Oates, 2004; Khalsa, Shorter, Cope, Wyshak, & Sklar, 2009;

Lazarus & Abramovitz, 2004; Nagel, 2010; Neftel et al., 1982; Powell, 2004; Schneider & Chesky, 2011; Spahn et al., 2010; Studer, Danuser, Hildebrandt, Arial, & Gomez, 2011; Studer, Gomez, Hildebrandt, Arial, & Danuser, 2011; van Kemenade, van Son, & van Heesch, 1995; Walker & Nordin-Bates, 2010; Wesner, Noyes, & Davis, 1990).

Fear is a natural reaction to a stressful situation, and there is a fine line between emotional excitation and perceived threat (real or imagined). The job of a performer is to convey to an audience through vocal production, physical gestures, and facial expression a most heightened state of emotion. Otherwise, why would audience members pay money to sit for two or three hours for a mundane experience? Not only is there the emotional conveyance of the performance, but also the internal turmoil often experienced by the singers themselves in preparation for elite performance. It is well-documented in the literature that even the most elite performers have experienced debilitating performance anxiety. MPA is defined on a continuum with anxiety levels ranging from low to high and has been reported to comprise four distinct components: affect, cognition, behavior, and physiology (Spahn et al., 2010). Affect composes feelings (e.g., impending doom, panic, anxiety) and can result in altered levels of concentration. This sense of fear creates behavioral components that result in postural shifts, quivering, and trembling, and finally physiologically the body's ANS system will activate the "fight or flight" response. In recent years, researchers have been able to define two distinct neurological pathways for MPA. The first pathway happens quickly and without conscious input (ANS) resulting in the same fear stimulus as if a person were put into an emergent, life-threatening situation. In those situations, the brain releases adrenaline resulting in physical changes of: increased heart rate, increased respiration, shaking, pale skin, dilated pupils, slowed digestion, bladder relaxation, dry mouth, and dry eyes, all of which severely affect vocal performance. The second pathway that has been identified results in a conscious identification of the fear/threat and a much slower physiologic response. With the second neuromotor response, the performer has a chance to recognize the fear, process how to deal with the fear, reassess the situation, and respond accordingly.

Treatment modalities to address MPA include psychobehavioral therapy (including biofeedback) and drug therapies (Gates et al., 1985; Khalsa et al., 2009; Nagel, 2010; Neftel et al., 1982; Powell, 2004; Spahn et al., 2010). Elite physical performance athletes have been shown to benefit from visualization techniques and psychological readiness training, yet within the performing arts community, stage fright may be considered a weakness or character flaw precluding readiness for professional performance. On the contrary, vocal athletes, like physical athletes, should mentally prepare themselves for optimal competition (auditions) and live performance. Joanna Cazden's (2009) CD, "Visualization for Singers," is specifically designed to help singers learn to mentally focus for performance. Learning to convey emotion without eliciting an internal emotional response that would potentially negatively affect the systems of singing by the vocal athlete may take the skill of an experienced psychologist to help change ingrained neural pathways. Ultimately, control and understanding of MPA enhances performance and prepares the vocal athlete for the most intense performance demands without vocal compromise.

References

Anderson, L. (2011). Myself or someone like me: A review of the literature on the psychological well-being of child actors. *Medical Problems of Performing Artists, 36*(3), 146-149.

Belin, P., Zatorre, R. J., Lafaille, P., Ahad, P., & Pike, B. (2000). Voice-selective areas in human auditory cortex. *Nature, 403,* 309-312.

Brantigan, C., Brantigan, T., & Joseph N. (1982). Effect of beta blockade and beta stimulation on stage fright. *American Journal of Medicine, 72*(1), 88-94.

Brown, S., Martinez, M., Hodges, D., Fox, P., & Parsons, L. (2004). The song system of the human brain. *Cognitive Brain Research, 20,* 363-375.

Brown, S., Martinez, M., & Parsons, L. (2006). Music and language side by side in the brain: A PET study of the generation of melodies and sentences. *European Journal of Neuroscience, 23,* 2791-2803.

Brugués, A. (2011a). Music performance anxiety—Part 1. A review of treatment options. *Medical Problems of Performing Artists, 26*(2), 102-105.

Brugués, A. (2011b). Music performance anxiety—Part 2. A review of treatment options. *Medical Problems of Performing Artists, 26*(3), 164-171.

Cazden, J. (2009). *Visualization for singers* [CD]. Amazon/Voice of Your Life.

Chanel, P. (1992). Performance anxiety. *American Journal of Psychiatry, 149*(2), 278-279.

Chartrand, J. & Belin, P. (2006). Superior voice timbre processing in musicians. *Neuroscience Letters, 405*(3), 164-167

Chen, J., Penhune, V., & Zatorre, R. (2008). Listening to musical rhythms recruits motor regions of the brain. *Cerebral Cortex, 18,* 2844-2854.

Drinkwater, E., & Klopper, C. (2010). Quantifying the physical demands of a musical performance and their effects on performance quality. *Medical Problems of Performing Artists, 25*(2), 66-71.

Fehm, L., & Schmidt, K. (2006). Performance anxiety in gifted adolescent musicians. *Journal of Anxiety Disorders, 20*(1), 98-109.

Fredrikson, M., & Gunnarsson, R. (1992). Psychobiology of stage fright: The effect of public performance on neuroendocrine, cardiovascular and subjective reactions. *Biology Psychology, 33*(1), 51-61.

Gaser, C., & Schlaug, G. (2003). Brain structures differ between musicians and nonmusicians. *Journal of Neuroscience, 23,* 9240-9245.

Gates, G., Saegert, J., Wilson, N., Johnson, L., Shepherd, A., & Hearne, E. (1985). Effect of beta blockade on singing performance. *Annals of Otology, Rhinology, and Laryngology, 94*(6 Pt. 1), 570-574.

Jones, J., & Keough, D. (2008). Auditory-motor mapping for pitch control in singers andnonsingers. *Experimental Brain Research, 190,* 279-287.

Jürgens, U. (2002). Neural pathways underlying vocal control. *Neuroscience Biobehavioral Reviews, 26,* 235-258.

Jürgens, U. (2009). The neural control of vocalization in mammals: A review. *Journal of Voice, 23,* 1-10.

Kenny, D., Davis, P., & Oates J. (2004). Music performance anxiety and occupational stress amongst opera chorus artists and their relationship with state and trait anxiety and perfectionism. *Journal of Anxiety Disorders, 18*(6), 757-777.

Khalsa, S., Shorter, S., Cope, S., Wyshak, G., & Sklar, E. (2009). Yoga ameliorates performance anxiety and mood disturbance in young professional musicians. *Applied Psychophysiology Biofeedback, 34*(4), 279-289.

Kleber, B., Veit, R., Birbaumer, N., Gruzelier, J., & Lotze, M. (2010). The brain of opera singers: Experience-dependent changes in functional activation. *Cerebral Cortex, 20*(5), 1144-1152.

Kriegstein, K., & Giraud, A. (2004). Distinct

functional substrates along the right superior temporal sulcus for the processing of voices. *Neuroimaging, 22*(2), 948–955.

Lazarus, A., & Abramovitz, A. (2004). A multimodal behavioral approach to performance anxiety. *Journal of Clinical Psychology, 60*(8), 831–840.

Murbe, D., Pabst, F., Hofmann, G., & Sundberg, J. (2004). Effects of a professional solo singer education on auditory and kinesthetic feedback—A longitudinal study of singers' pitch control. *Journal of Voice, 18*, 236–241.

Nagel, J. (2010). Treatment of music performance anxiety via psychological approaches: A review of selected CBT and psychodynamic literature. *Medical Problems of Performing Artists, 25*(4), 141–148.

Neftel, A., Adler, R., Käppeli, L., Rossi, M., Dolder, M., Käser, H., . . . Vorkauf, H. (1982). Stage fright in musicians: A model illustrating the effect of beta blockers. *Psychosomatic Medical Journal, 44*(5), 461–469.

Ozdemir, E., Norton, A., & Schlaug, G. (2006). Shared and distinct neural correlates of singingand speaking. *NeuroImage, 33*, 628–635.

Pa, J., & Hickok, G. (2008). A parietal-temporal sensory-motor integration area for the human vocal tract: Evidence from an fMRI study of skilled musicians. *Neuropsychologia, 46*, 362–368.

Pantev, C., Engelien, A., Candia, V., & Elbert, T. (2001). Representational cortex in musicians: Plastic alterations in response to musical practice. *Annals of the New York Academy of Sciences, 930*, 300–314.

Powell, D. (2004). Treating individuals with debilitating performance anxiety: An introduction. *Journal of Clinical Psychology, 60*(8), 801–808.

Schneider, E., & Chesky, K. (2011). Social support and performance anxiety of college music students. *Medical Problems of Performing Artists, 26*(3), 157–163.

Schulz, G. M., Varga, M., Jeffires, K., Ludlow, C., & Braun, A. (2005). Functional neuroanatomy of human vocalization: An $H_2^{15}O$ PET study. *Cerebral Cortex, 15*, 1835–1847.

Spahn, C., Echternach, M., Zander, M., Voltmer, E., & Richter, B. (2010). Music performance anxiety in opera singers. *Logopedica Phoniatrica Vocolology, 35*(4), 175–182.

Studer, R., Danuser, B., Hildebrandt, H., Arial, M., & Gomez, P. (2011). Hyperventilation complaints in music performance anxiety among classical music students. *Journal of Psychosomatic Research, 70*(6), 557–564.

Studer, R., Gomez, P., Hildebrandt, H., Arial, M., & Danuser, B. (2011). Stage fright: Its experience as a problem and coping with it. *International Archives of Occupational Environmental Health, 84*(7), 761–771.

van Kemenade, J., van Son, M., & van Heesch, N. (1995). Performance anxiety among professional musicians in symphonic orchestras: A self-report study. *Psychology Reports, 77*(2), 555–562.

Walker, I., & Nordin-Bates, S. (2010). Performance anxiety experiences of professional ballet dancers: The importance of control. *Journal of Dance Medicine Science, 14*(4), 133–145.

Wesner, R., Noyes, R., & Davis, T. (1990). The occurrence of performance anxiety among musicians. *Journal of Affect Disorders, 18*(3), 177–185.

Zarate, J., & Zatorre, R. (2005). Neural substrates governing audiovocal integration for vocal pitch regulation in singing. *Annals of the New York Academy of Sciences, 1060*, 404–408.

Zarate, J., & Zatorre, R. (2008). Experience-dependent neural substrates involved in vocal pitch regulation during singing. *NeuroImage, 40*, 1871–1887.

Zatorre, R., Belin, P., & Penhune, V. (2002). Structure and function of auditory cortex: Music and speech. *Trends in Cognitive Sciences, 6*, 37–46.

Zatorre, R., Chen, J., & Penhune, V. (2007). When the brain plays music: Auditory-motor interactions in music perception and production. *National Review of Neuroscience, 8*(7), 547–558.

5

Resonance and Vocal Acoustics

Introduction

Perhaps one of the most important components of the vocal mechanism for commercial music singers is the filter (resonance) as it allows the singer to "mix" his or her own sound source by altering the three-dimensional spaces above the vocal folds. These modifications in the resonators allow the singer an infinite number of vocal timbres and qualities unique to that individual. Like a painter with a palette, by adding a bit more lightness or darkness or mixing one color with another, you have a rainbow of interesting possibilities. The complexities of understanding acoustics and resonance can be daunting for many singers, but this chapter aims to provide the commercial music singer with a basic understanding of terminology and concepts related to resonance and how these principles may apply to the vocal athlete.

Resonators and Resonance

When the vocal folds vibrate, they generate a spectrum of sound frequencies depending on the length and tension of the vocal folds and the air pressure provided. Once that frequency is produced, the sound wave travels above (and below) the vocal folds into spaces that we call resonators.

There are seven vocal resonators: two subglottic (chest and trachea), the laryngeal vestibule, the pharynx (further broken into oropharynx, nasopharynx, and laryngopharynx), the oral cavity, the nasal cavity, and the sinus cavities (Figures 5–1,

> Fundamental frequency (F_0)—the pitch that you sing (A4 = 440 Hz, or 440 cycles per second).

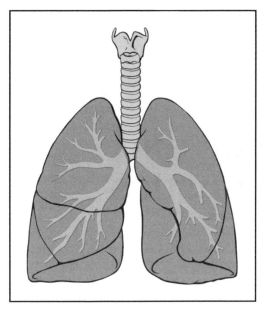

Figure 5–1. Anterior view of respiratory tract. Courtesy of Wikimedia Commons.

5-2, 5-3, 5-4, 5-5, and 5-6). Each of these should be air-filled spaces (which is why when you get fluid in the sinuses or swelling in the nasal passages, it changes the resonance or you feel things differently). Of the resonators above, some primarily provide sensory feedback to the singer and are not manipulated in terms of size and shape to modify the sound (chest, trachea, nasal cavity, sinuses). However, the laryngeal vestibule, pharynx, oral cavity, and to some degree the nasal cavity are vital components in shaping the timbre (brightness/darkness) and amplitude (loudness) of the sound. *Resonance* can be defined in simple terms as the enhancement or amplification of specific frequencies. How resonance affects vocal production warrants a brief description of sound waves, harmonics, partials, and formants.

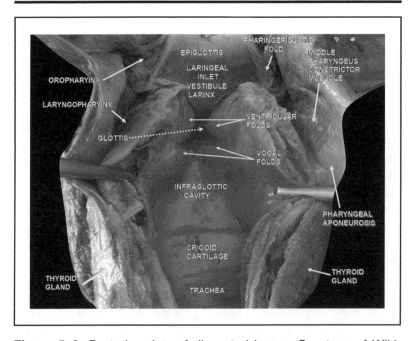

Figure 5–2. Posterior view of dissected larynx. Courtesy of Wikimedia Commons.

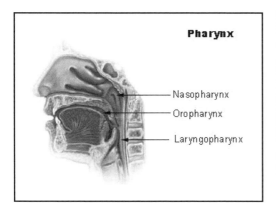

Figure 5–3. Lateral view of the pharynx. Courtesy of Wikimedia Commons.

Sound Waves

When the vocal folds vibrate at a given frequency, they produce a sound wave. This wave travels above (supraglottically) and below (subglottically) into the resonating chambers discussed above. Resonators will either enhance a part of the sound wave or damp a part of the wave. When this sound wave encounters bigger or smaller spaces

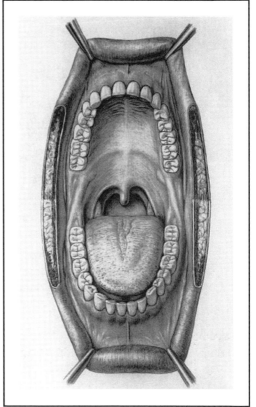

Figure 5–4. Frontal view of the oral cavity. Courtesy of Wikimedia Commons.

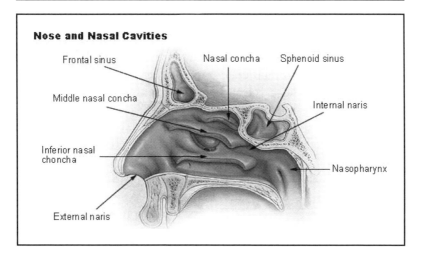

Figure 5–5. Lateral view of the nose and nasal cavities. Courtesy of Wikimedia Commons.

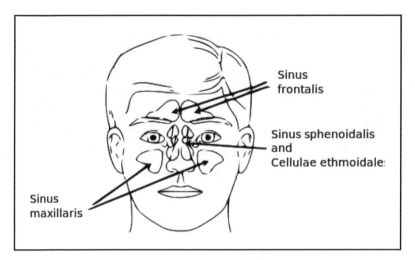

Figure 5–6. Anterior view of paranasal sinuses. Courtesy of Wikimedia Commons.

(think about singing into tubes of various diameters and/or lengths) or soft or hard tissue, these changes alter the wave.

Harmonics

A harmonic is an equally spaced frequency that is an integer multiple of the fundamental frequency (e.g., fundamental frequency (F_0 = 200 Hz, first harmonic (H1) = 400, H2 = 600, H3 = 800, etc.). Timbre is in part determined by the strength of the harmonics. Harmonics become strengthened when they are near formants. Research and theory related to how singers manipulate their vocal tract to strengthen harmonics is discussed further in Chapter 17.

Partials

A partial includes any overtone of the sound spectrum, including the fundamental frequency, and the harmonics. (The harmonic series does not include the fundamental frequency.) All harmonics of a fundamental frequency are also partials because they are part of the spectrum of frequencies; however, a partial is only considered a harmonic if it is an integer multiple of the F_0.

Formants

The word formant simply means a resonance of the vocal tract. Formant tuning occurs when there is a boost of vocal intensity because either the fundamental frequency or one of its harmonics matches exactly with a formant frequency.

Formants Versus Harmonics

The concept differentiating formants and harmonics is sometimes confusing to singers. It is helpful to remember that formants are linked to and define the vowel, and harmonics are linked to the fundamental frequency, or pitch. It is possible to alter one without the other. For example, consider the scenario where you sing a consistent vowel but vary the pitch. In this case, the formant structure remains primarily unaltered because the vowel has not been changed and the cross-sectional dimensions of the vocal tract remain relatively constant, but the harmonics have shifted because you have altered the fundamental frequency, or pitch. Now take the opposite example where the pitch remains the same, but you are changing the vowel while singing a steady frequency (F_0). In this scenario, the vocal tract shape has changed, and therefore formants have shifted (so that we perceive different vowels); however, the harmonics are largely the same because the frequency was steady and unchanged.

Vocal Tract as the Filter of Sound

Sung and spoken text is comprised of consonants and sounds with vocal fold vibration as a carrier for voiced consonant and vowels creating sound pressure waves via oscillation of the vocal folds. During sung vowels, the vocal folds create a spectrum of acoustic energy, with overtones and frequencies that travel through the vocal tract. Some frequencies will resonate more than others. Larger spaces (e.g., oral cavity/pharyngeal space) will resonate lower frequencies, and smaller spaces will tend to enhance higher frequencies. The first two formant frequencies (F1 and F2) define the vowels. The first formant F1 (throat/pharynx) is altered by the opening the jaw or by pharyngeal constriction. A narrowing of the oral cavity will lower F1 (i.e., /u/), whereas a narrowing of the pharynx will raise F1 (i.e., /a/; Figures 5–7, 5–8, 5–9, and Table 5–1). The second formant F2 (mouth) is influenced primarily by posterior tongue position. F2 lowers with constriction in lips

or oropharynx and is raised with constriction in oral cavity (i.e., /i/; Behrman, 2007).

There are additional ways to alter formant frequencies within the vocal tract. Below are parameters that impact the location of formant frequencies (http://www.ncvs.org).

1. Formants decrease uniformly if the length of the vocal tract increases, and the formants will raise uniformly if the vocal tract length is shortened. There are two primary ways to alter the length of the vocal tract. First, lip spreading shortens the vocal tract, thus raising the formants and resulting in a brighter sound quality. Conversely, rounding the lips lowers all of the formants, resulting in a darker timbre. The vocal tract length can also be modified by altering laryngeal position. An elevated larynx shortens the vocal tract, and lowering the larynx lengthens the vocal tract.
2. Constriction in the oral cavity lowers F1 and raises F2, resulting in more space between these first two formants and creating a more diffuse vowel spectrum with more energy spread out over low and high frequencies (i.e., /i/).
3. Pharyngeal constriction raises F1 and lowers F2, resulting in less acoustic energy spread out (i.e., /a/).

Table 5–1 shows the general effect of vocal tract length and constriction on formant frequencies.

Vocal Tract Resonances as Amplifier

As singers increase proficiency at optimizing the source (vocal folds) and filter (resonance) interaction, they also begin to maximize and utilize their resonators to

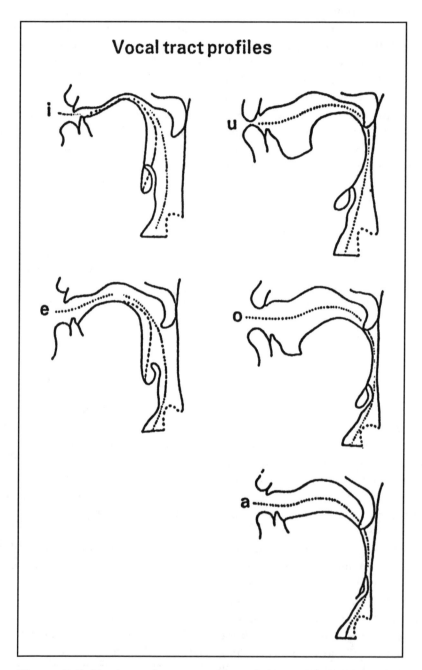

Figure 5–7. Tracings of x-ray profiles of the vocal tract showing articulatory configurations for some vowels. From R. T. Sataloff, *Vocal Health and Pedagogy: Science and Assessment* (2nd ed.), 2013, Plural Publishing. Reprinted with permission.

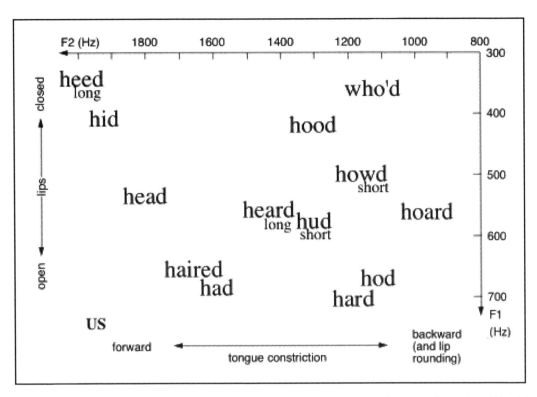

Figure 5–8. Vowel chart. From A. Ghonim, J. Smith, and J. Wolfe, *The Sounds of World English: A Vowel Perception Survey.* Sydney, Australia.

their advantage. Specifically, when vowels are "tuned" appropriately, the shape and response of the resonators behave in such a way that it helps provide an acoustical "boost" to the sound. One way to think of how the vocal tract is used to either boost or dampen acoustic energy is to imagine a child on a swing. When you swing, you need energy to keep swinging (either an external push or self-energy expenditure). If someone stands in front of the swing and blocks the ability to move forward and someone stands in back of you and blocks the ability to swing any farther back, your swing is very limited (damped). However, if those same two people stepped back, and each time you came to them, they gave you a little push, you would go higher and

higher (amplified). Although this is only an example of a simple wave, the swing example can provide a basis for understanding for amplification and damping of waves.

Within each of the resonating chambers, movements that narrow, widen, tense, or relax those spaces will damp or amplify the complex frequencies that come through them. Singers work to get the most "gain" with the least "output" so that maximum efficiency can be achieved. This is essential for all performance artists, but due to the many characters and styles that are required in commercial music, CCM singers must have excellent command of the source-filter interaction, so that they do not overdrive the vocal mechanism when increasing vocal intensity.

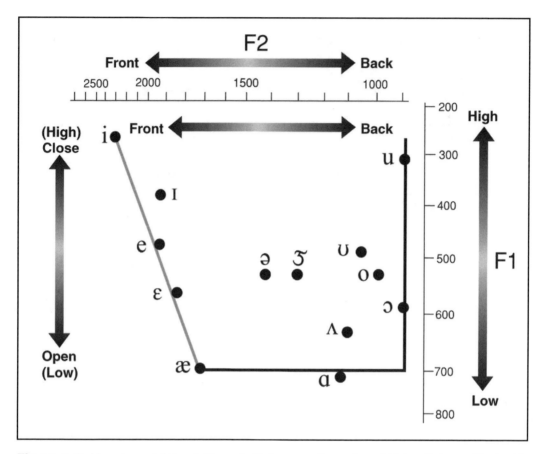

Figure 5–9. Vowel quadrilateral. From A. Behrman, *Speech and Voice Science* (2nd ed.), 2012. Plural Publishing. Reprinted with permission.

The "Singer's Formant"

Once a perfectly placed, focused tone has been achieved, the singer should experience a "ring" in the voice. The terminology "ring" is synonymous to singer's formant, but "ring" is used most commonly in the voice studio. Singers perceive the "ring" in the voice as an amplified overtone, which creates a ringing sensation in the head or mask of the face. From the voice teacher's standpoint, it is the production of a tone that helps the singer to be heard without amplification in a large auditorium over an orchestra. It is important to note that the majority of the operatic works performed today are done without personal amplification. However, musical theater utilizes body microphones on almost all of their cast members. This is evidenced even at the high school level of performance. Actors are also reported to have a similar boost ("speaker's formant") of acoustic energy with projected speech (Master, De Biase, Chiari, & Laukkanen, 2008).

The singer's formant is a clustering of acoustical energy at approximately 3000 Hz (Schutte & Miller, 1993; Sundberg, 1990; Titze, 1994). According to Sundberg

TABLE 5–1. General Effect of Vocal Tract Lengthening and Constriction of Formant Frequency

Formant Frequency	Increased Vocal Tract Length	Location of Constriction (Perturbation)					
		Hypopharynx	Pharynx	Oropharynx	Mid-Oral Cavity (palate)	Anterior Oral Cavity (alveolar ridge)	Lips
F1	Lowered	Raised	Raised			Lowered	Lowered
F2	Lowered	Raised		Lowered		Raised	Lowered
F3	Lowered	Raised	Lowered	Raised	Lowered	Raised	Lowered

Source: Behrman, A. (2013). *Speech and Voice Science* (2nd ed.). (Table 6–1, p. 229). San Diego, CA: Plural Publishing.

(1987), the singer's formant causes a peak in acoustical energy as a result of a clustering of the 3rd, 4th, and 5th formants. The amplitudes of the harmonics that determine these formants (F3, F4, and F5) will determine the amplitude of the singer's formant. The physiologic basis for the singer's formant may be demonstrated by envisioning the vocal tract as a series of tubes. Imagine a small quarter-wave resonator inside of a larger quarter-length resonator. Ideally, to achieve the singer's formant, the smaller tube inside of the vocal tract must be less than 1/6 of the entire vocal tract length (2.5–3.0 cm). Mathematically, the following would result: $Fn = 35,000$ cm/sec/$(4 \times 3.0$ cm$) = 35,000$ cm/sec/12 cm $= 2916.67$ Hz (Baken & Orlikoff, 2000). A spectrogram will demonstrate the increase of energy around 3000 Hz.

It is this increase in spectral energy that enables the singer's voice to carry over an orchestra. As vocal intensity increases, it has been shown that the singer's formant also increases (Sundberg, 1990). Sundberg (1990) further qualified this event as an increase in vocal intensity; "the overtones at high frequencies grow more quickly than those at low frequencies, which are responsible for the overall sound level" (p. 112). Sopranos have been shown in several studies to lack the singer's formant, although highly trained operatic sopranos do reveal some high frequency energy clusters (Sundberg, 1990; Sundberg & Skoog, 1998). Achieving the singer's formant is accomplished through learning to train the resonators to effectively enhance specific frequencies. Once the singer has experienced the singer's formant, often times a sensation of placement rather than auditory cues are relied upon to duplicate the phenomenon.

Ekholm, Papagiannis, and Chagnon (1998) found that the presence of the singer's formant in the classical voice correlated strongly with the perception of vocal beauty. Some recent research on the belt voice suggests a lack of the singer's formant, and an increase of spectral energy for F1 and F2 (Robison, Bounous, & Bailey, 1994). To further confuse the issue of the presence or absence of the singer's formant in the belt voice, Schutte and Miller (1993) concluded in a single subject design, the "chest" voice lacked the singer's formant, but the "pop" voice and the "classical" voice both maintained an increase in harmonics six to eight. No distinction was made in their study defining the difference between the "chest" voice and the "pop" voice, and many voice teachers consider these terms synonymous.

LeBorgne (2001) found that elite belters presented with a clustering of energy around 4000 Hz in the singers who were defined as elite (as compared with the average belters). This may indicate a slight shift of approximately 1000 Hz in the singer's formant for this group of female belters. The energy shift may also be because of the higher frequency of the fundamental in this group of singers.

Timbre

Tone color (timbre) as defined by William Vennard, both a musician and scientist, was a "subjective aspect of the harmonic structure of musical tone" (p. 235). In 1960, the American Standards Association defined timbre as "that attribute of auditory sensation in terms of which listeners can judge that sounds having the same pitch and loudness are dissimilar" (p. 847). Just as with an artist's color, the timbre of a voice, vowel, or instrument is a perceived event, distinguishable to the musically experienced ear. From the scientific standpoint, a bright sound is defined as "having high partials" (Vennard, 1967, p. 256). Vennard writes:

> *both colors and timbres awaken similar psychological responses. We may expect, therefore, that a timbre that is depressing because of its lack of partials would be called "dark," "dark brown," "gray," or "muddy." Analogies with the art of painting are used, like my mention of* pointillism. *Tones that are pleasing will be compared to pleasing colors; singers who produce them will be said to have "golden voices." High partial in a tone will be called "brilliance," "sparkle," "brightness." Many of these terms imply intensity of color more than hue. This is logical, since high partials tend to disappear in most musical tones when the intensity drops, and so we may expect ringing tones to be compared to colors of high intensity, and dull tones, to low. It is a good singer who can keep "2800" in his voice while singing softly. Those who get high partials at the expense of low ones are guilty of "white" production. The French Expression, "voix blanche," carries this connotation. (p. 151)*

Much terminology is available to describe timbre. Bloothooft and Plomp (1988) discerned 21 bipolar semantic pairs of descriptive terms for timbre that were actively used in the voice studio. These authors found that both trained and untrained listeners were able to discriminate even small changes in vocal timbre. Attempting to objectify their findings related to changes in timbre, they found that "a difference in timbre correlates with a difference in ⅓-oct spectrum for stationary vowels, at least up to 392 Hz" (p. 858). Of the 21 pairs of descriptive terms, only sharpness turned out

to be the term upon which both musically experienced, and the musically nonexperienced, significantly agreed. Objectively, sharpness was the only term that was found to relate to the spectral slope. "Listeners seem to relate a shallow spectral slope to tenor-voice timbre and a steep negative slope to bass-voice timbre type" (p. 859). Their experiment further noted that high-frequency energy appeared to correspond to a rating of a higher voice classification by the listeners.

Baken and Orlikoff (2000) expound on the notion of spectral slope as it corresponds to timbre. Specifically, the typical spectral slope has been measured at negative 12 dB slope per octave because of the attenuation of the harmonics at higher frequencies. When the spectral slope becomes more shallow (−6 dB per octave), the perceived sound is brighter. Conversely, a deeper slope (−18 dB per octave) would result in a perceptually darker sound.

A study by Sundberg, Gramming, and Lovetri (1993) examined the formant characteristics of the belt voice in comparison with the classically trained singer. One of the major limitations of this study was the sample size. Because of the sample size, it is difficult to determine if the findings related to acoustic output would generalize to a population of belters. Regardless, the findings revealed that belting showed a weak fundamental and relatively strong overtones in comparison with the classical singing style for the /i/ vowel. It is speculated by the present investigator that the increase in overtones may give the listener a perception of a "brighter" sound than the classical voice. This postulation needs to be further examined.

Similar to the previous study, Schutte and Miller (1993) found differences in harmonic and formant intensities across different singing styles. Again, this study had a relatively poor sample size with only one singer studied. Another drawback is the lack of definitions for the terms they used to describe the various modes of singing. Chest, middle, pop, and belt are all used, and it is unclear as to the exact differentiation. Many teachers consider these terms synonymous. However, Schutte and Miller's (1993) research provided some preliminary insight into the possible timbre differences noted between the classical and nonclassical singing styles. "The higher formant frequencies of the 'chest' register articulation, characteristic of more 'open' singing, are closer to the average speech values than are those of the more 'covered' sound of the 'classical' articulation" (Schutte & Miller, 1993, p. 145). They suggested that "the dominant H2 in the 'pop' example results from the impact of F1 located not far below the harmonic. In the 'classical' example, both F1 and F2 have moved lower, making the first two harmonics nearly equal in level and giving the sound a 'darker' and 'rounder' perceptual quality" (Schutte & Miller, 1993, p. 146). Although their study provided initial insight into possible acoustic explanations, continued research regarding the phenomenon of harmonic and formant differences among belters is warranted and has further been investigated with a larger sample size in several other studies (LeBorgne, 2001).

Focus and Placement

Within the singing world, the terms placement and focus are closely related but have slightly different connotations. Placement, a perceptual illusion, is associated with the "brilliance" or "mellowness" of a tone (Vennard, 1967). When taken literally, "placement" means to put something somewhere. One obviously cannot take the voice and put it "in the mouth, nose, or pharynx;" rather the singer gains a sense (possibly sympathetic vibrations) that the voice is actually resonating or "placed" within those cavities. The singing teacher may further qualify the term placement by discussing the term focus.

Focus has two meanings with respect to tone placement. First, singers refer to focusing a tone or vowel in order to intensify the brilliance of a given sound. This concept of focus is similar to the convergence of light rays via a magnifying glass used to burn a hole in a piece of paper. The singer's connotation of focus is derived from the scientific connotation, typically associated with light or heat. A lens or some other type of reflector will converge or diverge (focus) the light or heat waves. Singers learn that voice production is the result of a series of waves (compressions and rarefactions), and as such, one should be able to focus the sound waves generated by the vocal folds. Often, the singer envisions the convergence of sound waves at a given point. Vennard (1967) concluded that "there is no lens or reflector in the vocal mechanism . . . but if we hold to the figurative use of the word, we are able to grasp something valuable to the singers, a sensation, illusory perhaps, that when the tone is well produced it 'comes to a point'" (p. 150).

A second use of the term focus refers to the ability of the singer to remove excess breathiness from a tone (tone clarity). This connotation of focus is associated with the nature and degree of glottal closure. Placement, focus, and clarity are perceived events or mental illusions utilized by singing teachers to evoke a desired perceptual quality. Forward placement/focus, sharper focus, and back focus are some of the readily used terms in the voice studio.

These terms pervade both the classical and belting training. Through examination of forward placement/focus and back placement/focus, from the singer's perspective, one may gain further insight into the use of these terms.

Placement

Forward placement is typically associated with a "bright" (white, open, forward) timbre. Vowels that are typically used to elicit a forward placement are /i/ and /I/. When these vowels are sung correctly, a sensation of a predominantly oral/nasal resonance is experienced by the singer. The singer is most likely experiencing a sympathetic vibration created by the optimal tuning of the resonators for a given vowel. Although /i/ and /I/ are often used to promote a frontal focus when a tone quality is aesthetically perceived "too dark," the degree of frontal focus can be taken to an extreme resulting in an overly "bright" sound. McKinney (1982) believes that faults of resonance related to a vocal production that is "too bright," may be the consequence of: "(1) lack of space in the pharynx due to the action of the constrictor muscles and/or elevation of the larynx; (2) tension in the walls of the pharyngeal resonator making it too selective; (3) wrong tonal models; (4) exaggerated mouth opening, pulling the lips back in a forced smile; (5) excessive tension in the muscles of the lips, tongue, jaw, or palatal muscles" (p. 139). As one examines the vocal tract configurations for the acoustic output for the vowels /i/ and /I/, McKinney's theories of faulty resonance may be considered plausible possibilities.

Musical theater belters have often been accused of an overly bright timbre (Miles & Hollien, 1990; Sullivan, 1989). In addition, the limited research published on belting suggests a higher laryngeal placement than in classical singing (Estill, 1988; Miles & Hollien, 1990; Schutte & Miller, 1993; Sullivan, 1989; Sundberg et al., 1993). To further contrast McKinney's suggested vocal fault, Jan Sullivan (1989) suggested that her belters posture their lips, teeth, tongue, and jaw in such a way that the articulators are shaped like the bell of a trumpet. Belting, as implied by the literature, may resemble an overly bright, focused tone when compared with the classical voice.

In contrast to a "bright" sound, some singers often produce sounds that are considered too "dark" or placed too far "back." Vowels used to elicit a back placement are typically /ɑ/ and /ɔ/. McKinney (1982) cites five reasons for the singer producing a sound that is too far "back": "(1) overuse of the "yawning" muscles, with resulting spread throat and/or depressed larynx; (2) lack of oral space due to lip, jaw, or tongue position; (3) wrong tonal models; (4) flabby surfaces of pharyngeal walls (not enough muscle tone to give any character to the sound); (5) tongue pulled back into the pharynx" (p. 141).

Resonance of Tubes

From an acoustic standpoint, what is it about the vowels /i/ and /I/ that produces a perceived forward focus while the /ɑ/ and /ɔ/ produce a perceived back focus? To address this question, the quarter-wave resonating tube and the resulting acoustic phenomenon are discussed. The vocal tract is considered a quarter-wave resonating tube, closed at one end (glottis) and open at the other (mouth; Kent & Read, 1992; Titze, 1994). This type of tube presents with certain acoustic properties that can be applied to vocal tract resonances. The formula used to determine the resonance frequencies of a quarter-wave resonator is $Fn = (2n - 1)c/4l$ (Kent & Read, 1992). Assuming the length (l) of the average vocal tract is 17.5 cm, the speed of sound (c) is 35,000 cm/sec, and n is an integer (F1-first formant, F2-second formant, etc.), the resonant frequencies of the vocal tract can be calculated ($Fn = c/4l = 35,000\ cm/sec/4 \times 17.5cm = 500\ l/s\ or\ 500\ Hz$). If the tube length and diameter remain constant, the vocal tract in a neutral position /ʌ/ would produce formant frequencies of 500, 1500, 2500, 3500, and 4500 Hz. Lengthening the tube by lowering the larynx or rounding the lips would result in an overall lowering of the formant frequencies, whereas shortening the vocal tract would have the opposite effect. Measurement and observation of this phenomenon may be obtained through formant plotting on time spectrograms (Baken & Orlikoff, 2000).

Singing and speech require that the vocal tract be changed and shaped to produce different vowel sounds. Therefore, instead of a single quarter-wave resonating tube, the vocal tract is a series of several tubes used to achieve the acoustical phenomenon and resultant formant characteristics of different vowels. Each vowel is defined by the first and second formants. In most cases, the oral cavity can be considered one tube while the pharynx can be considered a second tube. The two-tube model will be used to discuss the formation of the /i/ and /ɑ/ vowels, in contrast with the one-tube neutral vowel /ə/.

Both /i/ and /I/ are considered high front vowels. Acoustically "high" vowels have a low F1 frequency and "front" vowels have a high F2 frequency in comparison with their low back counterparts. To achieve these ideal formants, adjustments of the vocal tract must be made to enhance certain partials of the fundamental frequency, resulting in this particular formant pattern. The typical vocal tract configuration for an /i/ vowel in comparison with a neutral vowel /ʌ/, which is that of a widened pharynx and narrowed oral cavity. Titze (1994) described the two-tube model for the /i/ vowel:

The first formant pressure pattern is nearly constant in the pharynx and shows a "virtual zero" pressure far to the right, acoustically elongating the tube and lowering F1. For the second formant, the mouth tube is the dominant resonator. An overall reduction in the pharynx moves the pressure zero toward the tube interface. The mouth tube then supports a half wavelength, approximately, because it has nearly two open ends. This raises F2 because the half wavelength of the mouth tube is shorter than the half wavelength of the neutral tube. (p. 152)

The acoustic principles governing F1 and F2 for a "bright" vowel, such as /i/, correspond to the type of perceived placement of the vocal tract speculated by McKinney (1982). An overly constricted pharynx, raised larynx, or pharyngeal wall rigidity most likely results in changes of F1 and F2 for the vowel /i/. The task of the singing teacher and the singer is to determine, via a well-trained ear, how a correctly "placed" /i/ feels in the mouth and pharynx. Phrases such as "think of a yawn" and "keep the tongue arched a little higher" are commonly used in the voice studio to elicit such vocal tract configurations. Coaching the singer with such images presumably changes the formant frequencies of a given vowel, so that they more closely resemble the formants of the target vowel. The degree of "brightness" or "darkness" is a personal aesthetic choice and will vary depending on society's taste regarding tone color and vocal genre performed.

In contrast with the front vowels, there are also perceived back vowels /ɑ/ and /ɔ/. To achieve the F1 and F2 for /ɑ/ and /ɔ/, the pharynx must narrow and the oral cavity widen. From an acoustic standpoint, these two vowels are considered midback in placement; F1 is high and F2 is low. There is usually less F1–F2 difference between back vowels than front vowels. The /ɑ/ vowel results in a higher F1 because of the narrowed pharynx in comparison with /ʌ/ (Titze, 1994). When the narrowed pharynx is coupled with the wider than normal oral cavity, the F2 is "acoustically lengthened because the mouth pressure is lowered" (p. 152).

Singers learn to adjust and manipulate their vocal tract, so that correct vowel placement becomes second nature. The image concept of placement and focus may seem rather odd to the scientist, but the terms must not be taken literally. Rather, the connotations of the terms placement and focus in the voice studio may be a result of the pharyngeal, oral, and nasal resonances (sympathetic vibrations, or changes in pressures) perceived by the singer when they have achieved optimal F1 and F2 for given vowels. The literature reviewed above suggests that belters may use a brighter, more forward tone placement than other types of singing. LeBorgne (2001) objectively quantified that elite belters indeed had a shallower spectral slope (brighter sound) than the average belters.

Focus

The ability to remove excess breathiness from a tone may also be described as focus. Focus in this sense relates directly to the sound source. If glottal closure is not complete, or if the open phase of the vibratory cycle predominates, the perceived tone is often considered "spread" or containing excess breath. A spectrogram analysis reveals "a loss of energy between 2 and 5 kHz and an increase of noise at frequencies exceeding 5 kHz" because of incomplete glottic closure or a considerably open glottis phase (p. 320; Rihkanen, Leinonen, Hiltunen, & Kangas, 1994). Singers must learn to balance breath pressure, degree of glottic closure, and tuning of the resonators in order to achieve a well-placed, focused tone. Hirano (1988) offered six points that help explain the ability of the human voice to maintain phonation for song:

(1) the human vocal fold has a unique structure that fits the task, (2) the vocal folds undergo delicate adjustments executed by the laryngeal muscles, and therefore, they can function as many different sound generators, (3) the vocal fold adjustments are precisely and delicately controlled by the central nervous system, (4) the respiratory behavior is appropriately controlled, (5) the resonance cavity shaping is adequately controlled, (6) the interaction between the sound source and the resonator is appropriately controlled (p. 51).

Nasality in Commercial Music Singing

Excessive nasality in singing or speaking voices is considered a vocal fault. Yet, the literature on belting suggests that increased nasality in tone production is often perceived (Estill, 1988; Miles & Hollien, 1990; Schutte & Miller, 1993; Sullivan, 1989). Increased nasal resonance results from an

Nasality versus Twang. Nasality and twang are unique entities. The term "twang" for the purposes of this text is based in the research of Sundberg and Thalen (2010). Twang is used in the CCM context to describe an acoustic result of a longer closed quotient during the vibratory cycle, H1–H2 is smaller than neutral singing, and F1–F2 is higher and F3 and F5 are lower in twang as compared with neutral singing.

incomplete closure of the velopharyngeal port resulting in an additional acoustic tube (Baken & Orlikoff, 2000; Kent, 1997; Kent & Read, 1992; Slawson, 1985). The consequence of the additional resonating tube is that it produces resonance frequencies independent of the oral cavity. As a result, the combined oral-nasal cavities produce oral formants (previously discussed), nasal formants, and nasal antiformants (Kent & Read, 1992). All three formants are combined to produce a complex spectral output, resulting in spectral envelopes with deep valleys and increased higher frequencies (Kent & Read, 1992; Slawson, 1985). Other than utility for stylistic or character choices, nasality is not a desired quality in commercial music (LeBorgne, 2001).

Formant Tuning and Belting

Schutte and Miller (1993) report that the first formant tended to track the second harmonic, resulting in a first formant frequency over 950 Hz, and LeBorgne (2001) found similar results when comparing elite and average belters. Specifically, LeBorgne found H2 of /ɑ/ in *star* (from the belted phrase *I'm the greatest star*) was greater in amplitude than H1 for all subjects, and the first spectral peak corresponded to this peak around 1200 Hz. Schutte and Miller (1993) also examined an /ɑ/ vowel sung by Barbra Streisand on D5. Ms. Streisand's production of D5 resulted in H2 dominance and the first formant reported at 1175 Hz. Understanding of why H2 tracks F1 is warranted for those teaching belting.

The explanation that Schutte and Miller provide for this phenomenon is that by raising the larynx, belters are able to maintain F1 very close to H2. Their rationale is supported by the fact that decreasing the size of the pharyngeal cavity will raise F1. Schutte and Miller (1993) write, "Part of the excitement of extending this technique upwards is the sense that one is on a collision course with a finite termination of the range. The listener is aware of the risk the singer is taking" (p. 147). It is the opinion of these authors that if belters were to maintain this high laryngeal position with primarily chest voice production (heavy mechanism, thyroarytenoid-dominant), over a period of time, vocal problems would most likely result because of collision forces and sheering stresses. Schutte and Miller (1993) suggest that good belters begin to mix the belt voice with their definition of "pop" voice. The "pop" voice maintains a higher than normal laryngeal position but not as long of a closed phase, thus decreasing the length of time of impact. Their theory is speculative at this time, as it has not yet been objectively evaluated. Sundberg et al. (1993) found that although the singer in their study maintained relatively consistent formant frequencies on isolated vowels, significant variability in the formant frequencies was noted during song.

A second theory relates to reported characteristics of the belt voice; specifically, an elevated larynx, the "bell-shaped lips," and formant tuning. Rothenberg, Miller, Molitor, and Leffingwell (1987) define formant tuning for the high pitches of the soprano voice as follows:

If the glottis—the space between the vocal folds-opens and closes regularly, with a complete, or nearly complete, closure between the open periods, and if the vocal tract tuning is such that the first formant is tuned to the voice fundamental frequency, the returning air pressure pulse from the previous glottal open periods is in such a phase as to oppose the airflow through the glottis and reduce airflow. This results in a louder voice being produced by means of a reduced airflow. (p. 263)

Formant tuning is used in high-frequency phonation to decrease the degree of vocal trauma, which has been documented throughout the literature (Carlsson & Sundberg, 1992; Sundberg, 1990; Sundberg & Skoog, 1998; Titze, 1994). This may be one reason many belters are able to maintain a long career. One of the ways in which singers accomplish formant tuning is by lowering the jaw, which in turn raises the first formant (Sundberg, 1990; Sundberg & Skoog, 1998). Not only does formant tuning help to reduce the glottic airflow, it also increases overall SPL. Personal experience and private instruction on the belting technique have also advocated an increased jaw opening, especially at higher frequencies. It is very common to see "belt mouth" at extreme frequencies. Specifically, when belting E_5, a jaw opening similar to the production of a C_6 in classical voice may be used.

In addition to the formant tuning accomplished by the lowered jaw, a shorter vocal tract will also affect F1 and F2. Sundberg (1990) reported that in one professional soprano, a shortened vocal tract (up to 30%) than average (13.5 cm) may result in first formant frequencies for an /ɑ/ to be in the range of 1300 Hz. He suggests that the shortened vocal tract would allow this singer to ascend in her range without significant timbre or articulatory changes. This raises an interesting point for belters. If certain persons naturally possess a shorter vocal tract, could they be at potentially lower risk for vocal injury than a person who physically elevates the larynx continually in order to maintain a shorter vocal tract when belting?

LeBorgne (2001) found an elite group of belters presented with frequency values significantly higher than expected for F1. Specifically, the first spectral peak strongly tracked H2–H3, again suggestive of possible formant tuning. This finding further supports the theory of formant tuning for elite belters, as all of the subjects presented with H1 as the strongest harmonic. More recent studies have continued to validate these findings (Bourne & Garnier, 2012; Björkner, 2006; LeBorgne, 2001; Sundberg et al., 1993; Sundberg, Thalén, & Popeil, 2012). Because the theories regarding formant tuning, jaw lowering, and elevated larynx continue to hold true, the resultant acoustic output helps to explain why belters are perceived as having brighter voices than classical singers. Altering the frequencies of the first and second formant will affect timbre.

Additional information on elite belters and average belter comparisons indicated that elite belters had higher noise to harmonics ratios and voice turbulence scores than average belters, signifying an increase in the degree of high frequency noise in the signal (LeBorgne, 2001). One possible theory for this phenomenon relates to tracheal coupling and the source/tract interaction (Klatt & Klatt, 1990; Titze & Story, 1997) report with regard to belting, "In high pitched operatic singing, belting, and twang singing, the narrow epilarynx seems to be the configuration of choice . . . This configuration provides the desirable inertive reactance to facilitate vocal fold oscillation. When the narrowed epilarynx is combined with a wide pharynx, the reactance never goes negative below about 3000 Hz, which means the acoustic load is inertive for all possible values of F_0" (p. 2243).

Vocal Tract Modifications for Classical Singers

In general terms, classical singers strive to sing with a generally low, stable laryngeal position, attempting to tune each vowel at each frequency for maximum beauty and output. That is not to say that the larynx is "stuck" or never moves, but the generally stable laryngeal position often provides the classical singer with an optimal resonating space above the vocal folds to shape the sound. Generally at high frequencies, vowels are modified to /a/ in order to minimize an interaction between the fundamental frequency being sung (perhaps A5–880 Hz). In order for the audience to understand that A5 is an /a/, the fundamental frequency (880 Hz in this case), has to be below the first formant for an /a/ vowel. Because the first and second formants define what vowel the listener perceives, if the fundamental frequency is above the first formant, we will perceive a different vowel. In classical singing, vowel integrity and beauty of the vocal line are

essential components for a professional career.

Vocal Tract Modifications for Commercial Music and Belting

Within the commercial music genre, understanding of text is paramount for the artist. It is the text that conveys or moves the story forward. Therefore, minimal vowel modification is acceptable in commercial music, which is why much of the music is written in a speech range. However, high-frequency belting can present a problem for singers because sometimes the fundamental frequency required is above the typical first formant for a given vowel. When that occurs, the singer must modify the vocal tract in order for the audience to perceive the correct text. Returning to what was just discussed regarding vowel modification, this may involve raising the larynx, dropping the jaw, or spreading the lips. Research has shown that belters often raise the F1 above and near the second harmonic (H2) to achieve the bright sound associated with belting. This can be achieved by shortening the vocal tract in two ways: (1) spreading the lips and (2) elevating the larynx. This raises the F1 to 1000 Hz in males and 1200 Hz in females and allows for a belt sound quality without solely using TA contraction. There is also a third way to raise the F1. Narrowing the pharynx and epilaryngeal tube also provides the bright, twang-like quality (Sundberg & Thalen, 2010; Titze, Bergan, Hunter, & Story, 2003).

In many ways, commercial music mimics the laryngeal movements of speech in that there is movement of the larynx up and down and millions of combinations of the articulators during a typical conversational exchange. The caveat is that many speakers, especially when speaking at a heightened state of emotion, tend to elevate the larynx and increase vocal intensity, resulting in unnecessary vocal tension and trauma. Commercial music singers must learn to convey heightened emotion in the most vocally "cost efficient" manner, which is further discussed in Chapter 17.

Chapter Summary

Understanding the basics of acoustics and shaping of the sound above the vocal folds is necessary for the commercial music artist. As each vocal athlete has a unique vocal mechanism, an appreciation of how many different vocal qualities can result from a single instrument are discussed. Effectively and efficiently manipulating the resonators can aid the singer in maximal output with minimal cost to the system.

References

Baken, R., & Orlikoff, R. (2000). *Clinical measurement of speech and voice* (2nd ed.). San Diego, CA: Singular Publishing.

Behrman, A. (2007). *Speech and voice science* (2nd ed.). San Diego, CA: Plural Publishing.

Björkner, E. (2006). Musical theater and opera singing—Why so different? A study of subglottal pressure, voice source, and formant frequency characteristics. *Journal of Voice, 22*(5), 533-540.

Bloothooft, G., & Plomp, R. (1988). The timbre of sung vowels. *Journal of the Acoustical Society of America, 84*(3), 847-860.

Bourne, T., & Garnier, M. (2012). Physiological and acoustic characteristics of the female music theater voice. *Journal of the Acoustical Society of America, 131*(2), 1586-1594.

Carlsson, G., & Sundberg, J. (1992). Formant frequency tuning in singing. *Journal of Voice, 6*(3), 256-260.

Ekholm, E., Papagiannis, G., & Chagnon, F. (1998). Relating objective measurements to expert evaluation of voice quality in western classical singing: Critical perceptual parameters. *Journal of Voice, 12*(2), 182-196.

Estill, J. (1988). Belting and classic voice quality: Some physiological differences. *Medical Problems of Performing Artists*, March, 37-43.

Hirano, M. (1988). Vocal mechanism in singing: Laryngological and phoniatric aspects. *Journal of Voice, 2*(1), 51-69.

Kent, R. (1997). *The speech sciences*. San Diego, CA: Singular Publishing.

Kent, R., & Read, C. (1992). *The acoustic analysis of speech*. San Diego, CA: Singular Publishing.

Klatt, D., & Klatt, L. (1990). Analysis, synthesis, and perception of voice quality variations among female and male talkers. *Journal of the Acoustical Society of America, 87*(2), 820-854.

LeBorgne, W. (2001). *Defining the belt voice: Perceptual judgments and objective measures* (Doctoral dissertation). University of Cincinnati. Retrieved from https://etd.ohiolink.edu/ap:10:0:NO:10:P10_ETD_SUBID:85293.

Master, S., De Biase, N., Chiari, B., & Laukkanen, A. (2008). Acoustic and perceptual analyses of Brazilian male actors' and nonactors' voices: Long-term average spectrum and the "actor's formant." *Journal of Voice, 22*(2), 146-154.

McKinney, J. (1982). *The diagnosis and correction of vocal faults*. Nashville, TN: Genevox Music.

Miles, B., & Hollien, H. (1990). Whither belting? *Journal of Voice, 4*(1), 64-70.

Rihkanen, H., Leinonen, L., Hiltunen, T., & Kangas, J. (1994). Spectral pattern recognition of improved vocal quality. *Journal of Voice, 8*(4), 320-326.

Robison, C., Bounous, B., & Bailey, R. (1994). Vocal beauty: A study proposing its acoustical definition and relevant causes in classical baritones and female belt singers. *The NATS Journal,* September/October, 19–30.

Rothenberg, M., Miller, D., Molitor, R., & Leffingwell, D. (1987). The control of airflow during loud soprano singing. *Journal of Voice, 1*(3), 262–268.

Schutte, H., & Miller, D. (1993). Belting and pop, nonclassical approaches to the female middle voice: Some preliminary considerations. *Journal of Voice,* 7(2), 142–150.

Slawson, W. (1985). *Sound color.* Berkeley, CA: University of California Press.

Sullivan, J. (1989). How to teach the belt/pop voice. *Journal of Research in Singing and Applied Vocal Pedagogy, 13*(1), 41–56.

Sundberg, J. (1987). *The science of the singing voice.* Dekalb, IL: Northern Illinois University Press.

Sundberg, J. (1990). What's so special about singers? *Journal of Voice, 4*(2), 107–119.

Sundberg, J., Gramming, P., & Lovetri, J. (1993). Comparisons of pharynx, source, formant, and pressure characteristics in operatic and musical theatre singing. *Journal of Voice,* 7(4), 301–310.

Sundberg, J., & Skoog, J. (1998). Dependence of jaw opening on pitch and vowel in singers. *Journal of Voice, 11*(3), 301–306.

Sundberg, J., & Thalén, M. (2010). What is twang? *Journal of Voice, 24*(6), 654–660.

Sundberg, J., Thalén, M., & Popeil, L. (2012). Substyles of belting: Phonatory and resonatory characteristics. *Journal of Voice, 26*(1), 44–50.

Titze, I. (1994). *Principles of voice production.* Englewood Cliffs, NJ: Prentice Hall.

Titze, I., Bergan, C., Hunter, E., & Story, B. (2003). Source filter adjustments governing the perception of vocal qualities twang and yawn. *Logopedics, Phoniatrics, and Vocology, 28,* 147–155.

Titze, I., & Story, B. (1997). Acoustic interactions of the voice source with the lower vocal tract. *Journal of the Acoustical Society of America, 101*(4), 2234–2243.

Vennard, W. (1967). *Singing: The mechanism and the technic.* New York, NY: Carl Fischer.

SECTION II

Vocal Health and Fitness

6

Impact of Phonotraumatic Behaviors on Vocal Health and Singing

Introduction

Most singers, at some point or other, have experienced voice difficulties for various reasons. These difficulties can result in a transient change in vocal function as the result of an acute illness such as an upper respiratory infection, or changes can become chronic for a variety of reasons. Singers, actors, teachers, and other high-level voice users, are at an increased risk for experiencing vocal difficulties or sustaining a phonotraumatic vocal injury, as these voices are typically used more frequently, and at a

> Phonotrauma—The result of a vocal behavior either volitional or involuntary, impacting vocal fold vibration in a manner that compromises vocal fold integrity.

higher level and demand (Hoffman-Ruddy, Lehman, Crandell, Ingram, & Sapienza, 2001; Korovin & LeBorgne, 2009).

This chapter provides a description of phonotrauma, its causes, and impacts on voice in general with specific reference to the singing voice. Phonotraumatic injuries commonly seen in singers and management strategies of diagnoses are included in this chapter. Information is provided regarding which vocal injuries are typically amenable to voice therapy with a speech language pathologist with expertise in voice, and which diagnoses are more commonly managed surgically under the hands of a skilled laryngologist who has expertise in treating singers. Current considerations on wound healing relative to phonotrauma will be reviewed with reference to existing research in this area. Finally, the importance of collaboration of the voice care team including the laryngologist, speech language pathologist with expertise in voice and singing, and the voice teacher when working with an injured singer are briefly discussed, with a more detailed discussion in the chapter on Multidisciplinary Voice Care (Chapter 11).

What Is Phonotrauma?

For the purposes of this book, we define phonotrauma as *the result of a vocal behavior either volitional or involuntary, impacting vocal fold vibration in a manner that compromises vocal fold integrity*. This can be a transient occurrence or a chronic behavior. To further define, we can categorize phonotraumatic behaviors into two very general categories: (1) nonphonatory behaviors, and (2) phonatory behaviors. Nonphonatory, phonotraumatic behaviors include actions such as throat clearing, persistent coughing, loud sneezing, weight-lifting with vocal strain, and grunting. In contrast, shouting, yelling, cheering, singing out of range, imitating sounds in a loud, pressed manner, are all considered to be phonatory, phonotraumatic behaviors. Distinguishing between the two types of phonotrauma (phonatory and nonphonatory) is vital because often the perception is that only inappropriate speaking and/or singing habits could result in laryngeal injury. However, it is not uncommon for nonphonatory phonotraumatic behaviors to contribute to vocal fold irritation and/or injury as well. That is not to say that engaging in a phonotraumatic behavior automatically results in vocal fold injury, especially in a vocally healthy singer. However, frequent use of any combination of phonotraumatic behaviors may lead to laryngeal irritation and possibly vocal injury.

When a patient with a voice complaint is seen for a voice assessment, one of the first things identified by the voice pathologist during the evaluation is appraising vocal behaviors and the level of awareness the patient has about these behaviors. Awareness is a critical factor in eliminating any behavior. Often patients have to be guided and educated about phonotrauma in order to identify, monitor, and track their vocal behaviors, resulting in reduction and ultimately elimination of potentially injurious actions. The speech pathologist, may have the patient log phonotraumatic behaviors in an effort to provide insight into how often they are engaging in that behavior, and in what environments. This information is then used to help the patient determine alternative strategies to replace their higher risk behavior with a healthier vocal choice. For example, if the patient weight trains but notices that they hold their breath at the onset of each sit-up, the verbal and mental cue to maintain an open airway through active breathing may provide a vocally healthier substitution. It is important for the patient and the voice pathologist to address each of the identified phonotraumatic behaviors and to work methodically to reduce and eliminate them. Each incident of a phonotraumatic behavior, whether it is a throat clear or a holler, increases vibratory collision, friction, and compression of the vocal folds over the course of the day. If you consider the analogy of counting calories when on a diet, and you have a limited number of calories you can consume in one day, you avoid higher calorie foods. Frequent moments of throat clearing by the end of the day add up to a lot of excessive vocal calories. Every vocal calorie that can be cut out of a singer's daily vocal diet will add up to a lot of saved voice use over time, paving the way back toward vocal health and optimal voice functioning. Cutting vocal calories should not be confused with complete vocal rest; rather it should be viewed as budgeting vocal use, and eliminating both phonatory and nonphonatory, phonotraumatic behaviors.

Risk for Phonotrauma

Several research studies have investigated the incidence of voice disorders among CCM singers. Studies that completed imaging on singers without vocal complaints have demonstrated approximately a 35% presence of vocal fold pathology (Elias, Sataloff, Rosen, Heuer, & Spiegel, 1997; Lundy et al., 1999). These findings suggest that perhaps these lesions in asymptomatic singers may be considered a "normal baseline." If a vocal athlete has adequate and consistent vocal stamina, power, flexibility, and agility to perform at the level that their career demands, regardless of vocal fold status, they may be considered functionally normal. Baseline information on the status of the vocal folds when asymptomatic can provide useful information regarding what risk factors might be relevant for that singer. Donahue, LeBorgne, Brehm, and Weinrich (2013) screened 188 incoming music theater freshmen entering a competitive, intensive conservatory musical theater training program. These singers underwent a videostroboscopic screening. Only 18.6% were deemed to have a "normal" laryngeal examination. The most common finding was dehydration as evidenced by thick secretions on the vocal folds (51.1%). Interestingly, reflux was the second most prevalent finding (35.1%) followed by vocal fold erythema (Donahue et al., 2013).

Data looking at teachers and occupational voice users have reported estimates of voice disorders to be as high as 58% (DeJong et al., 2006; Roy et al., 2004; Smith, Lemke, Taylor, & Kirchner, 1998b). Furthermore, voice, drama, and PE teachers are thought to have even higher risk (Smith, Kirchner, Taylor, Hoffman, & Lemke, 1998a; Thibeault, Merrill, Roy, Gray, & Smith, 2004). Singers in preprofessional, collegiate training programs reported engaging in phonotraumatic behaviors. Continued engagement in phonotraumatic behaviors may place these singers at higher risk for sustaining vocal injury (Hoffman-Rudy et al., 2001). This is particularly relevant given that some singers present with asymptomatic, yet abnormal laryngeal findings. The research has not yet established if specific laryngeal abnormalities may predispose further injury in the vocal athlete. In light of these factors, an understanding of how to minimize and prevent vocal difficulties and/or injury is imperative for anyone who trains or treats vocal athletes.

Impact of Phonotraumatic Behaviors on Voice and Singing

The impact of repeated phonotraumatic behaviors on the vocal folds can be thought of as a spectrum beginning with mild irritation and/or swelling (edema) leading all the way up to frank laryngeal pathology. The resultant effect on the speaking and singing voice becomes dependent on the degree, nature, and duration of impact of these behaviors on the microstructure of the vocal folds and their vibratory function. Recall from Chapter 3 that the microstructure of the vocal folds can be thought of as layers. The outermost layer is covered by a very thin mucosal layer. It is the most gelatinous and pliable, made up primarily of elastin fibers that stretch and elongate. The inner layers are primarily collagen fibers that are sturdier and less resistant to elongation. Finally, the TA muscle composes the innermost layer of the vocal fold. A detailed description of every laryngeal pathology and direct impact on the vocal folds is beyond the scope of this book. In general terms, lesions on the vocal folds will increase the overall mass of the vocal fold impacting and impeding vibration. Lesions on the free, vibrating edge of the vocal fold, even if small, will often impact vocal fold closure. Pathologies that extend into the deeper layers of the vocal fold will have a greater impact on vocal fold vibration. Generally speaking, the more the vocal fold is "weighed down" by a larger lesion or stiffened by the lesion that goes deeper into the vocal fold, the greater the impact on vocal fold vibration and singing. Any disruption in the vibratory function of the vocal folds can negatively impact voice production and quality.

When Is Vocal Rest Indicated?

There are multiple scenarios in which a singer might consider altering, reducing, or eliminating typical voice use. These might include a general upper respiratory tract infection, or laryngitis, a decline in vocal quality after prolonged use, or hyperfunctional use or after vocal fold surgery. All singers will encounter at least one of the scenarios above (illness, fatigue after heavy vocal load) at some point in their life and potentially multiple times in their singing career. Common sense typically prevails and singers self-limit voice use based on effort and discomfort until they are feeling well again. Singers can risk laryngeal injury

when pushing through an illness and placing high demands on the voice when ill.

Many singers are often told by doctors to rest their voice when they are having voice difficulties. In fact, sometimes singers are told to go on complete voice rest when vocal problems arise. This advice may be provided by a general practitioner or general ear, nose, and throat physician who does not specialize in voice. Unfortunately, the reversibility principle, which is discussed in Chapter 15, informs us that a singer can very quickly detrain or become deconditioned with lack of use. This, however, does not mean that a singer who is having difficulties should proceed with normal voice use and singing. The challenge is to balance the appropriate amount of voice rest with some variation of a vocal fitness regimen depending on the situation. However, the guidelines are not clear. Who guides the singer through this process? When should a singer go on complete voice rest? Is it advisable to sing when ill? How much is too much? How much is not enough? These are the questions that singers and teachers face often without any real guidance as to what would constitute an appropriate recommendation. The following section will provide an overview on what voice pathology and otolaryngology literature supports regarding voice rest.

Voice Rest and Vocal Fold Surgery

In the case of vocal fold surgery to manage vocal fold lesions, otolaryngologists on average prescribe approximately 1 week of complete vocal rest. However, there are no standard data-driven protocols for how and when to reintroduce voice use post-operatively, and surgeon protocols vary widely. Behrman and Sulica (2003) surveyed 1,208 otolaryngologists in the United States on opinions about voice rest post-surgically. Surgeons were queried specifically about complete vocal rest versus modified voice rest. Additionally, they were asked how long they prescribed voice rest after surgical management of vocal fold nodules, polyps, and cysts. A little more than one-half reported that they recommended complete voice rest postoperatively (51.4%) versus 62.3% who reported they prescribed modified voice rest. Approximately 15% of the surgeons polled did not make any postoperative recommendations regarding voice rest. The range for prescribed voice rest or modified rest was 0 to 14 days for complete voice rest, and 0 to 24 days for modified voice rest, with one week being the average recommendation. There was no trend toward one type of voice rest versus the other based on a specific diagnosis (Behrman & Sulica, 2003).

There are a handful of studies that have investigated optimal voice use guidelines postoperatively to maximize recovery. But, reported findings are difficult to generalize because the nature and complexity of phonosurgical techniques varies depending on diagnosis and surgical skill.

Koufman and Blalock (1989) looked retrospectively at 127 phonosurgical cases (not specifically singers) and the length that hoarseness persisted after surgery. Incidence of postoperative dysphonia lasting greater than 4 weeks after surgery was 37%. The authors identified several factors that may have accounted for prolonged dysphonia postoperatively. These included hyperfunctional voice use and smoking. Analysis of variables contributing to prolonged dysphonia revealed that "vocal abuse" in the

postoperative phase was the strongest variable. The authors did not endorse use of complete voice rest because aberrant voice behaviors are then simply temporarily avoided rather than remediated (Koufman & Blalock, 1989). This speaks to the importance of consideration of voice therapy pre- and postoperatively.

Although not all general otolaryngologists refer patients for pre- and postoperative voice therapy, these findings certainly support the notion that there is benefit for both pre- and postoperative voice therapy with a voice pathologist to guide the compliant and motivated patient toward productive postoperative voice recovery. The goal of preoperative voice therapy is to identify and remediate any deviant vocal behaviors, strengthen and balance the laryngeal mechanism, and provide information to the surgeon regarding the "readiness" of the patient for a good postoperative outcome. Phonosurgeons want their singers to come out of surgery significantly better than when the singer went into surgery. Therefore, the importance of preoperative voice therapy and collaboration with the surgeon is vital for optimal surgical outcomes. Additionally, the voice teacher should be part of the voice care team for a given student and have open communication with both the voice pathologist and laryngologist regarding voice use guidelines during the postoperative period.

Ideally, there would be clear-cut and standardized practice guidelines for all otolaryngologists whether specialized as a laryngologist or a general ENT regarding indications for voice rest and voice therapy pre- and postoperatively. Unfortunately, this is not the case, and singers presenting with voice complaints could receive varying recommendations and opinions depending on the voice care team. The above section has identified that clear-cut guidelines for voice rest and voice therapy do not appear to be globally present despite the fact that research has shown that there is benefit from voice therapy. This further highlights the need for singers and teachers to identify and collaborate with voice specialists in their area.

Wound Healing Physiology

Conventional wisdom suggests that limiting voice use after a phonotraumatic event is warranted in order to decrease friction, agitation, and stress and to allow for healing. Although there are certainly scenarios in which complete voice rest is appropriate, research from other fields such as orthopedics has demonstrated that a certain degree of controlled tissue mobilization could actually play a role in facilitating wound healing and reducing tissue edema, or swelling (Verdolini Abbot et al., 2012). In order to better understand the physiology behind why this might be applicable to the laryngeal mechanism, a general understanding of wound healing is needed. Readers seeking in-depth discussions about laryngeal wound healing are referred to the resources listed at the end of the chapter (Clark, 1996; Titze & Verdolini Abbot, 2012).

In general terms, the process of wound healing occurs in three primary phases ideally resulting in regeneration of healthy tissue that is biomechanically functional. Phase I is the inflammatory phase where blood and inflammatory cells are increased at the site of injury. The goal of this phase in wound healing is cleaning up and maintaining viability of the wounded area. Additionally, there are substances called growth factors and inflammatory proteins that play an essential role in this stage of wound healing. Disruption of this process could potentially impact the integrity of how the tissue heals. The events during Phase I have important implications for voice use, specifically with regard to benign vocal fold lesions such as nodules. Although a certain amount of inflammatory response is initially beneficial, too much inflammation for prolonged periods of time can impede healing and adversely impact voice production (Titze & Verdolini Abbot, 2012).

Phase II occurs approximately 3 to 5 days after initial injury. This phase involves the generation of collagen and other agents responsible for the formation of scar tissue. Improper reorganization of tissue during this phase of wound healing may impact vocal fold vibration because of stiffness and tethering of tissue between the vocal fold layers. Ideally, this phase in wound healing would be minimized with little or no formation of nonfunctional scar tissue. Phase III begins around day 14 after initial injury and can last up to a year. It is during this phase that tissue remodeling occurs. Collagen fibers are frequently turned over, ultimately creating areas of reinforcement around areas of injury. Ideally, these areas of replaced scaffolding of collagen fibers would align themselves in an organized fashion that promotes optimal biomechanical function versus a disorganized and random orientation of replacement fibers, which could have a negative impact on overall function. To summarize the goals of this process for the voice patient, ideally, there would be minimal inflammation during Phase I, and remodeling of replacement tissue would be "encouraged" toward functional biomechanical behavior (Titze & Verdolini Abbot, 2012). Table 6–1 provides readers with an overview of the entire wound healing process and time line.

TABLE 6–1. Summary of Normal Wound-Healing Mechanisms

Stage of Wound Healing	Time Course (Approximate)	Principal Molecular and Cellular Events
Hemostasis/Coagulation	Immediately to 1 day post-injury	Formation of fibrin clot at site of injury.
Inflammation	Immediately to 3 days post-injury	Vasoconstriction and vasodilation at site of injury. Presence of neutrophilis followed by macrophages whose function is to phagocytose bacteria and dead tissue and secrete enzymes for tissue breakdown.
Mesenchymal Cell Migration and Proliferation	2 to 4 days post-injury	Fibroblasts migrate into wound site and become predominant cell type. Some fibroblasts phenotypically change into myofibroblasts for tissue repair.
Angiogenesis	2 to 4 days post-injury	Formation of fewler larger blood vessels at site of the injury.
Epithelization	Hours to 5 days post-injury	Epithelial cell migration to form epithelium and BMZ.
Protein and Proteoglycan Synthesis	3 to 5 days to 6 weeks post-injury	Formation of ECM through production of proteins, proteoglycans, glycoaminoglycans by fibroblasts
Wound contraction and Remodeling	3 days to 12 months post-injury	Myofibroblasts and collagen mediate contraction. Scar remodeling consists of turnover for ECM proteins, proteoglycans, and glycoaminoglycans. Apoptosis of myofibroblasts and epithelian cells.

Source: From *Voice Science.* Sataloff, R. Plural Publishing, 2005. Reprinted with permission.

Vocal Rest Versus Vocal Exercise

A comprehensive review of scientific literature on vocal rest versus vocal exercise was undertaken (Ishikawa & Thibeault, 2008). These authors not only looked at scientific data on postoperative voice rest, they looked closely at orthopedic literature and the impact of rest versus exercises in orthopedic rehabilitation, which has been shown to promote active recovery. Ultimately, they determined that tissue differences between vocal musculature and ligaments and orthopedic structures were too great to infer complete application of orthopedic rehabilitation guidelines to post operative voice therapy guidelines. However, the general consensus was that voice rest facilitates wound healing during the immediate postoperative period compared with unregulated phonation (such as spontaneous speech).

An additional study by Verdolini Abbot, Li, Branski, Rosen, Grillo, Steinhauer, and Hebda (2012) investigated the effect of tissue mobilization tasks using gentle resonant voice exercises during observed periods of vocal fold edema. The rationale for this study was based on orthopedic literature, which has demonstrated that there are anti-inflammatory mediators reliant on tissue mobilization as a triggering mechanism. The authors separated the nonsinger subjects into three groups. All subjects were put through 3 cycles of a 15-minute vocal loading task (loud reading) followed by 5 minutes of vocal rest totaling 1 hour. Subsequent to the hour of rest, one group engaged only in resonant voice exercises for which they were trained prior to the vocal loading tasks. A second group went on complete vocal rest only, and the last group engaged in spontaneous speech after the vocal loading tasks. Results from this study indicated that the subjects in the resonant voice group appeared to have the most reduced inflammation markers when retested. The vocal rest group showed the next most reduced inflammation markers. However, the group who returned to spontaneous speech after the vocal loading tasks had significantly worse post-vocal loading measurements. In fact, the subjects in the spontaneous group's postloading measurements were worse than their initial baseline measurements up to 24 hours after the vocal loading task. The authors were cautious to endorse use of vocal exercises after acute vocal injury; however, they did endorse the use of resonant voice exercises as possible favorable options over complete vocal rest to help facilitate reduction of vocal fold edema for some cases of phonotrauma. These preliminary findings are potentially useful suggesting that the conventional practice of complete vocal rest after injury could possibly have a reduced impact on the wound healing cascade. And, like other body tissues, gentle tissue mobilization (e.g., resonant voice exercises) has been shown to potentially aid in the release of anti-inflammatory mediators helping to facilitate the wound healing process.

Management of Phonotrauma

Earlier, phonotrauma was defined as a vocal behavior (either volitional or involuntary), impacting vocal fold vibration in a manner that compromises vocal fold integrity. These behaviors can lead to vocal difficulties or even pathology; therefore, the laryngologist and voice pathologist should be and are often involved in management. When determining a specific management plan, a variety of factors are considered. First, and foremost, laryngeal imaging (stroboscopic, high-speed, kymography) will provide important information as to the presence of laryngeal pathology and the impact that pathology has on the vibratory mechanics of the vocal folds.

Results of the laryngeal imaging along with information obtained through a detailed case history, aerodynamic, and acoustic analyses allows the voice care team to: (1) identify presence or absence of vocal fold lesions and pathology, (2) determine the impact of the injury on the functional vibration and glottic closure patterns, (3) define phonotraumatic behaviors that may be contributing to voice difficulties, (4) rule out other more serious laryngeal conditions, and (5) determine the individualized plan of care. The voice care team designs a plan of care specifically to meet the needs of each patient. A vocal remediation plan can include any combination of surgical, pharmacological, and/or behavioral interventions.

Behavioral Intervention

Behavioral intervention may be the first course of action for benign (noncancerous) vocal fold lesions. Behavior modifications may include: compliance with vocal health and hygiene recommendations, elimination of phonotraumatic behaviors, conservative voice use, and adequate oral hydration. The information obtained in the initial patient history is used to identify instances of phonotraumatic behavior and suboptimal voice use patterns that are likely contributing to the existing pathology and/or voice

complaint. Identification of these behaviors early on in therapy is important, as simple modifications of behaviors can often make a notable difference during voice rehabilitation. Many singers are aware that yelling, screaming, talking loudly, and grunting may cause impact trauma (swelling, redness, lesions) on the vocal folds. Identification of when and where these instances occur, and then providing alternative strategies, may focus a positive approach on elimination and modifications related to vocal loudness. Utilization of vocal pacing, similar to the "vocal diet" concept previously discussed, involves increased consciousness of voice use patterns during the day and drawing attention to areas where unnecessary voice use can be reduced or eliminated. Strict compliance with vocal hygiene issues is generally incorporated into the behavioral modifications including appropriate use of amplification and monitoring, maintaining adequate systemic hydration, ensuring adequate levels of environmental hydration (monitoring humidity levels in living environment and/or performing environment), and complying with reflux recommendations (see Chapter 7) as warranted. The voice teacher provides an essential ally in helping, educating, and reinforcing students' adherence to the voice behavior modification recommendations. Table 6–2 provides an overview of factors and behaviors contributing to vocal fold irritation.

Direct Voice Therapy

In addition to identifying and modifying phonotraumatic behaviors, a primary goal in voice therapy, in order for a singer to return from injury to full performance

TABLE 6–2. An Overview of the Factors and/or Behaviors That May Result in Vocal Fold Irritation, Inflammation, and/or Disease, Considered to Be Representative of Poor Vocal Health

Factors and Behaviors	Effect	Suggestion	Why
Exposure to irritants (smoking, excessive alcohol, chemical fumes)	Irritates the delicate mucous lining of the nasal passages, throat, and larynx.	Avoid these irritants. Do not use tobacco products.	Minimizes vocal fold irritation and inflammation. Reduces potential incidence of cancer, emphysema, and other illnesses
Chronic cough, throat clearing	Causes the vocal folds to adduct forcefully.	Avoid overclearing the throat and excessive cough if possible. Use humming to clear the throat or soft swallow.	Minimizes vocal fold irritation.
Excessive talking, excessive use of vocal loudness	Vocal fold irritation, inflammation, overadduction, excess subglottal vibratory amplitude, and medial forces.	Avoid forceful speaking; Use a soft voice or a comfortable effort level voice.	Decreases the strain on the vocal folds.
Excessive strain resulting from talking while lifting weights, moving furniture, engaging in certain sports or aerobic exercise.	Excess pressure builds up within the chest during these activities; talking will cause excess pressure on the vocal folds.	Avoid overexertion or heavy lifting especially accompanied with talking.	Reduces excess pressure on the vocal folds.

Excessive caffeine	Caffeine has a dehydrating effect on the vocal folds.	Drink water or natural juice.	Reduces the drying effect on vocal fold mucosa and subsequent alterations to vocal quality.
Vocal fatigue	Overstraining may occur to compensate for vocal fatigue.	Take "vocal naps" during the day.	Allows time to rest the voice, optimizing vocal function.
Eating rich spicy foods, chocolate, carbonated beverages, etc.	May reduce pressure in the esophageal sphincter allowing stomach acid to flow up into the esophagus*	Avoid spicy food, especially near bed time.	Reduces reflux which is more active during sleep.
Singing without warming up	Minimizes vocal fold flexibility, reduces respiratory muscle activity, minimizes tongue and jaw flexibility and movement	Two octave pitch glides on /i/ or /u/ lip trill tongue trill Humming forward tongue roll *messa di voce***	Increases blood flow to the vocal fold structure, activates intrinsic laryngeal muscle activity to encourage vocal flexibility, loosens tongue and jaw

*Not everyone who eats spicy food will suffer from heartburn or reflux. Heartburn is a common condition and affects over 40% of all Americans at least once a month. Kaltenbach, Crockett, and Gerson (2006) provide a review of the impact of lifestyle measures and the effects in patients with gastroesophageal reflux disease.

**These exercises were suggested by Dr. Ingo Titze, and further information can be found on the National Center for Voice and Speech website, http://www.ncvs.org/ncvs/info/singers/warmup.html.

Source: Reprinted from *Voice Disorders*, by Sapienza and Hoffman Ruddy, 2013. Plural Publishing. Used with permission.

function, is to identify, modify, and replace aberrant voice production patterns with efficient, effective alternatives. Targeted vocal goals are established by the speech pathologist and are typically focused on recoordination, strengthening, and balancing of the respiratory, phonatory, and resonating subsystems used for voice production. A multitude of therapeutic tools and approaches can be used to achieve the desired vocal goals. Voice pathologists use a variety of initial therapeutic probes in order to determine the most effective approach to achieve the long-term goal of healthy, efficient voice use for daily needs. The voice pathologist specializing in the singer's voice may also incorporate specific goals and exercises related to the singing voice. If the patient has an established voice teacher, it is helpful for the voice pathologist and voice teacher to be in close communication regarding treatment goals. Many voice pathologists encourage and welcome voice teachers to attend therapy sessions of their students, as the teacher's insights can often be valuable during the therapy process, especially if modified voice lessons are concurrent with voice therapy.

Medical and Surgical Management

Based on professional medical opinion, a laryngologist may use pharmacological measures to inhibit or reduce inflammation of the vocal folds (i.e., oral steroids) and/or use antibiotics to treat an acute infection. There are a multitude of examples where an elite singer requires immediate pharmacological intervention in order to restore a certain level of voice function to fulfill contractual obligations and maintain the singer's livelihood. However, improper use and/or overuse of steroids can have adverse long-term effects, in addition to giving the singer a false sense of vocal wellness. All pharmacologic decisions should be made judiciously and only under the guidance of a laryngologist with expertise in working with singers.

Generally speaking, singers (or most surgeons) want to avoid vocal fold surgery if it is possible. But, there are instances where phonosurgery may be warranted to allow for continued vocal performance. Decisions regarding surgical and/or medical management are determined by the laryngologist, with input from the patient and voice care team, and can occur as either the primary intervention, or in conjunction with voice therapy depending on the nature of the diagnosis. Detailed description of the vocal pathologies and surgical intervention techniques are beyond the scope of this chapter. However, the postoperative recovery is typically related to the extent of the surgical intervention and the wound healing response of a given patient. For example, superficial lesions (that affect the epithelium) will often have a different postoperative healing window as compared to a lesion that involves the deeper layers of the vocal folds (intermediate and deep layers). Laryngologists who work with singers should be willing to have a thorough discussion, including anticipated outcome, rehabilitation time frame, and associated risks of medical or surgical interventions. Singers are always cautioned to ensure that the otolaryngologist from whom they are seeking medical advice or surgical consultation routinely treats singers. If the singer does not feel that he or she has been provided with detailed information regarding treatment options, it is not unreasonable to seek a second opinion. Additionally, it is helpful for singers and voice teachers to know who the laryngologist(s) and voice pathologist(s) are in their geographic area, understanding that some travel may be necessary for those in more remote areas to ensure they are getting the best voice care available.

Chapter Summary

Singers of all styles are at increased risk for sustaining vocal difficulties or even injury at some point during their singing careers. This chapter has defined phonotrauma, including possible contributing factors. Current research on vocal rest and wound healing were also discussed,, including indications and implications for both rest and controlled vocal exercise to facilitate optimal wound healing. Information on management of the results of phonotrauma including behavioral, therapeutic, medical, and surgical options was discussed. The roles of individuals on the voice care team were briefly identified here and are further discussed in Chapter 11. Ultimately, the process of identification of phonotraumatic elements and remediation from injury back to performance is multifactorial and requires input from multiple members of the voice care team.

References

Behrman, A., & Sulica, L. (2003). Voice rest after microlaryngoscopy: Current opinion and practice. *Laryngoscope, 12*(2), 2182–2186.

Clark, R. (1996). *Wound repair: An overview and general considerations*. New York, NY: Plenum Press.

DeJong, F., Kooijman, P., Thoman, G., Huinck, W., Graamans, K., & Schutte, H. (2006). Epidemiology of voice problems in Dutch teachers. *Folia Phoniatrica et Logopedica, 58*(3), 186–198.

Donahue, E., LeBorgne, W., Brehm, S., & Weinrich, B. (2013). *Prevelence of vocal pathology in incoming freshman musical theater majors: A 10-year retrospective study*. Paper presented at the Fall Voice Conference, New York City, NY.

Elias, M., Sataloff, R., Rosen, C., Heuer, R., & Spiegel, R. (1997). Normal strobovideolaryngoscopy: Variability in healthy singers. *Journal of Voice, 11*(1).

Hoffman-Ruddy, B., Lehman, J., Crandell, C., Ingram, D., & Sapienza, C. (2001). Laryngostroboscopic, acoustic, and environmental characteristics of high-risk vocal performers. *Journal of Voice, 15*(4), 543–552.

Ishikawa, K., & Thibeault, S. (2008). Voice rest versus exercise: A review of the literature. *Journal of Voice, 24*, 379–387.

Korovin, G., & LeBorgne, W. (2009). *A longitudinal examination of potential vocal injury in music theater performers*. Paper presented at the The Voice Foundation 36th Annual Voice Symposium: Care of the Professional Voice, Philadelphia, PA.

Koufman, J., & Blalock, P. (1989). Is voice rest never indicated? *Journal of Voice, 3*, 87–91.

Lundy, D., Casiano, R., Sullivan, R., Roy, S., Xue, J., & Evans, J. (1999). Incidence of abnormal laryngeal findings in asymptomatic singing students. *Otolaryngology-Head and Neck Surgery, 121*, 69–77.

Roy, N., Merrill, R., Thibeault, S., Parsa, R., Gray, S., & Smith, E. (2004). Prevelence of voice disorders in teachers and the general population. *Journal of Speech, Language, and Hearing Research, 47*, 281–293.

Smith, E., Kirchner, H., Taylor, M., Hoffman, H., & Lemke, J. (1998a). Voice problems among teachers: Differences by gender and teaching characteristics. *Journal of Voice, 12*(4), 328–334.

Smith, E., Lemke, J., Taylor, M., & Kirchner, H. (1998b). Frequency of voice problems among teachers and other occupations. *Journal of Voice, 12*(4), 480–488.

Thibeault, S., Merrill, R., Roy, N., Gray, S., & Smith, E. (2004). Occupational risk factors associated with voice disorders among teachers. *Annals of Otology, Rhinology, and Laryngology, 14*(10), 786–792.

Titze, I., & Verdolini Abbot, K. (2012). *Vocology: The science and practice of voice habilitation*. Salt Lake City, UT: The National Center for Voice and Speech.

Verdolini Abbot, K., Li, N., Branski, R., Rosen, C., Grillo, E., Steinhauer, K., & Hebda, P. (2012). Vocal exercises may attenuate acute vocal fold inflammation. *Journal of Voice, 26*(6), 814e811–814e813.

7

Laryngopharyngeal Reflux: What the Singer Needs to Know

ADAM D. RUBIN and MARIA CRISTINA JACKSON-MENALDI

Introduction

Reflux refers to the reverse or backward flow of contents from the stomach into the esophagus. The stomach secretes acid and enzymes to help aid in digestion of food. When food is ingested, it passes from the mouth through the throat and esophagus into the stomach. Acid secretion starts even when one thinks about food. When the acid and enzymes from the stomach move backward into the esophagus and throat, they can cause damage to the lining of these structures, inflammation, and irritation of nerve endings. This can result in a number of symptoms and complications.

The health of a singer's vocal folds is of paramount importance to his or her livelihood and happiness. Reflux is just one of many potentially negative agents that can compromise the health of the vocal apparatus. Even a singer who has never had any symptoms from reflux has to be aware of potential triggers. One badly timed reflux episode before a performance or audition can have a significant negative effect on voice quality. Chronic reflux exposure can lead to more serious vocal and health problems. The singer has no "case" in which to put his or her instrument for protection when not in use. He or she must practice good vocal hygiene at all times to keep the voice in top shape. Being aware of how to prevent and treat reflux is an important aspect of maintaining good vocal health.

Symptoms

A number of terms have been applied for acid reflux. The term "gastroesophageal

123

reflux" or "GERD" typically applies to the effect of reflux on the lining of the esophagus leading to symptoms such as heartburn The term "laryngopharyngeal reflux" or "LPR" refers to reflux into the upper aerodigestive tract potentially affecting the throat, larynx (including the vocal folds), lungs, and sinuses. Reflux is currently thought to be at least partially responsible for maladies traditionally felt to be attributed to other inflammatory mechanisms, such as allergies. Additional problems may include sinusitis, post-nasal drip, middle ear infections, and chronic sore throats. LPR has been described as a common cause of chronic hoarseness. Although reflux certainly can contribute to voice problems, the singer should never assume persistent hoarseness is solely due to reflux unless the vocal folds have been visualized with videostroboscopy, and other causes, such as vocal fold masses, have been ruled out by a laryngologist. Symptoms of classic GERD include heartburn, regurgitation of food, and acid brash. Swallowing may be affected as well. Symptoms that may be attributable to LPR include: hoarseness, cough (Lieder & Wilson, 2012), sinonasal problems, (Loehrl et al., 2012; Lupa & DelGaudio, 2012), breathing problems (Banaszkiewicz et al., 2013; Blumin & Johnston, 2011), eustachian tube dysfunction (feeling of ears needing to be "popped," or pressure in the ears; White, Heavner, Hardy, & Prazma, 2002), globus pharyngeus (Kirch, Gegg, Johns, & Rubin, 2013), and laryngospasm (Obholzer, Nouraei, Ahmed, Kadhim, & Sandhu, 2008). Such symptoms are often referred to as "atypical reflux symptoms" or "extraesophageal symptoms." It is important to note, many of these symptoms are not specific to reflux alone, but rather for chronic inflammation or irritation. Reflux is a potential cause of such inflammation, but other factors can contribute as well, such as allergies, vocal overuse or abuse,

smoking, medications, and neuralgia (nerve irritation).

Two symptoms that are most often attributable to reflux are laryngospasm and globus pharyngeus. Laryngospasm is a spontaneous closure of the vocal folds resulting in an inability to inspire (breathe in). The vocal folds close not only to produce voice, but also to protect the lungs from food or noxious substances entering. This protective closure is called the "adductor reflex" (Sun, Chum, Bautista, Pilowsky, & Berkowitz, 2011). One can think of spontaneous laryngospasm as an abnormal reflex or the reflex occurring at an inappropriate time. Spontaneous laryngospasm due to reflux typically will break (the airway will open back up), but sometimes it can lead to significant anxiety creating the sensation of breathing difficulties even after the episode. Although reflux is the most common cause, spontaneous laryngospasm can also be seen in neurologic disorders (Fourcade, Castelnovo, Renard, & Labauge, 2010; Sun et al., 2011).

Globus pharyngeus is the sensation of a lump or mucus in the throat. The most common cause of globus pharyngeus is reflux. This symptom can be particularly troublesome for the singer or professional voice user who is particularly sensitive to abnormal sensations in the throat. When a lump is felt, it often makes it difficult to initiate a swallow. When the sensation of mucus exists, it leads to strong urges to clear the throat, which is a potentially traumatic behavior for the vocal folds. Interestingly, many people often feel the need to clear the throat to "get their voice going." They feel mucus clinging to the vocal folds that is inhibiting vibration. This is sometimes observed during visualization of the larynx in the office setting while the patient sings or speaks. However, in the majority of cases, there is no visible mucus on the vocal folds. This suggests that the symptom is due to irritated nerves sending erroneous signals back to the brain, essentially "fooling" the brain to think there is mucus when in fact there is not.

Complications of Reflux

Esophageal complications of reflux include strictures (scarring causing narrowing, which can increase resistance for food to pass), Barrett's esophagus, and esophageal cancer. Barrett's esophagus refers to precancerous changes to the esophageal lining. If left untreated, Barrett's esophagus can progress to dysplasia, and eventually to adenocarcinoma (cancer) of the esophagus. It is important to recognize that esophageal symptoms, such as heartburn, are not required to develop esophageal findings, even cancer (Falcone, Garrett, Slaughter, & Vaezi, 2009; Reavis, Morris, Gopal, Hunter, & Jobe, 2004). In fact, studies have suggested that atypical reflux symptoms, such as cough, may be more common in patients with Barrett's esophagus and esophageal cancer. Adenocarcinoma of the esophagus has increased more rapidly than any other cancer in the United States over the last 30 years (Peery et al., 2012). Although singers are most concerned about the effects of reflux on their voices, the potential disastrous complications of reflux need to always be kept in mind.

Laryngeal complications of reflux are related to the inflammatory effects of the reflux contents on the vocal fold mucosa. The larynx lacks many of the inherent protective mechanisms against injury from acid that exists in the esophagus. Therefore, even small exposures may lead to symptoms (Remacle & Lawson, 2006). Some argue that it is not necessarily the acid that is the damaging agent. Pepsin, a digestive enzyme secreted by the lining of the stomach may be the culprit. Pepsin requires an acidic environment to be activated. Traditionally, it has been thought to be activated at a pH of 4. However, more recent studies of higher pH environments, even a neutral pH of 7, might still be sufficient for pepsin to cause damage (Ali, Parikh, Chater, & Pearson, 2013; Johnston, Wells, Samuels, & Blumin, 2010). Pepsin has even been suggested to potentially be a causative factor in laryngeal and throat cancer (Johnston et al., 2012).

Laryngeal complications of reflux exposure include inflammation of the vocal folds, causing hoarseness (chronic laryngitis), granulomas, dysplasia, and even laryngeal cancer (Doustmohammadian, Naderpour, Khoshbaten, & Doustmohammadian, 2011; Francis et al., 2011; Koufman, 1991). Inflammation of the vocal folds will impair vibration of the vocal folds and may contribute to some raspiness of the voice. The passagio is particularly sensitive to even slight impairment of vibration. A break in the passagio, particularly when singing softly signifies an impairment of vibration, which may be from inflammation related to reflux. In addition, vocal fold swelling increases the mass of the vocal fold, and therefore can result in lowering of the pitch and more difficulty reaching the upper register. Additional vocal strain because of underlying inflammation may ultimately lead to the development of traumatic vocal fold lesions, such as nodules, polyps, and scars. Patients who may have had no extraesophageal symptoms of reflux could develop lesions after causing injury to the vocal folds from vocal trauma.

One lesion often linked to reflux is a granuloma. Granulomas are growths of inflammatory tissue, which result from a response to injury. They can occur from trauma from an endotracheal tube after intubation, but when they occur spontaneously, they are thought to result from vocal trauma and reflux. Spontaneous granulomas will usually respond to aggressive reflux management, often in conjunction with voice therapy.

Dysplasia (precancerous changes) and laryngeal cancer may result from chronic reflux exposure as well. Dysplasia will usually present with white plaques (leukoplakia) on the vocal folds. These plaques can often lead to voice changes themselves if they extend onto the medial (contact) edge of the vocal fold. In the absence of smoking and human papilloma virus, leukoplakia of the vocal folds is likely attributable to reflux.

How Do I Know if I Have Reflux?

Because of the lack of specificity of many of the symptoms of laryngopharyngeal reflux, often an empiric trial of reflux medication is necessary to confirm the diagnosis. Another possible indicator of reflux is the Reflux Symptom Index (RSI). The RSI is a questionnaire that was developed to see if a patient was likely to have laryngopharyngeal reflux. It is suggested that a score <13 is normal (Belafsky, Postma, & Koufman, 2002). Its use is controversial and should not preclude or confirm the diagnosis using the RSI alone. It may be useful for following treatment effectiveness as well as in conjunction with laryngeal imaging. Other tests are available that may be useful in the diagnosis of LPR include:

Laryngeal Imaging

There are a number of ways to visualize the larynx including a laryngeal mirror examination, flexible laryngoscopy, and videostroboscopy. The singer should always try to have a videostroboscopy examination, particularly if hoarseness is a symptom. In addition to looking for signs of reflux, it is important to rule out other causes of hoarseness, such as masses and scar. Significant edema (swelling) of the vocal folds or the tissue in the posterior (back) aspect of the larynx are highly suggestive of reflux, particularly in the absence of other obvious causes, such as smoking. The "Reflux Finding Score" (Belafsky et al., 2002) is used by some otolaryngologists to try to grade the severity of the changes to the larynx. Although a noble attempt to quantify the visualized changes, its use is controversial and not required to make the diagnosis.

pH Probe Testing

pH probe testing measures the amount of acid reflux episodes during a 24- to 48-hour period. Traditional pH probe testing is done with a thin catheter placed through the nose that goes down the esophagus. Ideally, the probe has two sensors, one in the upper esophagus, near the larynx, and the other in the lower esophagus (near the stomach). The two sensors provide information of the amount of acid in both locations. It has long been considered the "gold standard" for reflux. There are several drawbacks including patient sensitivity to the probe and if the patient does not reflux within that 24- to 48-hour period, they are assumed to not have reflux. Yet, many patients who have LPR may only reflux occasionally.

The Bravo probe is an implantable pH monitor placed in the lower esophagus via an esophagogastroduodenscopy. It is more comfortable for the patient than the traditional pH probe; however, it only measures acid near the stomach. Therefore, it does not provide information about the amount of acid reaching the throat.

A new probe, by Restech sits in the throat above the larynx. It offers the advantage of being more comfortable than the traditional probe, while providing information to evaluate for LPR (Sun et al., 2009).

Impedance Testing

Impedance testing is also done with a probe passed through the nose down to the stomach. Impedance, unlike traditional pH probe testing, will show any material refluxed from the stomach, whether it is a liquid or gas, acidic, or basic. Sometimes impedance testing will be done while a patient is on reflux medications in conjunction with traditional testing to confirm if the medicine is controlling acidity, while also testing to see if reflux is present. Impedance testing might be useful in patients who fail aggressive PPI management to determine if they have nonacid reflux (Caroll, Fedore, & Aldahlawi, 2012). Studies have suggested that even one episode of LPR might be considered abnormal (Hoppo et al., 2012).

Esophagoscopy

Esophagoscopy is a test performed to evaluate the lining of the esophagus. Although an abnormal esophagoscopy with evidence of esophagitis or Barrett's esophagus supports the diagnosis of reflux, a normal esophagoscopy does not mean the patient does not have reflux. It only means the patient has not had any esophageal complications from reflux. Indications for esophagoscopy are controversial. Traditional esophagogastroduodenoscopy (EGD) requires sedation which creates risk of cardiovascular complications. It is significantly more costly as it requires the need of additional personnel

(e.g., nurses, anesthetist, recovery room). In-office, transnasal esophagoscopy (TNE) can be performed in the office setting in the unsedated patient. This is typically performed by an otolaryngologist. This involves less risk and expense than the traditional EGD. Given the high incidence of esophageal findings in patients presenting with atypical reflux symptoms and the recognition that esophageal cancer can develop in patients with only extraesophageal symptoms (Peery et al., 2012; Reavis et al., 2004), the use of TNE as a screening tool for Barrett's esophagus is gaining ground.

Modified Barium Swallow (MBS)

A modified barium swallow is an x-ray that follows the course of barium swallowed by the patient through the upper gastrointestinal tract. It is used by some to test for acid reflux, but a negative study does not mean the patient does not have LPR as it simply captures a moment in time. MBS can help identify esophageal motility disorders and can screen for strictures resulting from reflux.

In the authors' opinion, although esophagoscopy and laryngeal imaging are important in the evaluation of reflux, particularly to evaluate for complications of reflux, other objective testing is less frequently warranted. This is mainly due to the fact that criteria for a positive pH or impedance testing remains controversial. Unless the patient has absolutely no reflux episodes (which is quite rare) or a large number of reflux episodes, it is difficult to say if the study is truly positive or negative. Furthermore, even if a study is "positive," it does not necessarily mean that reflux is causing the symptoms with which the patient presented. The authors favor an empiric trial of high-dose reflux medications for at least 3 months to determine if symptoms are indeed caused by reflux. Other authors have supported a similar approach (Abou-Ismail & Vaezi, 2011).

Treatment

Treatment options for reflux include lifestyle and dietary behavioral modifications, medicine, and surgical intervention. Lifestyle and behavioral modification are a vital component of reflux prevention. Onstage singers may be at risk for reflux episodes because of rapid changes of subglottal and intra-abdominal changes resulting from techniques of breath support (Cammarota, Elia, Cianci, Galli, Paolillo, Montalto, & Gasbarrini, 2003). Nervousness and stress can also promote acid reflux. Offstage, the lifestyle of a singer or performer often lends itself to poor vocal hygiene habits such as late night eating and drinking, and poor dietary choices. As reflux prevention is just one element of vocal health, the performer's desire to enjoy other aspects of life, such as socializing after a show, having a few alcoholic beverages, and/or talking to fans, has to be balanced with the potential of causing damage to the vocal folds. One must recognize his or her own body's sensitivity and vulnerability and respect it. It is important for both the day-to-day health of the vocal folds, and for avoiding more serious health sequelae down the road.

What, When, and How?

It may take a while to adjust your diet and lifestyle, but you can change when and how you eat. A healthy diet can play a big role in reflux prevention and vocal health. Below is a nonexhaustive list of dietary and lifestyle recommendations that could help prevent reflux and promote vocal health.

1. Avoid spicy and acidic foods. This includes foods with tomato-based sauces, raw onions and garlic, fried and fatty foods, chocolate, peppermint, spearmint, citrus fruits, and fruit juices (particularly from fruits with many seeds). These foods have higher acidity content.
2. Strive for a high-protein, low-fat diet.
3. All meats should be lean and trimmed of visible fat. Meats may be boiled, broiled, roasted, or baked. Use a rack so that fat can drain.
4. Avoid fried foods, fatty foods may require more digestive acids to break down.
5. Try to prepare stews, soups, and mixed dishes ahead of time, so they may be chilled and skimmed of fat.
6. Limit your intake of coffee, tea, alcohol, and colas. All these drinks are quite acidic. Caffeine will increase acid production from your stomach. If you want coffee or tea, try to limit yourself to one a day. Wash it down with a glass of water to help "rinse" pharyngeal and esophageal tissues.
7. Eat slowly, and do not gorge yourself at mealtime. Small frequently timed meals are better than several large meals.
8. Avoid eating right before singing. Try to eat at least 3 hours prior to rehearsal or performance.
9. Watch your weight.
10. Wait at least 2 hours after eating prior to exercise.
11. Eat your evening meal or snack at least 3 hours before bedtime or lying down. Avoid bedtime snacks.
12. Do not smoke and avoid smoke-filled environments.
13. Elevate the head of your bed six to eight inches. Avoid too many pillows that

will make you bend at the waist and increase pressure on your stomach.

14. Limit the use of aspirin and ibuprofen.
15. Hydration is very important. Drink lots of water.
16. Throat clearing may result from irritation from reflux. Try to resist this behavior as it can cause damage to the vocal folds. Instead of clearing, tuck your chin and swallow, or take a sip of water. If necessary log the number of times you catch yourself clearing your throat in order to increase awareness and reduced the behavior.

Medication

Although dietary and behavioral modifications are critical, medicine is often necessary to treat and prevent reflux symptoms (Behlau & Oliveira, 2009; Toohill & Kuhn, 1997).When reflux symptoms are present, the singer should be evaluated by a physician (gastroenterologist). If extraesophageal symptoms are present, the singer should see an otolaryngologist. Although the range of medication possibilities is beyond the scope of this chapter, there are several classes of drugs used to treat reflux: antacids; histamine blockers (H-2); and proton pump inhibitors. Combination drugs that include both an H-2 blocker and proton pump inhibitor are also now on the market. Chapter 10 provides a table (Table 10–1) that details available reflux medications and potential side effects. Below, the reader finds a discussion of the indications and use of proton pump inhibitors (PPIs).

Proton Pump Inhibitors (PPI)

Because the larynx does not have the same protective mechanisms as the esophagus, aggressive reflux management is often necessary to ameliorate the symptoms of LPR.

Although studies are controversial, the consensus is treatment with twice a day PPI (Kahrilas, Shaheen, & Vaezi, 2008; Park, Hicks, & Khandwala, 2005). PPIs act to prevent the activation of acid pumps in the wall of the stomach and have been shown to be effective (Chiba et al., 2011). The majority of these medications need to be taken 30 minutes to 1 hour before breakfast and dinner for maximal effect. Failure to respond to this medication may be due to incorrect diagnosis, poor compliance (e.g., not taking medication appropriately timed with meals, poor diet, and behavioral habits), resistance to the medication, or symptoms due to nonacidic reflux. In the authors' opinion, failure to respond to medication and behavioral modifications in a compliant patient should prompt the physician to strongly consider other reasons for the symptoms.

A still unanswered question is how long to treat with PPI therapy. Most otolaryngologists do not consider empiric trial of medication a failure until the patient has been treated at least 3 months. If symptoms are resolved, attempts may be made to wean the patient off medication or at least to a lower dose. Consideration should be made to evaluate the esophagus to screen for Barrett's esophagus. Long-term high-dose PPI use has been shown to have some potential negative sequelae including decreased calcium absorption and increased risk of hip fracture. Therefore, efforts should be made to wean down to the lowest dose possible.

Targeting pepsin has recently been suggested given that pepsin may be one of the factors causing symptoms and tissue damage (Koufman & Johnston, 2012). Some suggest that voice therapy is a useful adjunct to antireflux therapy in helping patients with hoarseness related to reflux (Park et al., 2012). In our opinion, reflux is often not the sole cause for voice problems.

Even in the absence of any structural problems, often some element of vocal misuse or abuse is present contributing to the patient's symptoms, particularly if hoarseness is the main symptom.

Surgery

A number of surgical approaches are used to treat reflux. The majority of the procedures used currently are focused on tightening the lower esophageal sphincter, which acts as a barrier to keep stomach contacts from refluxing into the esophagus. Although other procedures have been described (Ganz et al.; Trad, Turgeon, & Deljkich, 2012), Nissen fundoplication is still the most commonly performed procedure for reflux. It is most effective in patients who respond to PPI management, and has been shown in some studies to be effective for extraesophageal symptoms (Iqbal, Batch, Moorthy, Cooper, & Spychal, 2009; Van der Westhuizen et al., 2011).

One could imagine that if nonacidic reflux is the etiology of symptoms, or if pepsin is the major offending agent (Wassenaar et al., 2011), that a Nissen could be useful in patients who do not respond to therapy. Studies have been conflicting concerning when a Nissen fundoplication is appropriate in nonresponsive patients (Koch et al., 2012). However, if surgery is considered in a nonresponder to PPIs, all other potential etiologies should be ruled out. Empiric treatment for other etiologies should be tried (e.g., gabapentin for neuralgia, allergy management, etc.) prior to surgery. Impedance testing should also be obtained first to confirm the presence of reflux. One should be aware of the potential complications or ramifications of the surgery as well, particularly inability or difficulty to belch or regurgitate, as well as swallowing difficulties.

Chapter Summary

Prevention of voice disorders for singers requires good vocal hygiene, which includes attention to preventing reflux. Maintaining a healthy environment for the vocal folds is critical. Prevention and treatment of reflux is a major component vocal health. Although reflux can contribute to voice disorders, one should never assume that reflux is the sole cause of persistent hoarseness. This chapter provides information for the singer on common evaluation and treatment options for reflux.

References

Abou-Ismail, A., & Vaezi, M. F. (2011). Evaluation of patients with suspected laryngopharyngeal reflux: A practical approach. *Current Gastroenterology Report, 13*(3), 213–218.

Ali, M. S., Parikh, S., Chater, P., & Pearson, J. P. (2013). Bile acids in laryngopharyngeal refluxate: Will they enhance or attenuate the action of pepsin? *Laryngoscope, 123*(2), 434–439.

Banaszkiewicz, A., Dembinski, L., Zawadzka-Krajewska, A., Dziekiewicz, M., Albrecht, P., Kulus, M., & Radzikowski, A. (2013). Evaluation of laryngopharyngeal reflux in pediatric patients with asthma using a new technique of pharyngeal pH-monitoring. *Advances in Experimental Medicine and Biology, 755*, 89–95.

Behlau, M., & Oliveira, G. (2009). Vocal hygiene for the voice professional. *Current Opinion in Otolaryngology & Head and Neck Surgery, 17*(3), 149–154.

Belafsky, P. C., Postma, G. N., & Koufman, J. A. (2002). Validity and reliability of the Reflux Symptom Index (RSI). *Journal of Voice, 16*(2), 274-277.

Blumin, J. H., & Johnston, N. (2011). Evidence of extraesophageal reflux in idiopathic subglottic stenosis. *Laryngoscope, 121*(6), 1266-1273.

Cammarota, G., Elia, F., Cianci, R., Galli, J., Paolillo, N., Montalto, M., & Gasbarrini, G. (2003). Worsening of gastroesophageal reflux symptoms in professional singers during performances. *Journal of Clinical Gastroenterology, 36*(5), 403-404.

Caroll, T., Fedore, L., & Aldahlawi, M. (2012). pH impedance and high-resolution manometry in laryngopharyngeal reflux disease high-dose proton pump inhibitor failures. *Laryngoscope, 122*(11), 2437-2481.

Chiba, T., Kudara, N., Abiko, Y., Endo, M., Suzuki, K., Sugai, T., . . . Sato, H. (2011). Effects of PPI in patients with laryngopharyngeal reflux disease. *Hepato-Gastroenterology, 58*(110-111), 1580-1582.

Doustmohammadian, N., Naderpour, M., Khoshbaten, M., & Doustmohammadian, A. (2011). Is there any association between esophogastric endoscopic findings and laryngeal cancer. *American Journal of Otolaryngology, 32*(6), 490-493.

Falcone, M. T., Garrett, C. G., Slaughter, J. C., & Vaezi, M. (2009). Transnasal esophagoscopy findings: Interspecialty comparison. *Otolaryngology-Head & Neck Surgery, 140*(6), 812-815.

Fourcade, G., Castelnovo, G., Renard, D., & Labauge, P. (2010). Laryngospasm as preceding symptom of amyotrophic lateral sclerosis. *Journal of Neurology, 257*(11), 1929-1930.

Francis, D. O., Maynard, C., Weymuller, E. A., Reiber, G., Merati, A. L., & Yueh, B. (2011). Reevaluation of gastroesophageal reflux disease as a risk factor for laryngeal cancer. *Laryngoscope, 121*(1), 102-105.

Ganz, R., Peters, J., Horgan, S., Bemelman, W., Dunst, C., Edmundowicz, S., . . . Taiganides, P. Esophageal sphincter device for gastroesophageal reflux disease. *New England Journal of Medicine, 368*(8), 719-727.

Hoppo, T., Sanz, A., Nason, K., Carroll, T., Rosen, C., Normolle, D., . . . Jobe, B. (2012). How much pharyngeal exposure is "normal"? Normative data for laryngopharyngeal reflux events using hypopharyngeal multichannel intraluminal impedance (HMII). *Journal of Gastrointestinal Surgery, 16*(1), 16-24.

Iqbal, M., Batch, A. J., Moorthy, K., Cooper, B. T., & Spychal, R. T. (2009). Outcome of surgical fundoplication for extra-oesophageal symptoms of reflux. *Surgery Endoscopy, 23*(3), 557-561.

Johnston, N., Wells, C. W., Samuels, T. L., & Blumin, J. H. (2010). Rationale for targeting pepsin in the treatment of reflux disease. *Annals of Otology, Rhinology & Laryngology, 119*(8), 547-558.

Johnston, N., Yan, J. C., Hoekzema, C. R., Samuels, T. L., Stoner, G. D., Blumin, J. H., & Bock, J. M. (2012). Pepsin promotes proliferation of laryngeal and pharyngeal epithelial cells. *Laryngoscope, 122*(6), 1317-1325.

Kahrilas, P. J., Shaheen, N. J., & Vaezi, M. F. (2008). American Gastroenterological Association Institute technical review on the management of gastroesophageal reflux disease. *Gastroenterology, 135*(4), 1392-1413,

Kirch, S., Gegg, R., Johns, M., & Rubin, A. (2013). Globus pharyngeus: Effectiveness of treatment with proton pump inhibitors and gabapentin. *Annals of Otology, Rhinology, and Laryngology, 122*(8), 492-495.

Koch, O. O., Antoniou, S. A., Kaindlstorfer, A., Asche, K. U., Granderath, F. A., & Pointner, R. (2012). Effectiveness of laparoscopic total and partial fundoplication on extraesophageal manifestations of gastroesophageal reflux disease: A randomized study. *Surgery Laparoscopy Endoscopy Percutan Techniques, 22*(5), 387-391.

Koufman, J. A. (1991). The otolaryngologic manifestations of gastroesophageal reflux disease (GERD): A clinical investigation of 225 patients using ambulatory 24-hour pH monitoring and an experimental investigation of the role of acid and pepsin in the development of laryngeal injury. *Laryngoscope, 101*(4 Pt. 2, Suppl. 53), 1-78.

Koufman, J., & Johnston, N. (2012). Potential benefits of pH 8.8 alkaline drinking water as an adjunct in the treatment of reflux disease. *Annals of Otology, Rhinology & Laryngology, 121*(7), 431-434.

Lieder, A., & Wilson, J. (2012). An evidence-based review of the assessment and management of penetrating neck trauma. *Clinical Otolaryngology, 37*(3), 1749.

Loehrl, T. A., Samuels, T. L., Poetker, D. M., Toohill, R. J., Blumin, J. H., & Johnston, N. (2012). The role of extraesophageal reflux in medically and surgically refractory rhinosinusitis. *Laryngoscope, 122*(7), 1425-1430.

Lupa, M., & DelGaudio, J. M. (2012). Evidence-based practice: Reflux in sinusitis. *Otolaryngologic Clinics of North America, 45*(5), 983-992.

Obholzer, R. J., Nouraei, S. A., Ahmed, J., Kadhim, M. R., & Sandhu, G. S. (2008). An approach to the management of paroxysmal laryngospasm. *Journal of Laryngology Otology, 122*(1), 57-60.

Park, J., Shim, M., Hwang, Y., Cho, K., Joo, Y., Cho, J., . . . Sun, D. (2012). Combination of voice therapy and antireflux therapy rapidly recovers voice-related symptoms in laryngopharyngeal reflux patients. *Otolaryngology-Head and Neck Surgery, 146*(1), 92-97.

Park, W., Hicks, D., & Khandwala, F. E. A. (2005). Laryngeopharyngeal reflux: Prospective cohort study evaluating. *Laryngoscope, 115*, 1230-1238.

Peery, A. F., Hoppo, T., Garman, K. S., Dellon, E. S., Daugherty, N., Bream, S., . . . Jobe, B. A. (2012). Feasibility, safety, acceptability, and yield of office-based, screening transnasal esophagoscopy. *Gastrointestinal Endoscopy, 75*(5), 945-953.

Reavis, K. M., Morris, C. D., Gopal, D. V., Hunter, J. G., & Jobe, B. A. (2004). Laryngopharyngeal reflux symptoms better predict the presence of esophageal adenocarcinoma than typical gastroesophageal reflux symptoms. *Annals of Surgergy, 239*(6), 849-856.

Remacle, M., & Lawson, G. (2006). Diagnosis and management of laryngopharyngeal reflux disease. *Current Opinions in Otolaryngology & Head and Neck Surgery, 14*(3), 143-149.

Sun, G., Muddana, S., Slaughter, J. C., Casey, S., Hill, E., Farrokhi, F., . . . Vaezi, M. F. (2009). A new pH catheter for laryngopharyngeal reflux: Normal values. *Laryngoscope, 119*(8), 1639-1643.

Sun, Q. J., Chum, J. M., Bautista, T. G., Pilowsky, P. M., & Berkowitz, R. G. (2011). Neuronal mechanisms underlying the laryngeal adductor reflex. *Annals of Otology, Rhinology & Laryngology, 120*(11), 755-760.

Toohill, R. J., & Kuhn, J. C. (1997). Role of refluxed acid in pathogenesis of laryngeal disorders. *American Journal of Medicine, 103*(5A), 100S-106S.

Trad, J., Turgeon, D., & Deljkich, E. (2012). Long-term outcomes after transoral incisionless fundoplication in patients with GERD and LPR symptoms. *Surgical Endoscopy, 26*(3), 650-660.

Van der Westhuizen, L., Von, S., Wilkerson, B., Johnson, B., Cob, J., & Smith, D. (2011). Impact of Nissen fundoplication on laryngopharyngeal reflux symptoms. *American Surgeon, 77*(7), 878-882.

Wassenaar, E., Johnston, N., Merati, A., Montenovo, M., Petersen, R., Tatum, R., & Oelschlager, B. (2011). Pepsin detection in patients with laryngopharyngeal reflux before and after fundoplication. *Surgery Endoscopy, 25*(12), 3870-3876.

White, D. R., Heavner, S. B., Hardy, S. M., & Prazma, J. (2002). Gastroesophageal reflux and eustachian tube dysfunction in an animal model. *Laryngoscope, 112*(6), 955-961.

8

The Singer's Guide to Anesthesiology and Voice

ANDREW ROSENBERG

Introduction

Singers and other vocal professionals are often faced with the possibility of requiring anesthesia at some point in their lives. These vocal athletes who require a medical procedure or operation often have questions and concerns about how the process of receiving an anesthetic may affect their voice. This chapter provides a general overview about different types of anesthesia, what happens during common anesthesia procedures, possible complications impacting the voice, and questions that singers may wish to ask their anesthesiologists before surgery. The intent of this chapter is to provide the vocal athlete with relevant information, so that they can have an informed conversation with the surgeon and anesthesiologist, should the need for anesthesia arise.

Basics of Anesthesia

Anesthesia is the field of medicine where the safety and comfort of a patient is provided while they undergo a variety of procedures from minor, office-based interventions to major hospital operations. Among the many tasks an anesthesiologist performs is evaluating a patient's medical history in relation to the operation for which he or she is scheduled. Subsequently, an anesthetic plan is developed, along with the patient and surgeon that is best suited for the procedure. For the singer, this should include attention to minimizing influences that can disturb their voice, understanding that safety is first and foremost priority.

Anesthesia is generally categorized into techniques that sedate (ensure calm, sleepy, and some degree of relaxed forgetfulness) while maintaining the patient's ability to respond and breathe/move on their own, and on the other end of the anesthesia spectrum is a general anesthetic where a patient is completely unconscious and fully asleep. A third option is to numb a particular area of the body with a regional block in addition to either sedation or in combination with a general anesthetic.

Sedation techniques are used for minor office-based procedures and diagnostic or screening exams using thin, flexible scopes or catheters (e.g., colonoscopy, upper endoscopy, bronchoscopy, sinus or airway exams, draining tubes, or heart catheterizations). Usually, an intravenous medication and a local numbing anesthetic, along with supplemental oxygen, are used for these procedures. Patients are able to protect their airway and breathe on their own, so devices that fit into the mouth/airway are typically not needed. Rarely, a procedure that starts as a sedation case may need to be converted to a general anesthetic, and if there is risk for this, the anesthesiologist should discuss this with the patient prior to the procedure.

General anesthesia is provided when a patient needs to be rendered unconscious using intravenous and/or inhaled medical gases so that the patient is: (1) completely unconscious, (2) unable to feel pain, (3) completely forgetful (amnestic), (4) not responding physiologically to painful stimuli (heart rate and blood pressure under control), and (5) unable to move. Consequently, once the patient is asleep, the airway needs to be supported and protected to ensure the patient receives enough oxygen and breathes off carbon dioxide, as well as prevents fluids getting into the lungs (aspiration). A common device to do this is a breathing tube known as an endotracheal tube (ETT). This is a thin, hollow tube much like a straw with a balloon near the end that provides a seal that circumfer-

entially prevents fluids and secretions from entering the trachea while the patient is sedated and lying flat on the procedure bed. The usual sequence of events for a general anesthetic after a patient is set up with monitors and oxygen in an operating room are: (1) being given a small dose of sedation/amnestic, (2) breathing pure oxygen from a mask, (3) receiving an intravenous medication to produce complete sleep/unconsciousness, (4) placing an ETT from the mouth into the trachea, and (5) maintaining general anesthesia with IV inhaled anesthetic gases delivered by an anesthesia ventilator. At the end of the case, when awake enough to breathe on one's own and protect the airway, removal of the breathing tube (extubation) occurs, and the patient is moved to the recovery room. More details and issues related to the airway are described later in the chapter.

Regional anesthesia is another method to reduce pain and distress for surgical procedures and uses very thin needles and local anesthetics such as used by dentists to block specific nerves that innervate a region of the body. These regional blocks are commonly performed for orthopedic and other procedures on the limbs. Usually only moderate sedation is then needed for a procedure, obviating the need for a general anesthetic and an ETT. Occasionally, a regional block may be used in combination with a general anesthetic. Therefore, not all cases where a regional block is used can be performed without some need for airway protection (e.g., shoulder, lower pelvic, and hip). Rarely, some regional blocks for the upper body will temporarily numb nerves that affect the vocal cords and result in brief hoarseness. This occurs because the recurrent laryngeal branch of the vagus nerve is very close to where the anesthetic solutions are injected in order to block the nerves to the upper and lower arm and neck. Depending on the solution used, the numbness can last for several hours. Unless an extraordinarily rare complication occurs due to a direct injection into the nerve, or when the nerve is otherwise bruised or cut, the numbness and hoarseness completely resolve when the anesthetic wears off.

Procedures That Require Airway Devices

Assuming that alternative anesthetic techniques are not deemed safe and appropriate for the surgery planned, all general anesthetics require the use of a device that supports and protects the airway. As described above, the most common of these is the ETT. Figure 8–1 shows a standard ETT. Because of the nature of the ETT tube coming into contact with the larynx and vocal folds, it is reasonable to ask the anesthesiologist about alternative options such as the absolute need for an ETT versus another airway device such as a laryngeal mask airway (LMA). Figure 8–2 shows

a laryngeal mask airway device. The ETT is used when patients cannot breathe on their own, or the risk of aspirating fluids from the stomach or mouth into the trachea precludes the use of an LMA. The fundamental difference between the two is that the ETT is inserted in between vocal folds, and a soft balloon is inflated below them to prevent secretions or fluids from going distally into the trachea. The LMA is essentially a small mask with a tube that fits over the glottis opening and is most often used when a patient is deeply asleep but still able to breathe on their own. The LMA design does not prevent fluids from getting into the airway as well as the ETT, but because it rests above the vocal cords, there is less opportunity for some vocal cord swelling to occur (Brimacombe, 1995).

Harris, Johnston, Collins, and Heath (1990) completed a double-blinded investigation on the use of LMA (Brain Laryngeal Mask Airway) compared with ETT on 27 singers. Presurgery voice measurements and laryngeal video stroboscopic measurements were taken on 27 singers who underwent anesthesia for an average of

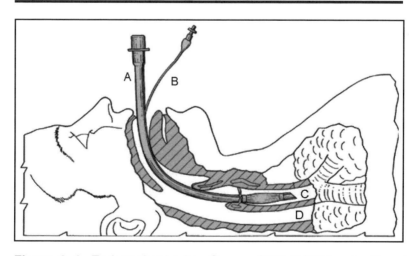

Figure 8–1. Endotracheal tube. *Source*: PhillipN/Wikimedia Commons /PD-US-patent-no notice.

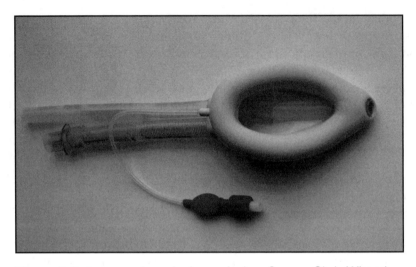

Figure 8–2. Laryngeal mask airway device. *Source*: Chris Wheatley, Senior Intensive care technologist/Wikimedia Commons/Creative Commons Attribution 3.0.

50 minutes. Ten subjects did not undergo postoperative measurement because of pain and discomfort in the throat postoperatively. Authors did not specify how many of these were from the ETT group compared with the LMA group. Postoperative measurements were taken on 17 subjects, 18 to 24 hours after their procedures. The six patients who were randomly assigned to ETT showed significant differences in postoperative laryngeal findings including edema (1), hematoma (1), pharyngeal laceration (1), and petechia (3), compared with the 11 patients who had LMA. In the LMA group, seven had no postoperative change, three had pharyngeal edema, and one demonstrated mucosal wave irregularity. The authors advocated the use of LMA when deemed a safe option from an anesthesiology standpoint. This study certainly promotes the use of LMA when feasible, but given the very small subject size, results should be interpreted with caution. Additionally, there were no additional follow-up examinations to see if laryngeal changes

had resolved or were lingering (Harris et al., 1990).

Rarely, singers will require an operation directly to their airway and/or vocal folds. These procedures are somewhat unique from an anesthesiology perspective in that a breathing tube is often placed by the anesthesiologist at the beginning of the case, and then either manipulated or even temporarily removed by the surgeon during the operation while the patient is still under general anesthesia. During these procedures, the patient's airway is often kept open with suspension tools that can potentially lead to some

Singers are always encouraged to disclose that they are a professional singer and to discuss their concerns with both the surgeon and anesthesiologist ensuring that extra care and concern will be given to help minimize anesthesia-related risk to the vocal folds.

degree of vocal fold swelling and/or pain. Airway and vocal tract issues unique to these operations are routinely discussed with the surgeon and not the anesthesiologist.

Singer Concerns

The following considerations are more nuanced and need to be placed in perspective with the other issues to ensure the safest care for a patient in a given operation. However, a singer who will be requiring general anesthesia may consider the following items to discuss. First, the size of the ETT may be a specific point to bring up with the anesthesiologist because the medical team usually considers placing the largest sized tube that would fit easily in an airway instead of the smallest sized tube that would still allow for easy breathing mechanics. This technical consideration often is not of great clinical consequence, and therefore, it is important to discuss with the anesthesiologist the intended size to be used.

Another point to discuss with the anesthesiologist might be the attention paid to extra care taken with the ETT balloon inflation pressures used during the operation. Rarely, (typically during longer cases) pressure on the mucosal lining of the trachea has been associated with temporary vocal fold weakness because of pressure on the recurrent laryngeal nerve, especially with neck operations occurring from 1.7% to as

high as 6%, and less than 1% for longer term paralysis (Apfelbaum, Mark, Kriskovich, & Haller, 2000; Ellis & Pallister, 1975). More commonly, the balloon pressure is the cause of postoperative sore throat (Sengupta, Sessler, Maglinger, Wells, Vogt, Durrani, & Wadhwa, 2004). It is possible for the anesthetist to periodically check the balloon inflation pressure during a procedure, and especially where the pressure may increase because of operative conditions in the neck or the use of nitrous oxide. After the surgery or procedure is complete, the airway is suctioned of any secretions, and the balloon of the ETT is deflated before removal to lessen risks of any mild injury to the vocal folds during extubation. Most patients do not remember this and simply wake up in the recovery room already extubated.

Airway and Vocal Tract Complications

Among the most common consequences of any form of airway supporting device during very deep sedation and general anesthesia are sore throat and some degree of hoarseness. Various studies have demonstrated wide-ranging incidence of some degree of vocal fold dysfunction after short-term intubation (Burgess, Cooper, Marino, Peuler, Wariner, 1979; Reber, Hauenstein & Echternach, 2007). Peppard and Dickens (1983) retrospectively examined 475 patients with no prior laryngeal pathology undergoing short-term intubation and found a 6% incidence of trauma including hematomas, lacerations to the vocal folds, false vocal folds and epiglottis, as well as 0.4% incidence of vocal fold paralysis (Peppard & Dickens, 1983). Loucks et al. (1998) has summarized various retrospective and prospective evaluations of patients who

> Asking the anesthesiologist to use the smallest sized tube that would still be safe and reasonable may help reduce some of the vocal cord swelling and postoperative complications.

received short-term intubation demonstrating a range of vocal process lesions as commonly as 73% to 80%, including visible edema, vocal fold hematoma, and other less common conditions such as ulceration and granuloma formation at the vocal processes (Loucks et al., 1998).

Although most of these complications are associated with ETTs, patients who have had an LMA used for anesthesia often have sore throat (Brimacombe, 1995). The LMA cuff, when fully inflated, presses on the tissues in the back of the throat and above the glottis opening, and this pressure routinely leads to some soreness in 6% to 34% of patients, usually lasting no more than several hours a day (Sue & Susanto, 2003). The ETT is associated with a greater likelihood for postoperative sore throat, from an incidence of 14% to at least 50%, due to the balloon's contact with the mucosal lining of the trachea (McHardy & Chung, 1999; Sue & Susanto, 2003). Furthermore, some degree of temporary, mild hoarseness is common after an ETT because of the contact between the plastic tube and the vocal cords during the procedure, as well as the tube also contacting the posterior portion of the tongue and throat during the procedure. Studies have demonstrated a wide range of this occurring (4% to 75%) and depending on the cause, it can last from several hours to a couple of days (Jones, Catling, Evans, Green, & Green, 1992). Unrelated to the ETT, other causes for vocal fold swelling are procedures that either directly involve the airway or those where the head is in a lower position (some neurosurgical procedures and back operations) as well as cases with significant fluid shifts.

Extubation is rarely the cause of injury to the cords or airway tissues, but occasionally, a patient, while still sedated, pulls the tube out of his own mouth with the balloon inflated, leading to some irritation of the cords and very rarely causing dislocation of the arytenoid cartilages. In addition, for long or complicated procedures, it is common for patients to go to the recovery room or an intensive care unit still under general anesthesia or deep sedation with the ETT still in place. Depending on the circumstances, the patient will have the ETT removed a day or several days later (e.g., cardiac, trauma, transplantation).

Some patients have physical features that make it difficult to place an ETT, and they are known as patients with a difficult airway. Causes of a difficult airway include limited mouth opening (less than the width of 3 adult fingers), very large front teeth, a small mouth, very short distance from the back of the mouth to the tip of the chin (thyromental distance less than the width of 3 adult fingers), a very short neck or limited ability to flex the neck, and very redundant or lax soft tissues in the back of the throat. Also, larger neck circumference and severe obesity (BMI >30 kg/m^2) may require the need to place an ETT using a variety of fiberoptic scopes (Shiga, Wajima, Inoue, & Sakamoto, 2005). This should not be viewed as a reason to not accept a general anesthesia, as general anesthesiologists relatively commonly perform these techniques.

Hoarseness associated with intubation is usually because of mild swelling of the vocal folds themselves, as described above from fluids and/or mild irritation from the airway devices used for general anesthesia (Loucks, Duff, Wong, & Finley-Detweiler, 1998). The devices used to assist in placing an ETT, known as a laryngoscopes, are rarely the cause of direct trauma to the cords or the arytenoid cartilages. However, when this occurs, it usually happens during unanticipated difficult intubations where placing the ETT is complicated by the inability to directly visualize the vocal cords. More significant swelling may occasionally be treated with anti-inflammatory agents including steroids on a case-by-case basis. When swelling or injury to the cords are more involved, the patient may have difficulty voicing when they wake up. In the more severe cases, patients may not be able to breathe properly because of swelling creating partial blockage of airflow and resulting in a loud inspiratory sound known as stridor. Stridor is treated with humidified oxygen and inhaled medications to reduce swelling (racemic epinephrine), and occasionally patients may need to be reintubated to allow for an adequate airway while the condition resolves. Direct injury to the vocal folds or the supporting structures also often heal on their own, but singers should have very little threshold for postoperative voice complications and should seek consultation from a laryngologist if symptoms persist for more than 2 weeks (Terris, Arnstein, & Nguyen, 1992; Sue & Susanto, 2003).

Less common complications occur because of direct irritation or damage to the vocal folds themselves. These include hematomas, or abrasions to the vocal folds, false vocal folds and surrounding tissues, arytenoid subluxation, delayed vocal cord immobility, and granuloma formation (Colice, 1992; Mendels, Brunings, Hamaekers, Stokroos, Kremer & Baijens, 2012; Santos, Afrassiabi, & Weymuller, 1994). These lesions result from either unavoidable contact with the devices used to intubate the patient, the artificial airways themselves (especially if left in for several weeks after an operation), overinflation of the airway balloon, or inappropriate technique of the anesthetist. Similar problems occur if patients have been intubated and placed on a

ventilator for serious medical illness (such as pneumonia). In the case of prolonged intubation (more than 4 days), issues mentioned above may also occur, as well as the formation of granuloma, usually secondary to ulcerations on the vocal processes.

These issues occur rarely, reported to range from 0.01% to 3.5%, and should be primarily considered in sick patients who have been intubated in an ICU on prolonged mechanical ventilation and have hoarseness lasting beyond a week (Stauffer, Olson, & Petty, 1981). Although hoarseness may be present immediately, symptoms tend to develop over 4 to 6 weeks as the granuloma formation matures and tend to resolve spontaneously from 8 to 14 weeks depending on the presence of other risk factors such as gastroesophageal reflux and voice abuse (Sue & Susanto, 2003). In very rare circumstances, narrowing of the trachea below the level of the cords (tracheal stenosis) may occur, but as described above, tends to be only in patients who were intubated for more than 6 days (<2%). There is a 12% incidence in patients intubated greater than 11 days (Whited, 1992). Fortunately, these conditions are extremely rare, and specific treatments at specialized voice centers are usually available.

For singers, among the most dreaded complications to the vocal cords is temporary or permanent paralysis of the cord (Cavo, 1985). The most common (yet rare) reasons for this are due to direct injury to the nerves that innervate the vocal cord (Lim, Chia, & Ng, 1987). The operations where this complication may occur tend to be those involving the thyroid organ and other neck operations, as well as those in the upper chest. The incidence of recurrent laryngeal nerve injury is approximately 2% to 3%, many of which are temporary (Apfelbaum et al., 2000; Shindo & Chheda,

2007). Less common are direct injuries from the endotracheal intubation itself. Spontaneous recovery and the best prognoses were seen among patients whose injuries were associated with the endotracheal tube intubation, and spontaneous voice recovery in all patients with cord paralysis occurred in over 76% of patients (Yamada, Hirano, & Ohkubo, 1983).

Frequently Asked Questions for Anesthesia

1. Do I need a general anesthetic?
   A. If you are going to need to be completely unconscious and not moving at all during an operation, you will likely need some form of very deep sedation or general anesthesia and will require an airway device to support your breathing and protect your airway. Sometimes, a procedure could be accomplished with a regional block and moderate sedation, and it may be possible to avoid an airway tube. You should ask if these techniques are possible for your procedure. In general, these combination procedures usually only work for operations on extremities.

2. Are there alternatives to an endotracheal tube?
   A. Yes. A laryngeal mask airway is inserted in the mouth into the back of the throat and rests just above the vocal folds. In general, it is used in procedures where the patient is still able to breathe automatically on their own, so the number of bigger operations for which this technique is possible is limited. There are pros and cons to using this device

in longer and more involved procedures, which you should discuss with your anesthesiologist.

3. I've been told I am a difficult airway. What does that mean?
   A. Some patients have physical features of their mouth, neck, or internal airway that make it difficult to place an endotracheal tube or provide a mask to support breathing without using special equipment.

4. What are the risks of vocal problems?
   A. The majority of patients who have had an ETT or LMA will have 1 to 2 days of throat or vocal-related symptoms, usually due to mild edema or irritation of the vocal process. These are:
      - Sore throat (14% to 45% for ETT, and 6% to 35% for LMA)
      - Hoarseness (4% to 75%)
      - Ulceration/granuloma (0.01% to 3.5%)
      - Vocal cord paresis (<2% in high risk operations (e.g., Thyroid surgery), and significantly less in general surgeries)
      - Arytenoid subluxation/fracture
      - Glottic stenosis (narrowing of the glottis) (1% to 20% in patients on prolonged mechanical ventilation)
      - Tracheomalacia (softening of the trachea)

5. What can the anesthetist do to reduce complications to my voice?
   A. Most importantly, notify the anesthesia team member that you are a singer and/or use your voice professionally. There may be some choice in what airway to use or even the possibility to do a procedure without the need for a general anesthesia. Particular care to the size of the airway tube, balloon inflation pressures throughout the procedure, humidification of

air/gases used in the procedure, and care when removing the tube.

6. I have hoarseness after my surgery; what I should I do?

   A. The vast majority of postintubation hoarseness is due to mild edema, and it will resolve. However, maintaining adequate hydration and avoiding extensive voice use and yelling is warranted. Additionally, active singing is not indicated until normal voicing functioning has returned. Gentle warm-ups such as lip trills and hums may be helpful during this period.

7. What should I do if my surgeon or anesthesiologist tells me I had a problem involving my vocal cords during an operation?

   A. Feel comfortable to ask for the specific issues that occurred. The anesthesiologist may offer or be able to produce a letter detailing the issues for you to keep and take to a voice specialist if needed. If voice change persists for more than 2 weeks, seek an evaluation from a laryngologist, even if the surgeon or anesthesiologist does not suggest or recommend it.

Chapter Summary

This chapter has provided a general overview of basic anesthetic procedures including intubation. There are some voice risks associated with undergoing anesthesia, and these have been discussed. The singer is always encouraged to make very clear the fact that they sing professionally. This will help ensure that extra care and concern are given to determining the size of ETT, monitoring pressures of the tracheal balloon, and controlling the process of extubation. While mild hoarseness and sore throat may typically occur directly after surgery, singers should consider laryngeal examination if voice symptoms persist two weeks after their surgery or procedure.

References

Apfelbaum, R. I., Mark, D., Kriskovich, M. D., & Haller, J. R. (2000). On the incidence, cause, and prevention of recurrent laryngeal nerve palsies during anterior cervical spine surgery. *SPINE, 25*(22), 2906–2912.

Brimacombe, J. (1995). The advantages of the LMA over the tracheal tube or facemask: A meta-analysis. *Canadian Journal of Anaesthesia, 42*, 1017–1023.

Burgess, G. E., 3rd, Cooper, J. R., Jr., Marino, R. J., Peuler, M. J., & Warriner, R. A., 3rd. (1979). Laryngeal competence after tracheal extubation. *Anesthesiology, 51*(1), 73–77.

Cavo, J. W. (1985). True vocal cord paralysis following intubation. *Laryngoscope, 95*, 1352–1358.

Colice, G. L. (1992). Resolution of laryngeal injury following trans laryngeal intubation. *American Review of Respiratory Disease, 145*, 361–364.

Ellis, P. D. M., & Pallister, W. K. (1975). Recurrent laryngeal nerve palsy after endotracheal intubation. *Laryngology Otology, 89*, 823–826.

Harris, T., Johnston, S., Collins, C., & Heath, M. (1990). A new general anesthetic technique for use in singers: The brain laryngeal mask airway versus endotracheal intubation. *Journal of Voice, 4*(3), 81–85.

Jones, M. W., Catling, S., Evans, E., Green, D. H., & Green, J. R. (1992). Hoarseness after tracheal intubation. *Anesthesia, 47*(3), 213–216.

Lim, E. K., Chia, K. S., & Ng, B. K. (1987). Recurrent laryngeal nerve palsy following endotracheal intubation. *Anaesthesia & Intensive Care Medicine, 15*, 342–345.

Loucks, T. M., Duff, D., Wong, J. H., & Finley-Detweiler, R. (1998). The vocal athlete and endotracheal intubation: A management protocol. *Journal of Voice, 12*(3), 349–359.

McHardy, F. E., & Chung, F. (1999). Postoperative sore throat: Cause, prevention and treatment. *Anaesthesia, 54*, 444–453.

Mendels, E. J., Brunings, J. W., Hamaekers, A. E., Stokroos, R. J., Kremer, B., & Baijens, L. W. (2012). Adverse laryngeal effects following short-term general anesthesia: A systematic review. *Archives of Otolaryngology-Head & Neck Surgery, 138*(3), 257–264.

Peppard, S., & Dickens, J. (1983). Laryngeal injury following short-term intubation. *Annals of Otology, Rhinology, & Laryngology, 92*, 327–330.

Reber, A., Hauenstein, L., & Echternach, M. (2007). Laryngopharyngeal morbidity following general anaesthesia. Anaesthesiological and laryngological aspects. *Anaesthesist, 56*(2), 177–189, 190–191.

Santos, P. M., Afrassiabi, A., & Weymuller, E. A. (1994). Risk factors associated with prolonged intubation and laryngeal injury. *Otolaryngology-Head & Neck Surgery, 111*(4), 453–459.

Sengupta, P., Sessler, D. I., Maglinger, P., Wells, S., Vogt, A., Durrani, J., & Wadhwa, A. (2004). Endotracheal tube cuff pressure in three hospitals, and the volume required to produce an appropriate cuff pressure. *BMC Anesthesiology, 4*, 8.

Shiga, T., Wajima, Z., Inoue, T., & Sakamoto, A. (2005). Predicting difficult intubation in apparently normal patients: A meta-analysis of bedside screening test performance. *Anesthesiology, 103*(2), 429–437.

Shindo, M., & Chheda, N. N. (2007). Incidence of vocal cord paralysis with and without recurrent laryngeal nerve monitoring during thyroidectomy. *Archives of Otolaryngology-Head & Neck Surgery, 133*(5), 481–485.

Stauffer, J. L., Olson, D. E., & Petty, T. L. (1981). Complications and consequences of endotracheal intubation and tracheotomy. A prospective study of 150 critically ill adult patients. *American Journal of Medicine, 70*(1), 65–76.

Sue, R. D., & Susanto, I. (2003). Long-term complications of artificial airways. *Clinics in Chest Medicine, 24*(3), 457–471.

Terris, D. J., Arnstein, D. P., & Nguyen, H. H. (1992). Contemporary evaluation of unilateral vocal cord paralysis. *Otolaryngology-Head & Neck Surgery, 107*, 84–90.

Whited, R. E. (1992). A prospective study of laryngotracheal sequelae in long-term intubation. *American Review of Respiratory Disease, 145*, 361–364.

Yamada, M., Hirano, M., & Ohkubo, H. (1983). Recurrent laryngeal nerve paralysis: A ten-year review of 564 patients. *Auris Nasus Larynx, 10*(Suppl.), 1–15.

9

The Life Cycle of the Singing Voice

Overview

There were slightly over 42,000 Equity actors who paid dues during the 2011–2012 season. Unfortunately, there was not a breakdown of ages publically reported for those years, but during the 2004–2005 year, the age range of the majority of Equity actors was between 31 to 50 years, with 80 members under the age of 10 and 38 members over the age of 90 (http://www.actors equity.org/docs/about/AEA_Annual_11-12 .pdf). Perhaps because of physical demands, physical appearance, or simply the fact that between the mid-teen years through mid-thirties our bodies are best able to handle training, neuromotor memory, and generally have quick recovery, the majority of commercial music singers (and many professional athletes) are under age 40. The commercial music world demands a marketable package at a young age. This is in contrast to the classical singer, who may not even be considered for young artist programs until their late twenties. The height of the classical singer's career is typically in the 35- to 60-year-old range. Because of the significant demands on young voices, the majority of this chapter focuses on the pediatric and adolescent singer. Natural changes will occur in the voice that may affect performance in the older singer, and a portion of this chapter also focuses on the typical aging of the voice.

The Pediatric Performer: Considerations for Vocal Performing in Children Through Adolescence

Understanding the pediatric and adolescent performing voice warrants unique consideration. Although most children begin vocalizing naturally at a young age through singing and imitating songs and melodic variations they hear, it is often a child's exposure to vocal music in a choral situation (church, school, or community) that sparks an interest to further train their instrument. However, it is occasionally the child's parent who actively pursues vocal training for the child, hoping to generate the next "star." Within the current pop culture, children and parents are inundated with unrealistic expectations of what young girls and boys should sound like without a full understanding of the demands placed on this type of performing and the potential injury risk associated with it. Professional young vocal athletes are like elite Olympic gymnasts, and issues related to their physical, emotional, and cognitive development must be understood by voice professionals who prevent, evaluate, and treat vocal injury in this population. This section of the text outlines historical pedagogical training of young voices, age- and development-specific considerations, and concerns for vocal injury within this subset of performers.

Historical Vocal Pedagogy of Young Singers

The "appropriate age" for a child to begin vocal training remains controversial in the singing community. Historically, voice teachers have debated the minimum age to begin private vocal training. Some teachers believe that no child is too young to begin training, while others believe that training should not begin until after puberty. The American Academy of Teachers of Singing endorsed training young voices by qualified voice teachers in 2002 (American Academy of Teachers of Singing, 2002). Boy choir singing (within the church) may be some of the earliest professional youth vocal performances and dates back to the late Middle Ages in the Viennese Court. Vocal prodigies have been present throughout the centuries, just as with athletics, but with today's

popular media culture, very young child performers are often exploited for their talents. Parents seek out vocal teachers to train young voices often without knowledge or understanding of technical voice training.

There are multiple possibilities for exposing a young child to vocal music without enrollment in an intensive vocal training program. Musical stimulation in children should be encouraged but never forced. Parents of preschool-aged children should encourage their children to sing along with music from shows such as Sesame Street, Veggie Tales, and Blue's Clues. Organized music programs that specifically target children, such as Kinder-music, are excellent resources for introducing music appreciation and ear training to infants and toddlers. In addition, many churches begin children's choirs as early as age three. Choral singing in a group environment provides the young child an outlet to sing with other children their age (Atkinson, 2010; Hook, 1998; Phillips, 1992; Rutkowski & Miller, 2002; Siupsinskiene & Lycke, 2011; Welch, 1988). These types of venues provide age-appropriate music and are typically limited in vocal range and musical complexity. School-aged children are exposed to vocal music as part of the school's curriculum. Music education in the schools typically involves both vocal and instrumental training. A child's participation in choirs and/or musical presentations may be a young singer's first exposure to public performance. If a child of elementary school age demonstrates an aptitude and eagerness to further involve themselves in singing, one may consider private or group lessons. Professional children's choirs can provide children the opportunity to learn decent vocal techniques within a group situation. Community and professional theater productions often have roles for children. The classical singing world has generally more limited roles for children, but the Metropolitan Opera maintains an active children's vocal program where students in the program are used in choral and solo roles.

Unlike speech pathology or music educators within the educational system, there is no formal certification or education required to become a private vocal instructor. Vocal pedagogues historically worked in a master-apprentice relationship. In order to be considered for acceptance into a given vocal studio, the student must have passed a rigorous audition process that included natural vocal talent, good looks, willingness/ability to train, commitment to training, and a lack of vocal flaws (Appelman, 1967; Miller, 1996, 2000, 2009; Sataloff, 1999; Vennard, 1967). Once a student was accepted into a studio, it was often a 2- to 5-year process of vocal training working only on technique (no songs were allowed to be sung, only vocal exercises). Students were expected to be committed to daily vocal practice, adequately care for their vocal instrument and body, and should they not follow the directions of their teacher (or not make expected vocal progress), they were cut from the vocal studio.

Today's vocal training programs are often financially driven, and if a student is paying for voice lessons, a product (recital, performance, etc.) is typically expected within 3 months of initiation of vocal training. Collegiate level musical theater degree programs are growing rapidly, as it is an ever popular major. The above model may not provide enough basic vocal training for the pliable laryngeal musculature to develop appropriate motor patterns. Training neuromuscular patterns requires drill and repetition. Vocalises to train agility and flexibility should be fun and creative with young voices in order that they are willing to engage in daily practice. There is preliminary scientific evidence documenting the efficacy of singing voice training in prepubescent and pubescent voices (Andrews, 1997; Barlow & Howard, 2002, 2005; Edwin, 1997; Reilly, 1995; Skelton, 2007 Siupsinskiene & Lyke, 2011). Private instruction for the truly interested and talented child should include education regarding appropriate vocal hygiene; experimentation with high and low sounds (within a limited range); experimentation with loud and soft singing (within a musically acceptable range); and appropriate breathing techniques. When seeking out private vocal instruction, good teachers and studios should provide an initial consultation visit in order to determine if a child is ready for voice lessons physically, emotionally, and musically. Repertoire for the young child should be age- and range-appropriate and should be emotionally within their present life experiences. Tables 9–1 and 9–2 provide considerations for child roles in classical and music theater. Table 9–3 provides the reader with a listing of child stars (generally commercial music) who have continued their careers into adulthood.

Vocal Pedagogy for Young Voices

One current pedagogical approach to training children's voices is for the singing teacher to take on the role of "vocal parent." Edwin (1995, 1997, 2001) advocates singing with different colors to help the child experiment with timbre (i.e., "sing a hot pink /i/" or "sing a navy blue /u/"). One game called "The Human Boom Box" teaches children to alter timbre by having them "turn up the treble" or "boost the bass" in their voices. Ideally, these exercises will teach the vocal student they are capable of producing many different vocal sounds. It then becomes the goal of the voice teacher

TABLE 9–1. Operas with Roles for Children

A Mid Summer Night's Dream

Amahl and the Night Vistors

Alban Berg: Wozzeck

Attila

Let's Make an Opera (The Little Sweep)

Billy Budd

Boheme

Boito's Mephistopheles

Boris Godunov

Noye's Fludde

The Little Sweep

Golden Vanity

Carmen

Cavalleria Rusticana

Cunning Little Vixen

Der Rosenkavalier

Des Esel's Schatten

Die Frau ohne Schatten

La Damnation de Faust

Tosca

The Magic Flue

Turandot

Grendel

Fedora

Gianni Schicchi

Hansel and Gretel

Pollicino

I Pagliacci

TABLE 9–1. *continued*

Il Ritorno di Ulisse in Patria

Kovantchina

La Gioconda

La Vita Nuova (The New Life)

El Gato Montes

Mefistofele

Moses und Aaron

Opera delle Filastrocche

Otello

Pagliacci

Pagliacci/Cavaleri Rusticana

Parsifal

Pelleas & Melisande

Turn of the Screw

TABLE 9–2. Musicals with Roles for Children

Musical	*Roles*
Annie	Annie, Kate, Tessie, Pepper, and Molly, a chorus of orphans
A Christmas Story	Randy, Ralphie
Annie Get Your Gun	Nellie, Jessie, Young Jake
Anyone Can Whistle	Baby Joan
Assassins	Billy Moore
Beauty and the Beast	Chip
Big	Billy, Cynthia, Josh
Big River	Tom Sawyer, Huck Finn
Bye Bye Birdie	Randolph

continues

TABLE 9–2. *continued*

Musical	Roles
Caroline or Change	Young Noah
Children of Eden	Young Cain, Young Able
Chitty Chitty Bang Bang	Jemima, Jeremy
The Color Purple	Young Olivia, Young Celie
Falsettos	Jason
Fiddler on the Roof	Hodel, Chava, Motel, Tzeilel, Perchik, Fyedka, Bielke, Schprinze
The Full Monty	Nathan
Grease	Danny, Sandy, many roles originally written for teens
Gypsy	Baby June, Baby Louise
Honk	Ducklings
Into the Woods	Jack, Red Riding Hood
Joseph and the Technicolor Dreamcoat	Chorus of children
The King and I	Louis, Prince Chulalonghorn, royal children
Les Miserables	Young Eponine, Gavroche, Young Cosette
Lestat	Claudia
The Lion King	Young Nala, Young Simba
The Little Mermaid	Flounder
Matilda	Most of the cast
Mame	Young Patrick
Mary Poppins	Jane, Michael
Meet Me in St. Louis	Tootie, Agnes
Merrily We Roll Along	Frank Jr.
Miss Saigon	Tam
The Music Man	Tommy, Zaneeta, Amaryllis, Winthrop
Nine	Young Guido

TABLE 9–2. *continued*

Musical	Roles
Oklahoma	Teen dancers
Oliver	Oliver, Artful Dodger, Bette, Orphans
Peter Pan	Wendy, Michael, John, Lost Boys
Pippin	Theo
Ragtime	Small boy
Ruthless	Tina
The Secret Garden	Collin, Mary, Dicken, Martha
Seussical	Baby Kangaroo, Jojo
The Sound of Music	Brigitta, Kurt, Gretl, Marta, Freidric, Liesl, Rolf
Sweeney Todd	Tobias (Toby)
South Pacific	Gerome, Ngana
Spring Awakenings	Cast of adolescents
Tarzan	Young Tarzan
Tommy	Tommy Age 10, Tommy Age 4, Young Sally
The Wizard of Oz	Dorothy, Munchkins
Thirteen	Cast of young boys

to influence the child's perception of good singing by maintaining a balanced, even vocal production throughout the vocal range. Providing good vocal models in the studio and suggesting appropriate role models in the "pop" culture and classical world will also help to influence young singers in a positive way. Many young vocal students successfully emulate the vocal style of unhealthy vocal techniques (hard glottal attacks, breathy voices, glottal fry phonation, and singing too high and out of range) demonstrated in the pop world.

In some popular singing styles, dysphonia is considered a desired quality. Unique voices (not always perfectly healthy) get hired. Vocal professionals should strive to promote a healthy, efficient singing voice including adequate agility and flexibility in the musculature to perform various vocal tasks with ease in order to minimize or prevent injury.

TABLE 9–3. Child Commercial Artist Examples

Classical Female	Classical Male	Commercial Music Artists
Charlotte Church—Pie Jesu (Age 11)	Vienna Boys Choir—Any Recording	Judy Garland (Age 2)
		Donny Osmond (Age 4)
		Michael Jackson (Age 5)
		Janet Jackson (Age 7)
		Beyonce Knowles (Age 9)
		Stevie Wonder (Age 11)
		Tanya Tucker (Age 13)
		LeAnn Rimes (Age 11)
		Taylor Swift (Age 16)
		Celine Dion (Age 12)
		Britney Spears (Age 12)
		Christina Aguilera (Age 12)
		Miley Cyrus (Age 12)
		Justin Bieber (Age 13)

This provides the reader with examples of professional young voices and the age which they turned professional. Many of these voices have continued to perform through puberty and adulthood. Searching iTunes should provide listeners with audio examples of professional young voices. The listener is reminded that because the more contemporary artists are often recorded in a high-tech studio setting, many of the voices are pitch corrected and may not actually reflect the raw voice of the singer. Live recordings of artists will provide the listener with the most accurate representation of the voice.

Considerations for Singing during Puberty

Vocal training during puberty is an additional source of controversy among singing teachers, and pedagogical literature on vocal training during puberty is mixed (Brown, 1996; Sataloff, 1998). Improved scientific understanding of the physiologic and acoustic developmental markers during puberty may provide a basis for improved research in the area of vocal training through puberty (Boseley & Hartnick, 2006; Fatterpekar, Mukherji, Rajgopalan, Lin, & Castillo, 2004; Fitch, & Giedd, 1999; Hartnick & Boseley, 2008; Hartnick, Rehbar, & Prasad, 2005; Hasek, Singh, & Murry, 1980; Kahane, 1978; McAllister, Sederholm, Sundberg, & Gramming, 1994; McAllister & Sundberg, 1998; Mecke & Sundberg, 2010; Reilly, 1995; Sergeant & Welch, 2009; Trollinger,

2007; Whiteside, Hodgson, & Tapster, 2002; Yarnell, 2006). If the adolescent performer is singing in a public or professional arena, the voice teacher can provide insight, education, and reassurance to the singer who is experiencing a significant vocal transformation. The voice pathologist or singing teacher may alleviate anxiety through education on physiological laryngeal changes that occur during puberty. With male students, discussion regarding the often drastic and audible vocal change may be beneficial. Research on the implications of male adolescent voice change has been well-documented with many studies involving members of boy choir ensembles (Cooksey, 1999; Harries, Walker, Williams, Hawkins, & Hughes, 1997; Hollien, 2011; Pedersen, Møller, Krabbe, & Bennett, 1986; Willis & Kenny, 2008). Similarly, female students should be made aware of vocal changes that may occur around their menstrual cycle and hormone fluctuations (Abitbol, Abitbol, & Abitbol, 1999; Cooksey, 1999; Decoster, Ghesquiere, & Van Steenberge, 2008; Williams, Larson, & Price, 1996). An attempt to answer all questions parents and students may pose regarding their voice change requires an understanding of the laryngeal physiological maturation process.

If a singer plans (or is required) to continue singing during puberty, general parameters for ongoing vocal training are warranted. First, heavy voice use during vocal mutation may be avoided. For the professional adolescent singer (specifically males), this may mean taking 6 months to a year off from a heavy performance schedule. Second, the endurance of the vocal mechanism may be limited. Therefore, voice lessons should never last longer than a half-hour, and practice sessions should be short in duration (15 to 30 minutes, 2 times per day). Third, all singing should be done in a comfortable mid-range at a medium vocal intensity level. This "comfortable" range may vary from week to week or even day to day, especially in the male voice. With a respected singer/teacher/voice pathologist relationship, the adolescent singer should learn to respect and identify their comfortable voice during puberty.

As the singing voice begins to stabilize and develop, the voice teacher considers vocal training as vocal building. Teachers must ensure that the singer can "crawl" before they "walk," and "walk" before they "run." Anyone who has observed children knows that younger children are always attempting to emulate what the older kids are doing (and sometimes get hurt in the process). Building the voice slowly over time (range, flexibility, stamina, power) toward specific goals (auditions, roles, collegiate training program) will incorporate respiratory, vocalises, and repertoire with increasing physical and technical difficulty. There are no perfect exercises for every singer, but a balanced voice (with head, mix, and chest) with coordinated registration is vital. Emergence of knowledge and skills on maximizing and utilizing appropriate respiration and resonance strategies depends on the vocal demands of a given performance. Even the young singer is exposed to microphones and pitch correction due to the readily available (and highly marketed) home systems. A discussion and understanding of how to use microphones and monitors with this student population is important.

In addition to the above-mentioned considerations for the adolescent voice, a special mention regarding the young, breathy female voice is in order. A breathy vocal quality is often considered a vocal flaw in a professional singer. However, breathy voices, especially in young females, are typical and have been shown to increase in the degree of breathiness following the onset of menstruation (Miller, 1995; Williams et al.,

1996). The breathy vocal quality exhibited by young female singers is typically the result of a large posterior glottic gap in conjunction with discoordination of the muscles of respiration, phonation, and resonance. If a voice teacher attempts to eliminate all of the normal breathiness by increasing vocal fold adduction in a forced manner, it may have long-term detrimental effects on the voice by creating laryngeal hyperfunction. The ability to distinguish the difference in breathiness and hoarseness, especially at high-frequency phonation is necessary. Excessive breathiness and the absence of improvement over several months may indicate a pathologic condition, which warrants a referral for evaluation.

Singing through adolescence without vocal difficulty is possible if appropriate considerations regarding the mutational voice change are followed. A study that lends support to private vocal study for high school students who are active performers examined eight high school leads in a musical theater production, pre-rehearsal and post-performance (Lee, Pennington, & Stemple, 1998). No vocal disorders were found among this group of singers prerehearsal or post-performance. All of the leads in this study had at least one year of private vocal instruction, and they were double cast, requiring a decreased (and manageable) amount of performance time. These findings suggest that, if the vocal demands of a young singer are reasonable (double casting) and appropriate singing technique is employed (private training), then they may maintain a healthy laryngeal mechanism.

Pedagogical debates regarding training of the adolescent voice will continue to persist in the voice community until empirical studies are able to document the efficacy of specific training modalities. Vocal training must include an adequate comprehension about the nature and function of the laryngeal mechanism. Specifically, physical, cognitive, emotional, and musical abilities must be realistically assessed in each child. This assessment should provide the basis for early vocal training with the understanding that each child must be trained on an individual basis with techniques appropriate for the young and changing voice. Empirical studies documenting the efficacy of vocal training continue to be needed.

The Triple Threat Young Performer

Not only are these young voices required to traverse their entire range with apparent ease and artistry, but the elite commercial singer must also be able to dance and act equally well. The physical development of a singer/actor/dancer will require the integration and muscle memory of multiple skill sets simultaneously. This can be confusing for the performer and the performer's body. Add to that, physical growth spurts and hormonal fluctuations, and the risk for development of less than optimal technique and/or injury due to trauma or repetitive strain increases. Therefore, it becomes the job of the teacher, parent, or voice pathologist to successfully assess and manage this delicate performer. Pending the skill set of the performer and the level of performance (as we have 12-year-old multiplatinum artists), a discussion of short- and long-term career goals is warranted. Every performer is replaceable. There will always be a new rising star. In young performers, if they are imitating what they hear, they are emulating what "has been." Singers should always be encouraged to find what is unique about their own instrument and market that uniqueness so that others wish to emulate them.

Laryngeal Pathology in the Pediatric Performer

Unlike the literature available on the physiologic, anthropometric, and psychological development and understanding of elite young physical athletes that provides insight into injury prevention and treatment, there are limited studies regarding parallel parameters in young vocal athletes (Reilly, 1995; Verduyckt, Remacle, Jamart, Benderitter, & Morsomme, 2011). Therefore, the research on vocal injury within the professional singing population is limited primarily to the late adolescent, college student, and adult populations (Hoffman-Ruddy, Lehman, Crandell, Ingram, & Sapienza, 2001; Lundy, Casiano, Sullivan, Roy, Xue, & Evans, 1999; Tepe, Deutsch, Sampson, Lawless, Reilly, & Sataloff, 2002). Similar to perceptual assessment in the adult, concerns such as dysphonia, loss of frequency range, throat pain, resonance abnormalities, or any abnormal vocal symptom in the young singer warrant a referral to an otolaryngologist to rule out any possible laryngeal pathology. A voice pathologist's assessment of aerodynamic, acoustic, and stroboscopic parameters are also warranted as subtle changes in mucosal flexibility, glottic closure patterns, and/or technical voice assessment; are vital for a complete understanding of the impact of the vocal problem; and provide insight for adequate treatment planning. When investigating the vocal difficulties of young choral performers (ages 3–25), Tepe et al. (2002) reported 55.8% had some vocal problems, and the late adolescent group was most at-risk for vocal difficulty. Research studies that provide preliminary insights into common vocal pathologies of professional voice users include overuse injuries, vocal fold lesions from phonotraumatic behaviors, and

reflux. However, pediatric vocal performers cannot be considered small adult performers, and the majority of the literature regarding habits, injuries, and findings cannot be transferred without adequate quantitative evidence.

Aspects of the Aging Voice and the Nonclassical Singer

The vocal mechanism is dependent on the physical state of the body and mind. As such, the voice will have physiological change associated with aging. Physiologic and histologic studies on the aging larynx have provided a basis for knowledge, and the classical singing world has provided some additional insights into performing through pregnancy and menopause in the female and the loss of androgen in the male. Readers are advised to access articles in the chapter references for further considerations into these changes, but a brief overview is provided here.

What Happens to the Laryngeal Mechanism as We Age?

Aging is not always a graceful process. The reality is that we are living longer as a human race, and some of the issues from cognitive decline and to ossification of hyaline cartilages and joint stiffness are unavoidable. The vocal mechanism does not escape the impact of aging. Genetics play a role for each of us in how we will age, including the voice. As a society, Americans spent over $20 billion annually on antiaging products. With everything from bioidentical hormones to "voice lifts," we inject and ingest products to make us look and feel younger, but to date no fountain of youth can stop the process (Reeves, 2005; http://abcnews.go.com/GMA/DrJohnson /story?id=127887&page=1).

From a respiratory standpoint, as we age, the elasticity of the lung tissue itself decreases, resulting in a decreased ability to inflate and deflate the lungs. Also, the costal cartilages (which attach the ribs to the sternum and allow for some movement/ expansion) begin to ossify, or they may get some arthritis in the joints, resulting in decreased rib cage expansion. The diaphragm and other inspiratory muscles will begin to lose strength as well. These changes begin as early as the third decade of life (Sharma & Goodwin, 2006; Table 9–4).

From a laryngeal standpoint, the cartilaginous framework of the larynx begins to ossify beginning in your twenties, with the arytenoids ossifying somewhat later (thirties). Some authors have proposed that this ossification may actually aid in stabilization of the larynx with increased vocal demands (Abitbol, 2006a). The length of newborn vocal folds is 6 to 8 mm. During puberty, the male vocal folds may increase as much as 60% in length, resulting in average vocal fold length in adult males of 17 to 23 mm. Female vocal folds will also increase in size during puberty to an average of 12 to 17 mm in length (Sataloff, Spiegel, & Rosen, 1998).

Histologically, the vocal folds change with age, resulting in a change in the anatomy and function of the laryngeal muscles (presbylaryngus). There is a breakdown of the elastin and collagen fibers, resulting in a "looser" cover and an inability of the lamina propria to have the flexibility of a younger mechanism. From a muscular standpoint, there are changes in the ability of the muscle fibers to regenerate and repair themselves, resulting in atrophy and thinning of the thyroarytenoid muscle. The result of

these changes leads to a gradual decrease in fundamental speaking frequency of the female voice and a gradual rise in fundamental frequency in the male voice after age 50 (Abitbol, 2006a; Malmgren, 2005; Sataloff, Spiegel, & Rosen, 1998; Stemple, Glaze, & Klaben, 2000).

Hormonal Factors on the Voice Post-Puberty

Males

Beginning with the tradition of boy choirs in Leipzig, the average age of voice break between 1727 to 1749 was assessed to occur around 18 years (Daw, 1970). The age of voice change in males has lowered throughout the centuries and during the 1960s and 1970s in Europe was estimated to occur between 14.2 to 15.5 years. The downward trend has continued with the most recent reporting (1994–2003) estimating the average age of puberty at 14 years (Juul, Magnusdottir, Scheike Prytz, & Skakkebaek, 2007; Juul, Teilmann, Scheike, Hertel, Holm, Laursen, Main, & Skakkebaek, 2006). This particular study retrospectively examined average age of voice break in 463 boys within the Copenhagen Royal Boychoir using a BMI comparison. Their findings indicate that a higher BMI prepuberty correlated to an earlier age of voice break. It is suspected that the age of onset of puberty in the United States is between 9 to 12 years.

Androgens are the hormones responsible for the masculinization of the voice. Abitbol (2006b) also suggests that androgens increase muscle performance by increasing blood flow to the laryngeal mechanism, resulting in power and strength of the adult male voice (which is present in many species beyond humans). As men age, the production of androgens decreases, resulting in decreased muscle tone, change in timbre,

TABLE 9–4. Anatomic and Physiologic Changes of Respiratory System with Aging

Anatomic	Air Space Size: Increased
Compliance	Chest wall compliance: Decreased Lung compliance: Increased to unchanged Total respiratory system compliance: Decreased
Muscle strength	Maximal inspiratory pressure (MIP): Decreased Trans diaphragmatic pressure (Pdi): Decreased Maximum voluntary ventilation (MVV): Decreased
Lung function	FEV1: Decreased FVC: Decreased TLC: Unchanged Vital capacity: Decreased Functional residual capacity: Increased Residual volume: Increased DLCO/VA: Decreased
Exercise capacity	VO2 max: Decreased Dead space ventilation: Increased
Immunology	Bronchial fluid Neutrophils %: Increased Ratio of CD4 +/CD8+ cells: Increased Epithelial lining fluid antioxidants: Decreased

DLCO, diffusing capacity of carbon monoxide; *FEV1*, forced expiratory volume in one second; *FVC*, forced vital capacity; *TLC*, total lung capacity; *VO2*, oxygen consumption; *VA*, alveolar volume.

and lack of vocal power. The suggestion for maintaining the voice as long as possible in males is continued practice and use of the mechanism (if you don't use it, you lose it). Because of the risk of possible changes in the prostate, androgen replacement therapy is generally not recommended for men (Abitbol, 2006b).

Females

The female voice is seemingly more complex due to the impact that three hormones may have on the female voice (androgens, estrogen, and progesterone). The balance of these three hormones throughout the adult lifespan is diverse. Abitbol (2006b), in his book *The Odyssey of Voice* discusses many of the hormone changes that affect the voice throughout a lifespan. Current research has been done on the menopausal voice in elite singers (Caprilli, 2013). In general terms, Abitbol (2006a) suggests that estrogen results in a slight thickening of the mucosal membrane, resulting in increased amplitude of vibration (voice is more flexible). The effect of estrogen may also impact the ossification of laryngeal cartilages as it alters the metabolism of calcium. Estrogen also counterbalances androgens, and estrogen must be present for progesterone to do its job. Progesterone is unique to females and is only present premenopausally. The job of progesterone is to allow the mucus membranes of the uterus to have an egg attach to it. Somewhat parallel, the effects of progesterone on the female vocal folds results in a sloughing off of the mucus membranes of the vocal folds (desquamation). In order for this to happen, Abitbol reports a thickening of laryngeal mucus secretions resulting in laryngeal dryness, throat clearing, decreased vocal agility, and loss of frequency range (typically 4 days before menstruation). It may also create a change in the way the small blood vessels (capillaries) maintain fluid during this time frame. If there is an imbalance of progesterone, there is potential risk for increased vocal fold edema and possible vocal fold hemorrhage. Androgen secretion in women is generally reported to be very small (150µg/dl). Too much androgen will result in permanent change in the female voice. Female singers should be alert to medications or foods that contain androgens. Research on both acoustic and respiratory changes in the female voice are documented (Awan, 2006; Higgins & Saxman, 1989; Sapienza & Dutka, 1996).

Singing During Pregnancy

From a hormonal standpoint, there is a lot going on in the female body during pregnancy. Varying levels of estrogen, progesterone, and androgens may be present at different stages of the pregnancy and can affect the vocal folds. Specifically, fluid retention in the vocal folds has been indicated to increase the collision threshold pressure and the phonation threshold pressure (Adrian, 2012; Babtista-La & Sundberg, 2012; Jahn, 1999). There are also obvious physical changes. Respiration is obviously affected as the pregnancy progresses. Reflux can also become a problem. Those changes may impair the ability of the commercial music singer to perform at an acceptable level. Many women are able to sing through much of their pregnancies up to the mid-portion of the third trimester. Postpartum, singers should be expected that as the body recovers and the hormones re-regulate, there will be both stamina and flexibility rebuilding of the voice.

Singing Through and Beyond Menopause

Overall interest in the physical (and vocal effects) of menopause are relatively new in that a large majority of women prior to the twentieth century typically did not live long enough to warrant study of or interest in menopausal changes. From a hormone standpoint, progesterone, estrogen, and androgen levels all drop off significantly, and if the male hormones overbalance the female hormones, some masculinization of the female voice may occur. There is potential thickening and atrophy of the vocal fold epithelial tissue in women (Abitbol, 2006a, 2006b; Oyarzún, Sepúlveda, Valdivia, Roa, Cantin, Trujillo, Zavando, & Galdames, 2011). Also, because of the drop in progesterone levels, the nerve that innervates the vocal fold may have slower conduction due to demyelinization (Benninger & Murry, 2006). This slowed down rate of nerve conduction has been suggested as a possible reason for a change/slowing of vibrato rate (Benninger & Murry, 2006). There are several excellent discussions on how menopause changes the female classical voice and the singer's response to these changes (Bernstein, 2005; Boulet &

Oddens, 1996; Caprilli, 2013; D'haeseleer, Depypere, Claeys, Wuyts, DeLey, & Van Lierde, 2011; Heman-Ackah, 2004; Leden & Alessi, 1994). Although there are no specific articles that explore commercial music singers voices during menopause, it is suspected that similar findings would emerge. The musical theater genre has, however, written a comedy about it called: *Menopause.*

Chapter Summary

The commercial music world is primarily a young person's profession, so those who train the performers must have an understanding of the volatile nature of the child and adolescent voice. With understanding and guidance, many of these performers can be allowed the opportunity to perform well into adulthood. The effects of hormones before, during, and after puberty can affect physiologic and histologic aspects of the voice. Considerations by the singing teacher and voice pathologist on possible implications of voice change based on age and stage of training are imperative.

References

Abitbol, J. (2006a). Normal voice maturation: Hormones and age. In M. Benninger, & T. Murry (Eds.), *The performer's voice* (pp. 33–50). San Diego, CA: Plural Publishing.

Abitbol, J. (2006b). *Odyssey of the voice* (P. Crossley, Trans.). San Diego, CA: Plural Publishing.

Abitbol, J., Abitbol, P., & Abitbol, B. (1999). Sex hormones and the female voice. *Journal of Voice, 3*(3), 424–446.

Actor's Equity Association. (2011–2012). *Theatrical Season Report: An Analysis of Employment, Earnings, Membership and Finance.* Retrieved from http://www.actorsequity.org/docs/about/AEA_Annual_11-12.pdf.

Adrian, S. (2012). The impact of pregnancy on the singing voice: A case study. *Journal of Singing, 68*(3), 265–271.

Andrews, M. (1997). The singing/acting child: A speech-language pathologist's perspective. *Journal of Voice, 11*(2), 130–134.

Appelman, R. (1967). *The science of vocal pedagogy: Theory and application.* Bloomington, IN: Indiana University Press.

Atkinson, D. (2010). The effects of choral formation on the singing voice. *Choral Journal, 50*(8), 24–33.

Awan, S. (2006). The aging female voice: Acoustic and respiratory data. *Clinical Linguistics & Phonetics, 20*, 171–180.

Babtista-La, F., & Sundberg, J. (2012). Pregnancy and the singing voice: A case study. *Journal of Voice, 26*(4), 431–439.

Barlow, C., & Howard, D. (2002). Voice source changes of child and adolescent subjects undergoing singing training: A preliminary study. *Logopedics Phoniatrics Vocology, 27*(2), 66–73.

Barlow, C., & Howard, D. (2005). Electrolaryngographically derived voice source changes of child and adolescent singers. *Logopedics Phoniatrics Vocology, 30*(3), 147–157.

Benninger, M., & Murray, T. (2006). *The performer's voice.* San Diego, CA: Plural Publishing.

Bernstein, T. (2005). Is the opera house hot or is it just me? (Effects of menopause on the voice). *Classical Singer, 18*, 26–29.

Boseley, M., & Hartnick, C. (2006). Development of the human true vocal fold: Depth of cell layers and quantifying cell types within the lamina propria. *Annals of Otology, Rhinology & Laryngology, 115*(10), 784–788.

Boulet, M., & Oddens, B. (1996). female voice changes around and after menopause—An initial investigation. *Maturitas, 23*, 15–21.

Brown, O. (1996). *Discover your voice: How to develop healthy vocal habits.* San Diego, CA: Singular Publishing.

Caprilli, B. (2013). *The effects of menopause on the elite singing voice: Singing through the storm* (D.M.A, Dissertation). Shenandoah Conservatory.

Cooksey, J. (1999). *Working with adolescent voices*. St. Louis, MO: Concordia Publishing House.

Daw, S. (1970). Age of boys' puberty in leipzig, 1727-1749, as indicated by voice breaking in J. S. Bach's choir members. *Human Biology, 42*, 87-89.

Decoster, W., Ghesquiere,S., & Van Steenberge, S. (2008). Great talent, excellent voices-no problem for pubertal girls? *Logopedics Phoniatrics Vocology, 33*(2), 104-112.

D'haeseleer, E., Depypere, H., Claeys, S., Wuyts, F., De Ley, S., & Van Lierde, K. (2011). The impact of menopause on vocal quality. *Menopause: The Journal of the North American Menopause Society, 18*(3), 267-272.

Edwin, R. (1995). Vocal parenting. *Journal of Singing, 51*(1), 53-56.

Edwin, R. (1997). The singing teacher as vocal parent. *Journal of Voice, 11*(2), 135-137.

Edwin, R. (2001). Vocal exercises for children of all ages. *Journal of Singing, 57*(4), 49-51.

Fatterpekar, G., Mukherji, S., Rajgopalan, P., Lin, Y., & Castillo, M. (2004). Normal age-related signal change in the laryngeal cartilages. *Neuroradiology, 46*(8), 678-681.

Fitch, W. T., & Giedd, J. (1999). Morphology and development of the human vocal tract: A study using magnetic resonance imaging. *The Journal of the Acoustical Society of America, 106*(3), 1511-1522.

Harries, M., Walker, J., Williams, D., Hawkins, S., & Hughes, I. (1997) Changes in the male voice at puberty. *Archives of Disease in Childhood, 77*, 445-447.

Hartnick, C., & Boseley, M. (2008). *Pediatric voice disorders: Diagnosis and treatment*. San Diego, CA: Plural Publishing.

Hartnick, C., Rehbar, R., & Prasad, V. (2005). Development and maturation of the pediatric human vocal fold lamina propria. *The Laryngoscope, 115*(1), 4-15.

Hasek, C., Singh, S., & Murry, T. (1980). Acoustic attributes of preadolescent voices. *Journal of Acoustic Society of America, 68*(5), 1262-1265.

Heman-Ackah, Y. (2004). Hormone replacement therapy: Implications of the women's health initiative for the perimenopausal singer. *Journal of Singing, 60*(5), 471-475.

Higgins, M., & Saxman, J. (1989). Variations in vocal frequency perturbation across the menstrual cycle. *Journal of Voice, 3*(2), 233-243.

Hoffman-Ruddy, B., Lehman, J., Crandell, C., Ingram, D., & Sapienza, C. (2001). Laryngostroboscopic, acoustic, and environmental characteristics of high-risk vocal performers. *Journal of Voice, 15*(4), 543-552.

Hollien, H. (2011). On pubescent voice change in males. *Journal of Voice, 26*(2), 1-12.

Hook, S. (1998). Changing voice and middle school music: An interview with John Cooksey and Nancy Cox. *Choral Journal, 39*(1), 21-26.

Jahn, A. (1999). Pregnancy: Singing your way through. *Classical Singer, 12*(12), 22-23.

Juul, A., Magnusdottir, S., Scheike, T., Prytz, S., & Skakkebæk, N. (2007) Age at voice break in Danish boys: Effects of prepubertal body mass index and secular trend. *International Journal of Andrology, 30*, 537-542.

Juul, A., Teilmann, G., Scheike, T., Hertel, N. T., Holm, K., Laursen, E. M., Main, K. M., & Skakkebaek, N. E. (2006). Pubertal development in Danish children: comparison of recent European and US data. *International Journal of Andrology, 29*, 247-255.

Kahane, J. (1978). A morphological study of the human prepubertal and pubertal larynx. *American Journal of Anatomy, 151*(1), 11-19.

Leden, H., & Alessi, D. (1994).The aging voice. In M. Benninger, B. Jacobson, & A. Johnson (Eds.), *Vocal arts medicine: The care and prevention of professional voice disorders*. New York, NY: Thieme Medical Publishers.

Lee, L., Pennington, E., & Stemple, J. (1998). Leading roles in a high school musical: Effects on objective and subjective measures of vocal production. *Medical Problems of Performing Artists, 13*(4), 167-171.

Lundy, D., Casiano, R., Sullivan, P., Roy, S., Xue, J., & Evans, J. (1999). Incidence of abnormal laryngeal findings in asymptomatic singing students. *Otolaryngology-Head and Neck Surgery, 121*, 69-77.

Malmgren, L. (2005). Cellular and Molecular mechanisms of aging of the vocal fold. In R. Sataloff (Eds.), *Voice science* (pp. 115-123). San Diego, CA: Plural Publishing.

Mcallister, A., Sederholm, E., Sundberg, J. & Gramming, P. (1994). Relations between voice range profiles and physiological and perceptual voice characteristics in ten-year-old children. *Journal of Voice, 8*(3), 230-239.

Mcallister, A., & Sundberg, J. (1998). Data on subglottal pressure and SPL at varied vocal loudness and pitch in 8- to 11-year-old children. *Journal of Voice 12*(2), 166-174.

Mecke, A., & Sundberg, J. (2010). Gender differences in children's singing voices: Acoustic analysis and results of a listening test. *Journal of the Acoustical Society of America, 127*(5), 3223-3231.

Miller, R. (1995). Breathy young female voices. *Journal of Singing, 51*(5), 37-39.

Miller, R. (1996). *The structure of singing: System and art in vocal technique.* New York, NY: Schirmer Books.

Miller, R. (2000). *Training soprano voices.* New York, NY: Oxford University Press.

Miller, R. (2009). Voice pedagogy: In the beginning: The genesis of the art of singing. *Journal of Singing, 66*(1), 45-50.

Oyarzún, P., Sepúlveda, A., Valdivia, M., Roa, I., Cantin, M., Trujillo, G., Zavando, D., & Galdames, I. (2011). Variations of the Vocal fold epithelium in a menopause induced model. *International Journal of Morphology, 29*(2), 377-381.

Pedersen, M., Møller, S., Krabbe, S., & Bennett, P. (1986). Fundamental voice frequency measured by electroglottography during continuous speech. A new exact secondary sex characteristic in boys in puberty. *International Journal of Pediatric Otorhinolaryngology, 11*, 21-27.

Phillips, K. (1992). *Teaching kids to sing.* Los Angeles, CA: Schirmer.

Reeves, K. (2005). Hormone therapy for the female performing artist. *Medical Problems of Performing Artists, 20*(1), 48-51.

Reilly, J. (1995). The three ages of voice: The "singing-acting" child: The laryngologist's perspective. *Journal of Voice, 11*(2), 126-129.

Rutkowski, J., & Miller, M. (2002). A longitudinal study of elementary children's acquisition of their singing voices. *Update: Applications of Research in Music Education, 22*(1), 5-14.

Sapienza, C., & Dutka, J. (1996). Glottal airflow characteristics of women's voice production along an aging continuum. *Journal of Speech & Hearing Research, 39*(2), 322-328.

Sataloff, R. (1996). The effects of menopause on the singing voice. *Journal of Singing, 54*(2), 39-42.

Sataloff, R. (1998). *Vocal health and pedagogy.* San Diego, CA: Singular Publishing.

Sataloff, R. (1999). *Vocal health and pedagogy.* San Diego, CA: Singular Publishing.

Sataloff, R., Spiegel, J., & Rosen, D. (1998). The effects of age on the voice. In R. Sataloff (Eds.), *Vocal health and pedagogy* (pp. 123-131). San Diego, CA: Singular Publishing.

Sergeant, D., & Welch, G. (2009). Gender differences in long-term average spectra of children's singing voices. *Journal of Voice, 23*(3), 319-336.

Sharma, G., & Goodwin, J. (2006). Effect of aging on respiratory system physiology and immunology. *Clinical Interventions in Aging, 1*(3), 253-260.

Siupsinskiene, N., & Lycke, H. (2011). Effects of vocal training on singing and speaking voice characteristics in vocally healthy adults and children based on choral and nonchoral data. *Journal of Voice, 25*(4), 177–189.

Skelton, K. (2007). The child's voice: A closer look at pedagogy and science. *Journal of Singing, 63*(5), 537–544.

Stemple, J., Glaze, L., & Klaben, B. (2000). *Clinical voice pathology: Theory and management* (3rd ed.). San Diego, CA: Singular Publishing.

Tepe, E. S., Deutsch, E. S., Sampson, Q., Lawless, S., Reilly, J. S., & Sataloff, R. T. (2002). A pilot survey of vocal health in young singers. *Journal of Voice, 16*(2), 244–247.

The Latest in Plastic Surgery: The "Voice Lift." (2013, April 22). *ABC News.* Retrieved from http://abcnews.go.com/GMA/DrJohnson /story?id=127887&page=1.

Trollinger, V. (2007). Pediatric vocal development and voice science: Implications for teaching singing. *General Music Today, 20*(3), 19–25.

Verduyckt, I., Remacle, M., Jamart, J., Benderitter, C., & Morsomme, D. (2011). Voice-related complaints in the pediatric population. *Journal of Voice, 25*(3), 373–380.

Vennard, W. (1967). *Singing, the mechanism and technique.* New York, NY: Carl Fischer.

Welch, G. (1988). Beginning singing with young children. *Journal of Singing, 45,* 12–15.

Whiteside, S., Hodgson, C., & Tapster, C. (2002). Vocal Characteristics in preadolescent and adolescent children: A longitudinal study. *Logopedics Phoniatrics Vocology, 27*(1), 12–20.

Williams, B., Larson, G., & Price, D. (1996). An Investigation of selected female singing—and speaking—voice characteristics through a comparison of premenarcheal girls to a group of post-menarcheal girls. *Journal of Singing, 52*(1), 33–40.

Willis, E., & Kenny, D. (2008). Relationship between weight, speaking fundamental frequency, and the appearance of phonational gaps in the adolescent male changing voice. *Journal of Voice, 22*(4), 451–471.

Yarnell, S. (2006). Vocal and aural perceptions of young singers aged ten to twenty-one. *Journal of Singing, 63*(1), 81–85.

10

Medicine, Myths, and Truths

Introduction

Singers are typically focused on general health and well-being. This attention to health is not surprising given that the singer's instrument is their body, and peak performance is dependent on vocal and physical fitness. Consequently, the vocal athlete must take measures to insure overall health, and singers often have a multitude of practices and habits to help prevent illness and promote wellness. These practices include over-the-counter and prescription medications as well as complementary and alternative medicine (CAM) including herbs, supplements, and alternative therapies.

The use of medications (prescribed and over-the-counter) to treat a variety of ailments from the common cold to life threatening disease have both benefits and associated risks. Similarly, supplements, vi-

tamins, and herbs are not without risk, but are widely and commonly used without full knowledge of the possible side effects of the drugs (Ernst, 2002). The concept that herbs are a "natural" substance whereas chemical compounds are not, has resulted in a huge increase in both the purchase and use of herbal remedies in the last 10 years resulting in a $22 billion industry (Gupta, 2008).

Surrow and LoVetri (2000) surveyed 142 singers on the kinds of alternative medical therapies (AMT) they used and under what circumstances. Of the singers surveyed, slightly over 70% endorsed use of AMT. Half of those claimed they used AMT daily. The most commonly reported AMT vitamin supplements included vitamins C, E, and zinc. About 45% of the singers reported using high dose vitamins. Echinacea, Goldenseal, and Ginkgo were the more commonly reported herbal supplements used in this group of surveyed singers. Singers were most likely to resort to using AMT in the presence of a cold or upper respiratory infection (URI); however, they were less likely to do so if hoarseness or voice change presented as a symptom of their illness.

In addition to vitamins and herbal supplements, singers also reported using body work modalities including massage, yoga, Alexander Technique™, and Feldenkrais®. Meditation and other similar modalities were also reported to be used frequently among the survey participants. The results of this study indicated that singers often did not discuss the decision to engage in AMT with their physician or receive physician-guided recommendations regarding use of AMT. This survey highlights the desire for singers to use AMT, but also brings to light the need for education and guidance as to potential risks and harmful interaction associated with many of these unregulated treatment modalities.

By no accounts is this chapter exhaustive of all of the drugs, vitamins, and herbal substances that exist, nor does it substitute for pharmacological advice. Rather, it provides singers with an overview of some of the most common classes of medications (prescribed and over-the-counter) that may impact vocal performance as well as some commonly used herbal supplements and remedies singers use. Vocal athletes, like many high professional athletes, have rituals and routines before performances that they believe make them perform better. The potential benefits/risks of some of the most common customs (steaming, teas, honey, lemon, scarves around the neck, gargling) are clarified for the singer. Several of these remedies reviewed have little or no data either supporting or refuting benefit to vocal health, and yet singers use these therapies by virtue of conventional wisdom and tradition passed down from teachers. Some of the practices/rituals do have

some degree of data supporting their use, and these references are provided when available.

The lists of medicines and practices are not exhaustive, so various websites and sources are provided for the reader seeking more specific information about medicines and herbs. As with prescription medicines, introducing a holistic regimen into daily practice should be discussed with a physician as many herbs and vitamins are contraindicated for various health issues. Herbs and vitamins can interact with some medicines reducing their effectiveness, or creating an adverse reaction. Therefore, readers are always cautioned to seek medical advice before starting new medicines and herbs, even if they are over-the-counter.

Medications and the Voice

Drying Medications

Unfortunately, many over-the-counter and prescription medications have drying effects. Laryngeal mucosal dryness, regardless of the source, results in increased effort to phonate, potentially creating an environment for increased tendency toward laryngeal pathology (Chan & Tayama, 2002; Miri, Barthelat, & Mongeau, 2012; Tanner, Roy, Merrill, Muntz, Houtz, Sauder, Elstad, & Wright-Costa, 2010). Listed below are several classes of drugs that singers may have to use for an extended period of time to treat medical conditions, which can result in laryngeal dryness.

Antihistamines

These medicines are often used to treat allergies and multiple over-the-counter versions in addition to prescription varieties are readily available. Antihistamines work by blocking the histamine response (the body's response to allergies or irritants) and may also cause drowsiness. These drugs may reduce edema and pain related to allergic symptoms, but they also increase viscosity of secretions creating a significant drying effect (Lawerence, 1987). The systemic drying has impact on voice output secondary to general dehydration of vocal fold tissue. Laryngeal mucosa dehydration impacts efficiency of vibration requiring higher subglottal pressures to maintain vibratory function (Verdolini-Marston, Titze, & Drucker, 1990). Additionally, when mucosa tissue of the respiratory tract is dry, a cough can be triggered.

Decongestants

These medicines reduce secretions and mucous production by shrinking mucosal membranes. They come in oral forms (pills and liquids) as well as nasal sprays (for nasal decongestants). A decongestant is often found in "daytime" cold medications because it may keep you awake. Decongestants can also create dryness and possible dry cough. Over-the-counter cold medicines containing the letter D (e.g., Allegra-D; Claritin-D, etc.) after the name contain a decongestant, and singers should be aware of the potential drying effects. This class of drugs may also affect the heart rate and in addition to keeping people awake, may cause cardiac issues.

Diuretics

These medicines are used to reduce and eliminate systemic swelling, or edema by increasing urination. Though shown to reduce swelling, these are not indicated for use with laryngeal swelling and may negatively impact voice because they can draw water out of the vocal folds (Verdolini Abbot et al., 2002). If diuretics are warranted for medical reasons, singers should be aware of potential systemic drying effects and carefully monitor vocal effort for possible signs of "vocal fold dehydration" (Sataloff, Hawkshaw, & Anticaglia, 2006).

Antihypertensives

This classification of drugs is used to treat high blood pressure. Depending on the medication and dosing, it has the potential to induce laryngeal dryness as a side effect. Obviously, the benefits of maintaining a healthy blood pressure are essential for overall health. If you suspect that the antihypertensive you have been prescribed may be causing excessive laryngeal dryness, it is advised that you discuss this side effect with the prescribing physician regarding safe alternative therapies to minimize dryness and maximize benefits. Within the class of antihypertensive drugs are ACE (angiotensin-converting-enzyme inhibitor) inhibitors. ACE inhibitors have been known to cause a nonproductive, chronic cough. Patients are advised to consult with their physician regarding alternative medications if a chronic cough begins after beginning an ACE inhibitor.

Antidepressants/Antianxiety/ ADHD Medications/Other Psychoactive Drugs

Depression, performance anxiety, and other mental health issues may be treated using antidepressants, antipsychotic, selective serotonin reuptake inhibitors, beta-blockers, psychostimulants (often used to treat ADD/ADHD and narcolepsy), and selective norepinephrine reuptake inhibitors (nonstimulant used to treat ADHD). Depending on the drug and use, oral, pharyngeal, and laryngeal dryness may result. The importance of effective treatment for any psychological or mental health condition trumps the side effects of the prescribed medication. However, working with the prescribing physician to find effective dosing and counterbalancing potential side effects with increased hydration, room humidification, and/or elimination of other drying agents is recommended.

Oral Acne Medications

Physical appearance in the performing arts is vital for casting and sustained performance. Acne is a common problem for many performers. Treatment of acne ranges from topical medications to antibiotic therapy to oral contraceptives to Isotretinoin. The oral acne medications carry the risk of dryness as a side effect. Isotretinoin can have significant mucosal drying effects, and if you are taking this drug, you should be closely monitored by your physician for a variety of potential serious side effects. U.S. brand names associated with Isotretinoin are: Absorica, Accutane, Amnesteem, Claravis, Myorisan, and Sotret.

Inhaled Corticosteroids

These drugs are often used to treat asthma by decreasing inflammation in the respiratory system. As adequate breath is necessary for sound production (and sustaining life), the benefits of use for singers who require corticosteroids to manage respiratory problems must be weighed with medication side effects to voice. There are known laryngeal mucosal changes, increased phonation threshold pressures, and dysphonia associated with the use of inhaled corticosteroids (Erickson & Sivasankar, 2010; Gallivan, Gallivan, & Gallivan, 2007; Lavy, Wood, Rubin, & Harries, 2000; Sahrawat, Robb, Kirk, & Beckert, 2013).

Mucolytics

These medicines are sometimes paired with a decongestant to offset the drying effect, although they do not substitute hydration and need to be taken with plenty of water. Guaifenesin is among the more popular mucolytic agents. It is considered to thin mucosal secretions and act as a vasoconstrictor and expectorant (Sataloff et al., 2006). Studies on mucolytic agents have not yet robustly demonstrated significant thinning effects on secretions; however, these drugs continue to be marketed for this purpose and have not necessarily demonstrated adverse effects (Titze & Verdolini Abbot, 2012).

Hormones

Hormones can affect the voice in both positive and negative ways. Generally speaking, standard birth control pills used for contraception do not have adverse impact on voice unless they contain high levels of progesterone, as low levels of natural (not synthetic) progesterone are not reported to adversely impact voice (Sataloff et al., 2006). For readers seeking more information regarding the effects of birth control pills on singers, there are several recent studies examining possible voice impact (Benninger & Murry, 2006; Lã, Sundberg, Howard, Sa-Couto, & Freitas, 2012; Lã, Ledger, Davidson, Howard, & Jones, 2007). Androgens are sometimes used to treat endometriosis and also in treatment for certain types of cancer. Treatment of these disorders are paramount, but androgens can permanently lower pitch range (Titze & Verdolini Abbot, 2012). For the aging singer, hormone replacement and specifically estrogen is sometimes used to balance effects of aging on the voice (Benninger & Murry, 2006). Women approaching menopause should balance these choices with a knowledgeable physician who understands potential impact on voice as well as overall health risks of a given individual. Different than traditional hormone replacement therapy, popular media has touted the positive benefits of bioidenical hormone therapy and testosterone pellet therapy from increased libido to improved muscle mass. Efficacy related to these therapies and both the short-term and long-term effects on voice and general health are unknown. Singers are advised with caution to discuss all potential risks and benefits of these therapies with their physician.

Systemic Corticosteroids

Uses for systemic corticosteroids are vast because they act as an immune suppressor as well as an anti-inflammatory. The use of systemic steroids to treat vocal fold inflammation due to a variety of reasons is efficacious in appropriate medical situations and conditions (Benninger & Murry, 2006). Decisions on how and when to use steroids in a singer should be left to the discretion of the singer's otolaryngologist. The continued and repeated use of steroids as a means to keep performing through a chronic vocal problem (as opposed to fixing the problem) may be ill-advised in the professional vocal athlete.

Recreational Drugs

Epidemiologic reports on substance abuse in the United States regarding the incidence and prevalence indicate the use of legal and illegal drugs is problematic. There are no specific reports on recreational drug use in singers, but the media has publicized the deaths of many elite performers due to drug overdose from Elvis Presley to Cory Monteith. A recent article in *Today* reports on the drug and alcohol issues classical singers face (http://www.today.com/id/20394770/ns/today-today_entertainment/t/pressure-driving-opera-singers-alcohol-drugs/#.UhkMhz91Nc4). Effects of recreational drugs vary depending on how they are administered and substance used, ranging from edema and erythema of the mucosal lining of the respiratory track and larynx to incapacitation and ultimate death. In the fast and furious world of performance, attending parties, maintaining energy, and masking underlying emotional conditions often results in actors and singers resorting to drug or alcohol abuse. The National Alcoholism and Substance Abuse Information Center provides a state-by-state listing of help and treatment centers for all income levels (http://www.addictioncareoptions.com/).

Reflux Medications

Medications to treat acid reflux fall in three general categories: antacids, H2 blockers, and proton pump inhibitors. There are now combination drugs that include both an H2 blocker and proton pump inhibitor. A complete discussion on how reflux may affect the voice is covered in Chapter 7. Table 10–1 provides an overview of the types of available reflux medications by category and possible benefits and risks associated with each class of drugs.

Herbal Supplements and Vitamins

The Food and Drug Administration has set forth a policy in 2006 on defining complementary and alternative medicine (CAM)

TABLE 10–1. Reflux Medications

Drug	How It Works	Contraindications
ANTACIDS		
Alka-Seltzer*, BromoSeltzer (Sodium bicarbonate antacid) *also contains aspirin	Neutralizes acid	Do not use if you have high blood pressure or a salt-restricted diet; Check for possible drug interactions
Tums, Alka-Mints (Calcium carbonate)	Neutralizes acid	Constipation Check for possible drug interactions
Amphojel (Aluminum-based antacid)	Neutralizes acid	May cause calcium loss. Do not use if you have kidney problems; Check for possible drug interactions
Phillips Milk of Magnesia (Magnesium compound)	Neutralizes acid	Diarrhea; Check for possible drug interactions
Maalox, Mylanta, Riopan (Aluminum-magnesium antacids)	Neutralizes acid	Check for possible drug interactions; kidney disease
Gaviscon (Alginic acid-a seaweed derivative)	Acts as a floating barrier that helps keep gastric juices from entering the esophagus	Check for possible drug interactions
H2 BLOCKERS		
Axid (nizatidine) Tagamet (cimetidine) Pepcid (famotidine) Zantac (ranitidine)	Decrease acid production in the stomach by preventing histamine from triggering the H2 receptors to produce more acid	May increase blood-alcohol level when drinking; Check for possible drug interactions

TABLE 10–1. *continued*

Drug	How It Works	Contraindications
PROTON PUMP INHIBITORS (PPI's)		
Nexium (esomeprazole) Prevacid (lansoprazole) Protonix (pantoprazole) AcipHex (rabeprazole) Prilosec (omeprazole) Dexilant (dexlansoprazole)	Decreases acid production by blocking the last step in gastric juice secretion (H+/ K+ATPase)	May inhibit B-12 absorption Long-term use may impact bone density
COMBINATION DRUGS		
Zegrid (Sodium bicarbonate + omeprazole)		

to include the use of herbal supplements and vitamins (http://www.fda.gov/OHRMS /DOCKETS/98FR/06D-0480-GLD0001 .PDF). Additionally, the National Institutes for Health provides an excellent online resource for many of the most common herbs that can be downloaded to smartphones and tablet devices for easy reference: http:// nccam.nih.gov/health/herbsataglance .htm. Another resource for both herbs and vitamins is: http://www.nlm.nih.gov/med lineplus/druginfo/herb_All.html. Cautionary risks when using AMT includes the potential of triggering hormonal activity, vitamin toxicity, effect on blood pressure, and anticoagulation effects are documented in the literature with respect to singers (Surrow & LoVetri, 2000).

Herbs

Herbs and herbal supplements are plant derivatives and can come from any part of the plant (leaves, roots, stems, flowers, or seeds). Depending on the intended use, these plants can be sold as a whole or broken down and mixed with other substances (water, alcohol, solvents). Herbs are used in many forms (teas, pill forms, applied to the skin, used in bath water). Depending on the method used on how the chemicals are extracted from the plant, the end herbal product may contain: fatty acids, sterols, alkaloids, flavonoids, glycosides, and saponins (Bent, 2008). Therefore, consumers of herbs must be cautious and educated in the risks and benefits as best they can. Some considerations when using any herb, just as any medication includes benefits, risks, side effect, recommended dosing, allergic reaction, and knowledge of the manufacturer of the herb. Table 10–2 provides common herbs used within the United States (reprinted from Benninger & Murry, 2006), with Table 10-3 providing additional supplements reported to be often used by singers.

Vitamins and Minerals

Vitamin and mineral imbalance in the body (excess or deficiency) sometimes results in

TABLE 10–2. Herbs Used for Medicinal Purposes

Herbal Supplement	Indications	Actions	Contraindications	Side Effects	Interactions	Dosage
Echinacea	Treatment and prevention of the common cold and flu	Immunostimulant Enhances phagocytosis	Autoimmune or chronic illness Allergy to flowers of the daisy family	Minor gastrointestinal irritation Increased urination Mild allergic reactions	Immune suppressants (i.e., oral prednisone imuran methotrexate)	As powder extract: 300 mg cap/TID Alcohol tincture (1:5): 3–4 ml TID Juice: 203 ml TID Whole dried root: 100–200 g TID
Goldenseal	Topical antibiotic for wounds that are not healing well Mouth sores and sore throats	Strong activity against a wide variety of bacteria and fungi	Pregnancy	Gastrointestinal distress Increased nervousness		As cream, cover entire surface of the wound Tincture: swish or gargled Tea: 0.5–1 g in a cup of water
Ginseng	Tonic Stimulant Diuretic Diabetic impotence	Physiologic effects Lower blood pressure Depress CNS activity Stimulates immune system	Coagulopathy Diabetes Insomnia Schizophrenia Cardiac disease	Bleeding Hypotension Hypoglycemia Insomnia	Medications for: Psychosis Diabetes MAO inhibitors Stimulants Coumadin Caffeine	American: Root: 0.25–0.5 po BID Asian (Panax): 0.6–3 gm 1–3 times daily

Herb	Uses	Actions	Pregnancy	Side Effects	Interactions	Dosage
Black Cohosh	Menopause Astringent Diuretic Expectorant Vertigo Tinnitus	Estrogen-like action Oxytocic Luteinizing hormone suppression Binds to estrogen receptors	None known	Occasional GI upset, nausea, headache and dizziness in high doses	None known	Extracts w/ alcohol: 40–60% (v/v) corresponds to 40 mg drug
Garlic	Reduces levels of lipids in blood Prevents age-dependent vascular changes Lowers Cholesterol 10–12%	Antibacterial Antimycotic Lipid-lowering Inhibition of platelet aggregation Prolongation of bleed and clotting time Enhances fibrinolytic activity	None known	GI upset Allergic reactions Odor may pervade breath and skin	Anticoagulants Hypoglycemic	4 g fresh garlic (minced bulb and prep is taken orally)
Pulsatilla	Sedative, headaches Fluid in the ears	Antispasmodic Increases circulation Antibacterial	Avoid during pregnancy	GI upset Topically skin irritation Mild renal and urinary tract irritation	None known	120–300 TID
St. John's Wort	Dizziness, Tinnitus Mild to moderate depression Viral infections Would healing	Antidepressant Weak MAOI SSRI and dopamine agonist	Avoid in pregnancy	Photosensitivity	Anti-depressants MAOI Anti-seizure meds Birth control	300 mg TID

continues

TABLE 10-2. *continued*

Herbal Supplement	Indications	Actions	Contraindications	Side Effects	Interactions	Dosage
Ma Huang	Asthma Bronchial edema (weight loss—not an approved use) Stimulant	Sympathomimetic Bronchodilator	Cardiac problems Anxiety Hypertension Angle closure glaucoma Phoechromocytoma Thyrotoxcicant	Hypertension neurosis Insomnia Palpitations Hyperglycemia Death	Halothone Cardiac glycosides MAOI Guanethedine Oxytosh	15–30 mg total alkaloid Or 300 mg herb/day
Gingko Biloba	Dementia Improve cognitive, sexual, and GI functions Dizziness/tinnitus	Increased CNS blood flow Neuroprotective Free Radical Lowers capillary fragility	If the patient is on anticoagulants	Spontaneous bleeding (rare) Headaches and gastrointestinal irritation	Cyclosporine SSRIs MAO inhibitors Thiazide diuretics Anticoagulant properties may induce seizures, infertility	120–480 mg/day in 2–3 divided doses
Saw Palmetto	Anti-inflammatory Increases urinary flow Lowers symptoms of BPH	Inhibits dihydro-testosterone Diuretic Anti-androgenic	Do not take while on prescription BPH treatment	None	Caution with diuretics	160 mg BID

	Uses	Mechanism	Contraindications	Side Effects	Interactions	Dosage
Pygeum Africanum	Symptoms of BPH Anti-inflammatory Diuretic Lowers cholesterol	Anti-proliferative effect on fibroblast	None reported	Nausea and abdominal pain	None known	50–200 mg stand ext/day
Guarana	Stimulant Headache Increases energy	Sympathomimetic Caffeine-like activities	Cardiac problems Renal disease HTN or hyperthyroidism	Increased heart rate HTN Anxiety Arrhythmias	Avoid other stimulants	Not specified
Feverfew	Migraine Rheumatoid arthritis	Inhibits serotonin release	Aster family allergies Avoid during pregnancy	GI upset 6–15% first week of use	Anticoagulants (inhib cycloxgenic)	50 mg–1.2 gm/d equivalent to 0.2–0.6
Hawthorne	Atherosclerosis Arrhythmia	Improves cardiac output and coronary blood flow	Do not use with other inotropes	Mildly sedative	Digitalis Fox Glove	160–900 mg/day

Source: From Benninger, M., & Murry, T. (2006). *The Performer's Voice*, Plural Publishing. Reprinted with permission.

TABLE 10-3. Additional Herbs Commonly Used by Singers: Uses, Potential Benefits, Risks, & Side Effects

Herb	Use	Efficacy Data	Potential Side Effects
Grapeseed Extract	Heart, blood vessels, blood pressure, cholesterol, circulation, wound healing, cancer, vision, and nerve problems due to diabetes.	Clinical trials have been conducted on some aspects of this herb related to several of its compounds. Ongoing research continues. Findings indicated efficacy for reducing swelling after surgery, diabetic retinopathy, vascular fragility, prevention of cell damage caused by free radicals.	Has been used up to 8 weeks safely in clinical trials; side effects reported: nausea, itchy scalp, dizziness, headache, elevated blood pressure, hives, and stomach upset.
Papaya Enzymes (*Carica papaya*)	Digestion	Papain (one of the components of papaya) is a vegetable pepsin and research is unclear on whether it may improve healing related to digestive issues.	Liver, pancreas, do not take if allergic to latex. Other side effects reported: dizziness, rash, heartburn, chest pain, effortful swallow.
Peppermint Oil	Upset stomach/irritable bowel	May improve symptoms of IBS.	Allergic reactions and heartburn.
Ginger	Nausea	Effective for short-term use during pregnancy. Studies are mixed regarding benefits for nausea stemming from chemotherapy or motion.	Gas, bloating heartburn, nausea (most commonly reported when ginger was taken in powdered form).

Chamomile: German & Roman	Insomnia/upset stomach	Lacks human trials for efficacy data. Small studies report it may provide some healing of oral ulcers in patients following chemo or radiation therapy. Possibility of improving nausea when combined with other herbs.	Skin rashes, throat swelling, anaphylactic reaction; People allergic to plants in the daisy family (ragweed, chrysanthemum, marigolds, daisies) should not consume.
Green Tea	Cancer/mental alertness/weight loss/ skin protection	Mixed results on cancer. May reduce or slow cancer growth in certain types of cancers. Possible improvement in mental alertness due to caffeine.	Liver problems, caffeine may cause side effects, possible interaction with anticoagulant drugs.
Aloe Vera	Topical-wound healing Oral-laxative	Topical—Effective for light abrasions and burns. Not effective in deep surgical wound healing or radiation burns Oral—Strong laxative compound	Oral—diarrhea, abdominal cramps, may alter blood-glucose levels, link to large intestine tumors in rats (nondecolorized whole leaf extract)

Note: Since printing of Benninger and Murry text, Kava-Kava has been shown to cause liver toxicity.

unwanted physical manifestation. Similar to self-medicating with herbs, singers often take it upon themselves to add multivitamins or specific vitamins and minerals to their diet. Maximum safe dosing, indications for use, contraindications, interactions with other drugs, and foods where vitamins are naturally found for Vitamins A, B6, B12, C, D, E, and K can be found at The Office of Dietary Supplements at the National Institutes of Health (http://ods.od.nih.gov/). By eating a nutritionally balanced diet, most people in civilized nations will obtain the appropriate amount of vitamins and minerals to maintain health. Minerals that your body requires to function properly include: calcium, phosphorus, magnesium, sodium, potassium, chloride, sulfur, iron, manganese, copper, iodine, zinc, cobalt, fluoride, and selenium. The amount of each of these minerals your body needs varies and too much or too little can impact function of the body systems. Readers are again referred to The Office of Dietary Supplements at the National Institutes of Health (http://ods.od.nih.gov/) for full guidance on risks and benefits of many of these minerals. The three most commonly reported vitamins (C & E) and mineral (zinc) reported to be used by singers are briefly discussed with respect to singers.

Vitamin C

Ascorbic acid (Vitamin C) is often taken in large amounts to ward off a cold. The actual beneficial effects of taking vitamin C for the treatment of a common cold yield mixed results in the literature with studies indicating little-to-no impact on the treatment of the common cold (Hemilä & Chalker, 2013). If too much vitamin C is taken, it can have a dehydrating effect to the laryngeal mucosa because it causes frequent urination. Additionally, the acidic content when it is as high as it is dosed in certain over-the-counter cold prevention remedies can be problematic for singers who suffer from reflux (http://www.medicinenet.com/ascorbicacid-oral/article.htm).

Vitamin E

Providing immune health, supplying antioxidants, and improving the width of blood vessels to promote blood flow are some of the positive effects that a proper amount of vitamin E provides. Too much vitamin E may increase the risk of bleeding, specifically brain bleeds (intracranial hemorrhage). There is significant research on vitamin E regarding everything from its role in wound healing to immune boosting effects.

Zinc

Zinc is a necessary mineral for the body to have for fighting infection and wound healing. But, zinc deficiency in the United States is rare. The use of zinc lozenges to ward off a cold or reduce the length of a cold has been studied. Preliminary research indicates that zinc lozenges (not syrup or tablets) in doses ≥75 mg taken within 24 hours of the onset of cold symptoms may reduce severity and length of a cold (Singh & Das, 2013). However, appropriate dosing and long-term use are unproven and in people with potentially compromised immune systems or other health problems, may be contraindicated. Further research is warranted.

Myths and Truths about Dryness

Laryngeal and pharyngeal dryness as well as "thick, sticky, mucus" are often complaints of singers. Combating these concerns on how to maintain adequate viscosity of mucus for performance has resulted in some research on the topic. Specifically, there are many nonregulated products on the market for performers that lay claim to improving the laryngeal environment (Entertainer's Secret, Throat Coat Tea, Greathers Pastilles, Slippery Elm, etc.). Although there may be little detriment in using these products, quantitative research documenting change in mucosa is sparse. The following section will highlight some of the more popular choices singers use to combat dryness and/or promote vocal wellness.

Honey

Honey is a demulcent that has a long tradition of use in less Westernized medicine. There have been clinical studies demonstrating both antibacterial and anti-inflammatory effects of honey for cutaneous wounds such as burns. The chemical make-up of honey (low pH and high sugar content) reduces growth of microbes, and can stimulate wound-healing response. There are medical grade, therapeutic honeys that appear to have higher levels of antibacterial function (Lusby, Coombes, & Wilkinson, 2002; Mandal & Mandal, 2011). While these anti-inflammatory and antibacterial benefits have not been specifically rigorously studied on impact of oral and pharyngeal mucosa, there is potential for some benefit. Honey has also shown to be promising as an effective cough suppressant in the pediatric population (Shadkam, Mozaffari-Khosravi, & Mozayan, 2010). The dose of honey given to the children with cough that was found to be efficacious was 2 teaspoons. Efficacy of honey for reduction of adult cough has not been examined.

Slippery Elm

Found in Throat Coat tea and in lozenges, slippery elm bark contains mucilage that becomes a thick, gel-like coating when mixed with moisture. This then creates a coating on oral and pharyngeal mucosa, creating a feeling of lubrication. Additionally, antioxidant components in slippery elm are thought to create an anti-inflammatory response in addition to increase in mucus production (http://health.howstuffworks.com/wellness/natural-medicine/herba remedies/slippery-elm-herbal-remedies.htm).

Gargling

Gargling is sometimes used by singers to soothe a dry sore throat. There are numerous recipes and suggestions online for various types of gargling from lemon juice to "kill bacteria in the throat" to vodka to "loosen the vocal folds" to salt water to "exfoliate and clean your vocal folds." Of course, these effects have not been studied, and the current authors do not advocate these claims, as certainly one would not want their folds "exfoliated" (and nothing that is gargled actually touches the vocal folds in any capacity).

The use of salt water as a gargle has long been used as a remedy for sore throat. Traced back to China thousands of years ago, this salt water solution was used for treating gum disease because it was thought to have both analgesic (reduces pain) and antibacterial properties (http://health.howstuffworks.com/wellness/oral care/products/saltwater-as-mouthwash.htm). Oversaturation of the water solution with excess salt may act to draw water out of the oral mucosa, thus reducing inflammation. Among the more notable gargle recipes among singers is Dr. Wilbur Gould's gargle recipe. This recipe has been used by singers and the recipe is readily available online, with various descriptions and modifications. Below is the most basic recipe. The contents in the gargle are in small amounts and are not ingested (only gargled and then spit out). Ostensibly, the salt and baking soda are present for potential antibacterial components, and the syrup or honey for its coating and demulcent properties. To date, this specific combination of these ingredients has not been clinically proved to improve vocal functioning, but most likely, they are not harmful in these small amounts, and if singers perceive benefit then they can continue to use.

There are studies that have shown gargling to reduce URI symptoms compared to controls who didn't gargle. In a randomized controlled trial, on almost 400 volunteer subjects, the subjects who were instructed to gargle only water at least 3 times per day demonstrated 36% fewer episodes of URI compared with the group of subjects who did not engage in a gargling regimen. The authors attributed this to the facts that rhinovirus has an 8- to 12-hour incubation period. Therefore, frequent gargling of water rinses pathogens from oral and pharyngeal mucosa, reducing proliferation of these pathogens (Satomura et al., 2005).

Oral and Pharyngeal Moisturizers (Sprays and Teas)

Singers are often partial to herbal teas and sprays for additional oral and pharyngeal hydration. One study suggests that the use of Throat Coat tea (containing slippery

---

Dr. Gould's gargle recipe:
½ tsp sea salt (or kosher salt)
½ tsp baking soda
½ tsp corn syrup, honey, or maple
    syrup
1 cup warm water
Gargle silently, do not rinse for
    5 minutes

---

elm) when compared with a placebo treatment for pharyngitis did show a significant positive difference in soreness. Entertainer's Secret is also a popular over-the-counter throat spray used to increase oral and pharyngeal hydration. The long nozzle allows for delivery of glycerin in a mist form into the oral, pharyngeal, and nasal cavities. One study compared the use of Entertainer's Secret to two other nebulized agents and its possible effect on phonation threshold pressure (PTP). This study indicated there was no positive benefit in decreasing PTP by using Entertainer's Secret (Brinckmann, Sigwart, van Houten Taylor, 2003; Roy, Tanner, Gray, Blomgren, & Fisher, 2003). However, many singers empirically report benefit from use of such sprays, which may or may not be due to placebo effect.

Sinus Flushing and Nasal Rinsing

Neti pots and sinus flushes have become more popular over recent years for management of sinus and allergy related symptoms. Additionally, saline irrigation can be helpful when used in the short term to assist with mucociliary clearance (Brown & Grahm, 2004; Dunn, Dion, & McMains, 2013). However, a new study has reported that nasal saline irrigation when used daily for long periods of time (longer than 10 to 14 days, or 8 weeks if after sinus surgery) actually may wash away beneficial mucus that possesses infection-fighting, antifungal, and antiviral properties. Results from a study of 68 subjects showed that patients using long-term nasal saline irrigation had 62.5% more episodes of rhinosinusitis after they discontinued use. This information suggests that these techniques should be used during a cold or allergy episode, but perhaps not for longer than 10 days, as this could lead to additional problems with

Saline Sinus Rinse Recipe's (from American Academy of Allergy, Asthma, & Immunology)

1. Iodine-free salt (no anti-caking agents or preservatives)
2. Baking soda
3. Distilled or boiled water
4. Sterile jar/container

Mix 3 teaspoons of the salt with 1 teaspoon of baking soda and store in an airtight container.

Add 1 teaspoon of the above mixture into 8 ounces of lukewarm distilled/boiled (and cooled) water.

Use less of the salt/baking soda mixture if burning or stinging is noted

rhinosinusitis. Additionally, this professor of allergy/immunology highlighted the importance of keeping the nasal irrigation device very clean and dry; using distilled sterile, or boiled water. These guidelines may be important in preventing introduction of bacteria into the nasal mucosa, which can have harmful effects. He also recommends replacing the entire irrigation device every couple of months (Nsouli, 2009).

Hydration

The concept that singers need to be well-hydrated for optimal voice functioning is not only part of traditional conventional wisdom passed down from generations of voice pedagogues, but it has also now been scientifically studied and validated (Verdolini-Marston, Sandage, & Titze, 1994;

Verdolini-Marston, Titze, & Drucker, 1990). The exact amount of water needed to achieve adequate hydration needs will vary based on humidity, level of activity, sweat, and elevation. Dr. Van Lawrence popularized the phrase "Sing Wet, Pee Pale" as a gauge for his students to determine if they were adequately hydrated. As a general guideline, singers can use this as a gauge keeping in mind that certain medications and even vitamins may alter the color of urine. Due to the varying levels of physical and vocal activity of many performers, in order to maintain adequate oral hydration, the use of a hydration calculator based on activity level may be a better choice. These hydration calculators are easily accessible online and take into account the amount and level of activity the performer engages in on a daily basis. They are intended to provide a general guideline for intake based on activity level, but are not intended to take place of medical advise. In a recent study of the vocal habits of musical theater performers, one of the findings indicated a significantly under hydrated group of performers (Donahue, LeBorgne, Brehm, Weinrich, 2013, in press).

When pursuing the Internet, there are several recommendations that indicate that swallowing certain things will directly hydrate, or "clean" the vocal folds. This of course is inaccurate, as anything swallowed goes into the esophagus and bypasses the vocal folds completely unless the singer is choking on the substance. As a reminder of laryngeal and swallowing anatomy, nothing that is swallowed (or gargled) goes over or touches the vocal folds directly (or one would choke). The effects of systemic hydration are well-documented. There is evidence to suggest that adequate hydration will provide some protection of the laryngeal mucous membranes when they are placed under increased collision forces as well as reducing the amount of effort (phonation threshold pressure) to produce voice (Leydon, Sivasankar, Falciglia, Atkins, & Fisher, 2009; Leydon, Wroblewski, Eichorn, & Sivasankar, 2010; Sivasankar & Leydon, 2010; Verdolini-Marston, Sandage, & Titze, 1994; Yiu & Chan, 2003). These mechanisms are not fully understood, but there is enough evidence at this time to support that adequate oral hydration should be a component of every singer's vocal health regime to maintain appropriate mucosal viscosity.

Although very rare, overhydration (hyperhidrosis) can result in dehydration and even illness or death. An over indulgence of fluids essentially makes the kidneys work "overtime" and flushes too much water out of the body. This excessive fluid loss in a rapid manner can be detrimental to the body.

Steam and Humidifiers

Personal steam inhalers and/or room humidification to supplement oral hydration and aid in combating laryngeal dryness are used by many singers. There are several considerations for singers who choose to use external means of adding moisture to the air they breathe. Personal steam inhalers are portable and can often be used backstage or in the hotel room for the traveling performer. Typically, water is placed in the steamer, and the face is placed over the steam for inhalation. Because the mucus membranes of the larynx are composed of a salt water solution, one study looked at the use of nebulized saline in comparison with plain water and its potential effects on phonation effort in classically trained sopranos (Tanner et al., 2010). Data suggested that perceived effort to produce voice was less in the saline group than the plain water group.

In addition to personal steamers, other options of humidifiers come in varying sizes from room size to whole house humidifiers. When choosing between a warm air or cool mist humidifier, considerations include: personal preference and needs. One of the primary reasons warm mist humidifiers are not recommended for young children is due to the risk of burns from the heating element/hot water. Both the warm mist and cool air humidifiers act similarly in adding moisture to the environmental air. External air humidification may be beneficial and provide a level of comfort for many singers. Regular cleaning of the humidifier is vital to prevent bacteria and mold buildup. Also, depending on the hardness of the water, it is important to avoid mineral buildup on the device.

For traveling performers who often stay in hotels, fly on airplanes, or are generally exposed to other dry-air environments, there are products on the market designed to help minimize drying effects. One such device is called a Humidfly (http://www.humidiflyer.com/) and is purported to recycle the moisture in the person's own breath and replenish moisture on each breath.

Lemon

Lemon has a low pH, and therefore considered to have some antibacterial components. Although commonly used by singers in teas and gargles, there have not been extensive studies on impact of using lemon as part of a vocal hygiene regimen to maintain vocal health or reduced symptoms of upper respiratory infections. Additionally, those who have laryngopharyngeal reflux would be cautioned to consider the acidic impact of consuming excessive amounts of lemon.

Apple Cider Vinegar

Another popular home remedy reported by singers is the use of apple cider vinegar to help with everything from acid reflux to sore throats. Dating back to 3300 BC, apple cider vinegar was reported as a medicinal remedy and it became popular in the 1970s as a weight loss diet cocktail. Popular media reports apple cider vinegar can improve conditions from acne and arthritis to nosebleeds and varicose veins (http://www.healthline.com/natstandardcontent/apple-cider-vinegar). Specific efficacy data regarding the beneficial nature of apple cider vinegar for the purpose of sore throat, pharyngeal inflammation, and or reflux has not been reported in the literature at this time. Of the peer reviewed studies found in the literature, one discussed possible esophageal erosion and inconsistency of actual product in tablet form (Hill, Woodruff, Foote, & Barreto-Alcoba, 2005).

Neck Warmth (Scarves)

Singers are often seen in the heat of summer tightly wrapped in a neck scarf. The traditions of wrapping the neck are traced back to Northern European roots where the covering of the neck was used to keep the throat warm and protect it from the elements. No specific scientific data supporting or refuting this claim could be found. There is likely no harm in using a scarf, and using the scarf to cover the mouth and nose when in excessively cold temperatures may provide some comfort and warming of air as it is inhaled, but the claims of improved health and performance cannot be verified by independent scientific publications at this time.

Chapter Summary

Singers commonly use combinations of alternative medical therapies, over-the-counter medicines and herbs, and prescribed medicines to promote wellness and combat illness. These are often necessary to allow for singers to fulfill contracts and remain employed. Several regimens and remedies are relatively innocuous and though not scientifically proven, may provide the singer with a certain amount of mental and physical relief of symptoms. Other remedies, however, could have potential adverse effects on the voice or even general wellness due to potential interactions with other medicines or side effects. Therefore, singers should be cautioned to discuss with their physician all possible options of a wellness regimen, both AMT and prescription, in order to minimize any possible adverse effects. Singers should be aware of the many possible impacts of medicines on voice and discuss alternative options with the physician if medically appropriate. The references and websites included in this chapter provide the singer with general information keeping in mind that many of these modalities are not proven or regulated and should always be discussed with a physician.

References

Benninger, M., & Murry, T. (2006). *The performer's voice*. San Diego, CA: Plural Publishing.

Bent, S. (2008). Herbal medicine in the United States: Review of efficacy, safety, and regulation: Grand rounds at University of California, San Francisco Medical Center. *Journal of General Internal Medicine, 23*(6), 854–859.

Brinckmann, J., Sigwart, H., & van Houten Taylor, L. (2003). Safety and efficacy of a traditional herbal medicine (Throat Coat) in symptomatic temporary relief of pain in patients with acute pharyngitis: A multicenter, prospective, randomized, double-blinded, placebo-controlled study. *Journal of Alternative and Complementary Medicine, 9*(2), 285–298.

Brown, C., & Grahm, S. (2004). Nasal irrigations: Good or bad? *Current Opinion in Otolaryngology, Head and Neck Surgery, 12*(1), 9–13.

Chan, R., & Tayama, N. (2002). Biomechanical effects of hydration in vocal fold tissues. *Otolaryngology-Head & Neck Surgery, 126*(5), 528–537.

Donahue, E., LeBorgne, W., Brehm, S., & Weinrich, B. (in press). Reported vocal habits of first-year undergraduate musical theatre majors in a pre-professional training program: A ten-year retrospective study. *Journal of Voice.*

Dunn, J., Dion, G., & McMains, K. (2013). Efficacy of nasal symptom relief. *Current Opinion in Otolaryngology, Head and Neck Surgery, 21*(3), 248–251.

Erickson, E., & Sivasankar, M. (2010). Evidence for adverse phonatory change following an inhaled combination treatment. *Journal of Speech-Language-Hearing Research, 53*(1), 75–83.

Ernst, E. (2002). The risk-benefit profile of commonly used herbal therapies: Ginkgo, St. John's Wort, Ginseng, Echinacea, Saw Palmetto, and Kava. *Annals of Internal Medicine, 136*(1), 42–53.

Gallivan, G. J., Gallivan, K. H., & Gallivan, H. K. (2007). Inhaled corticosteroids: Hazardous effects on voice-an update. *Journal of Voice, 21*(1), 101–111.

Gupta, S. (2008, January 17). Herbal remedies' potential dangers. *Time,* http://www.time.com/time/specials/2007/article/.

Hemilä, H., & Chalker, E. (2013). Vitamin C for preventing and treating the common cold. *Cochrane Database System Review, 1*(Jan 31).

Hill, L., Woodruff, L., Foote, J., & Barreto-Alcoba, M. (2005). Esophageal injury by apple cider vinegar tablets and subsequent evaluation of products. *Journal of the American Dietetics Association, 105*(7), 1141–1144.

Lã, F., Ledger, W., Davidson, J., Howard, D., & Jones, G. (2007). The effects of a third generation combined oral contraceptive pill on the classical singing voice. *Journal of Voice, 21*(6), 754–761.

Lã, F., Sundberg, J., Howard, D., Sa-Couto, P., & Freitas A. (2012). Effects of the menstrual cycle and oral contraception on singers' pitch control. *Journal of Speech Language Hearing Research, 55*(1), 247–261.

Lavy, J., Wood, G., Rubin, J., & Harries, M. (2000). Dysphonia associated with inhaled steroids. *Journal of Voice, 14*(4), 581–588.

Lawerence, V. (1987). Common medications with laryngeal effects. *Ear Nose Throat Journal, 66*(8), 318–322.

Leydon, C., Sivasankar, M., Falciglia, D., Atkins, C., & Fisher, K. (2009). Vocal fold surface hydration: A review. *Journal of Voice, 23*(6), 658–665.

Leydon, C., Wroblewski, M., Eichorn, N., & Sivasankar, M. (2010). A meta-analysis of outcomes of hydration intervention on phonation threshold pressure. *Journal of Voice, 24*(6), 637–643.

Lusby, P., Coombes, A., & Wilkinson, J. (2002). Honey: A potent agent for wound healing? *Journal of Wound Ostomy Continence Nursing, 29*(6), 295–300.

Mandal, M., & Mandal, S. (2011). Honey: Its medicinal property and antibacterial activity. *Asian Pacific Journal of Tropical Biomedicine, April*(2), 154–160.

Miri, A., Barthelat, F., & Mongeau L. (2012). Effects of dehydration on the viscoelastic properties of vocal folds in large deformations. *Journal of Voice, 26*(6), 688–697.

Nsouli, T. (2009). *Long-term use of nasal saline irrigation: Harmful or helpful?* American College of Allergy, Asthma & Immunology (ACAAI) 2009 Annual Scientific

Meeting: Abstract 32. Presented November 8, 2009.

Roy, N., Tanner, K., Gray, S., Blomgren, M., & Fisher, K. (2003). An evaluation of the effects of three laryngeal lubricants on phonation threshold pressure (PTP). *Journal of Voice, 17*(3), 331–342.

Sahrawat, R., Robb, M., Kirk R., & Beckert L. (2013, April 9). Effects of inhaled corticosteroids on voice production in healthy adults. *Logopedics Phoniatrics Vocology.* Advance online publication.

Sataloff, R., Hawkshaw, M., & Anticaglia, J. (2006). Medications and the voice. In R. Sataloff (Ed.), *Vocal health and pedagogy—Advances assessment and treatment* (2nd ed.). San Diego, CA: Plural Publishing.

Satomura, K., Kitamura, T., Kawamura, T., Shimbo, T., Watanabe, M., Kamei, M., . . . Tamakoshi, A. (2005). Prevention of upper respiratory tract infections by gargling: A randomized trial. *American Journal of Preventative Medicine, 29*(4), 302–307.

Shadkam, M., Mozaffari-Khosravi, H., & Mozayan, M. (2010). A comparison of the effect of honey, dextromethorphan, and diphenhydramine on nightly cough and sleep quality in children and their parents. *Journal of Alternative and Complementary Medicine, 16*(7), 787–793.

Singh, M., & Das, R. (2013). Zinc for the common cold. *Cochrane Database System Review, 6.*

Sivasankar, M., & Leydon, C. (2010). The role of hydration in vocal fold physiology. *Current Opinion in Otolaryngology Head & Neck Surgery, 18*(3), 171–175.

Surrow, J., & LoVetri, J. (2000). Alternative medical therapy use among singers: Prevalence and implications for the medical care of the singer. *Journal of Voice, 14*(3), 398–409.

Tanner, K., Roy, N., Merrill, R., Muntz, F., Houtz, D., Sauder, C., Elstad, M., & Wright-Costa, J. (2010). Nebulized isotonic saline versus water following a laryngeal desiccation challenge in classically trained sopranos. *Journal of Speech Language and Hearing Research, 53*(6), 1555–1566.

Titze, I., & Verdolini Abbot, K. (2012). *Vocology: The science and practice of voice habilitation.* Salt Lake City, UT: The National Center for Voice and Speech.

Verdolini Abbot, K., Min, Y., Titze, I., Lemke, J., Brown, K., VanMersbergen, M., & Fisher, K. (2002). Biological mechanisms underlying voice changes due to dehydration. *Journal of Speech, Language, and Hearing Research, 45*, 268–281.

Verdolini-Marston, K., Sandage, M., & Titze, I. (1994). Effect of hydration treatments on laryngeal nodules and polyps and related voice measures. *Journal of Voice, 8*(1), 30–47.

Verdolini-Marston, K., Titze, I., & Drucker, D. (1990). Changes in phonation threshold pressure with induced conditions of hydration. *Journal of Voice, 4*(2), 142–151.

Yiu, E., & Chan, R. (2003). Effect of hydration and vocal rest on the vocal fatigue in amateur karaoke singers. *Journal of Voice, 17*, 216–227.

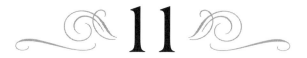

11

Multidisciplinary Care of the Vocal Athlete

LEDA SCEARCE

Introduction

For all people, the voice is intricately bound to personal identity, self-esteem, and self-image. The voice is our primary means of communication and expression, and it can be central to occupation, creativity, worship, and spirituality. This phenomenon becomes magnified for singers. For the singer, the voice is the source of livelihood and income, and artistic and creative expression. The voice is the vocal athlete's instrument, and unlike other instruments, it can never be replaced if irreparable damage occurs. A voice problem represents a crisis for the singer. Furthermore, the athleticism of singing and the demands of the singing career put vocal performers at high risk for developing a voice injury. When a voice injury occurs, it is essential that the singer receive comprehensive care that addresses all elements of their vocal health and that ensures efficient and effective outcomes so that they can return to performing at their optimal level as quickly as possible.

Voice problems are almost always multifactorial. Depending on the diagnosis and severity of the voice problem, the treatment plan may include surgical management, medications, lifestyle adjustments (e.g., changes in diet and sleep habits), optimizing vocal hygiene, improving vocal pacing (how much and how intensely one uses the voice and in what situations), and training to improve the efficiency of the speaking voice. For singers, the treatment plan becomes even more complex, as their rehabilitation will likely also include therapy that directly addresses the singing voice, including targeted rehabilitation exercises, counseling, and guidance in applying principles of voice efficiency into real-life performance situations. No single provider will have the education, training, experience, and qualifications to address all of these factors thoroughly, effectively, and efficiently. It takes a team to manage a singer's voice problem.

The Voice Care Team

The most important individual on the voice care team is the singer. The singer must know their own voice, must value their voice enough to seek care, must be dedicated enough to make the lifestyle changes necessary for recovery, and must commit to completing voice rehabilitation by attending therapy sessions and completing home practice regularly. Other key players on the singer's voice care team include the laryngologist, the speech-language pathologist, and the singing voice rehabilitation specialist. If the singer is currently taking voice lessons, the singing teacher is a critical member of the team as well. Depending on the nature of the voice disorder, referrals may be made to other physicians (such as neurologists, endocrinologists, gastroenterologists, pulmonologists, etc.) and/or to other health care providers such as physical therapists, dentists, or massage therapists. The team may also include nurses, nurse practitioners, physician assistants, and voice scientists (Benninger & Murry, 2006; Sataloff, 2006a, 2006b).

Credentials and Qualifications of the Voice Care Team

A laryngologist is an otolaryngologist who has specialized training in caring for voice problems. The laryngologist should be board certified in otolaryngology and fellowship trained in laryngology. However, it is important to keep in mind that the lar-

yngology fellowship was only established by the American Academy of Otolaryngology in 1990. Physicians who completed their residency prior to this date may not have completed a fellowship but may have achieved specialization in laryngology through other training paradigms (Sataloff, 2006a).

The speech-language pathologist who works with voice disorders should have his or her Certificate of Clinical Competence (CCC-SLP) from the American Speech-Language-Hearing Association and should be licensed by the state in which he or she practices (American Speech-Language-Hearing Association, 2001). Speech-language pathology is a very broad field, and training in evaluation and treatment of voice disorders is typically a very small part of the academic program. In most graduate speech-language pathology programs, students have a single course in voice disorders (sometimes only a half-semester course), and practical clinical experience may be limited to a single case. Some students complete their graduate program with no hands-on clinical experience in voice at all. Therefore, it is essential that the speech-language pathologist on the voice care team achieve specialization in voice beyond the minimum requirements. This can be achieved by seeking clinical internship experiences at a voice care center as part of their graduate training and through professional internship experiences and continuing education. This training should include in-depth study of the complete gamut of voice disorders; anatomy, physiology, and acoustics of voice; interpretation of laryngeal imaging including stroboscopy and high-speed video; execution and interpretation of instrumental voice measures, including acoustic and aerodynamic measures of voice and electroglottography (EGG); perceptual evaluation of voice; and administration and interpretation of self-assessment measures (Benninger & Murry, 2006; Roy, Barkmeier-Kraemer, Eadie, Sivasankar, Mehta, Paul, & Hillman, 2012).

Even though a clinician may be well prepared for rehabilitation of the speaking voice, singing voice rehabilitation is outside the realm of clinical practice for general speech-language pathologists. However, there are a small but growing number of speech-language pathologists/singing voice specialists who also have extensive experience as voice teachers and professional performers. Often they are "dual-trained," and most have at least a bachelor's or a master's degree in vocal performance/pedagogy in addition to their master's degree in speech-language pathology. According to many experts, this is the ideal background for the singing voice therapist (Sataloff, 2006b). Whenever possible, the vocal athlete should seek this specially trained clinical singing voice rehabilitation specialist to address their singing voice rehabilitation needs. There is currently no credentialing process or training program that specifically prepares one for clinical singing voice rehabilitation. However, there are degree programs in development, and it is likely that the coming decades will see increasing opportunities for those who seek this specialized training.

There are some voice centers that employ singing teachers who have sought extra knowledge in vocal health and voice disorders to provide singing voice rehabilitation in conjunction with a speech pathologist and laryngologist. In this situation, there are complexities in terms of how payment is made, as singing teachers are not able to bill insurance, as well as the concern of potential liability issues. In many cases, this arrangement works effectively, and the singing teacher works as part of the team with the physician and speech-language pathology providers (Sataloff, 2006a, 2006b).

Voice Care Team Collaboration

For optimal treatment results, the voice care providers should work as a team. This leads to a clearer diagnosis of the problem, a more comprehensive and integrated treatment plan, better monitoring of progress or identification of new problems, and better communication. This model also makes it easier for the singing patient to schedule their care. There are multiple models for how such collaborative team-management may be achieved. In some clinics, the laryngologist and speech-language pathologist and/or singing voice rehabilitation specialist may perform the evaluation simultaneously, making recommendations for medical, surgical, and behavioral components of the treatment plan together in the same visit. In other practices, the process occurs in a sequential or serial fashion, with the singing patient first seeing the laryngologist for medical evaluation and diagnosis. The laryngologist then refers the singer as needed to the speech-language pathologist and/or singing voice rehabilitation specialist, or to a singing teacher. These other providers may work in the same practice with the laryngologist or may work in a separate practice (Benninger & Murry, 2006; Sataloff, 2006a, 2006b).

The Voice Evaluation

The evaluation may also include use of a patient self-assessment tool of the impact of their voice complaint on their quality of life, such as the Voice Related Quality of Life (V-RQOL), Singer's Voice Handicap Index (*SVHI*), or Singer's Voice Handicap

The voice evaluation should include the following elements:

- Complete medical history and review of medications
- Complete head and neck examination
- Laryngeal imaging (videolaryngostroboscopy) completed by the laryngologist or speech pathologist
- Perceptual evaluation of speaking and singing voice (preferably including a standardized clinician administered assessment tool, such as the Consensus Auditory-Perceptual Evaluation of Voice (*CAPE-V*) or Grade, Roughness, Breathiness, Asthenia, Strain (*GRBAS*)
- History of the voice problem including onset and any associated precipitating factors
- Voice training history
- Assessment of voice use (speaking and singing)
- Assessment of vocal hygiene
- Acoustic and aerodynamic testing

Index-10 (*SVHI-10*). Some clinics are utilizing high-speed videography and videokymography in addition to videostroboscopy for laryngeal imaging, and some include electroglottography as part of the assessment. Following completion of the voice evaluation, the voice care team will make medical and communication diagnoses and recommendations for management and treatment plan, which may include surgical, medical, and/or behavioral intervention (Benninger & Murry, 2006; Hill-

man, 2013; Hirano & Bless, 1993; Roy et al., 2012).

Roles and Responsibilities of the Voice Care Team

All members of the vocal health team should provide vocal hygiene education (including recommendations for hydration, smoking cessation and avoidance, illness resistance, and minimizing infection risk) as well as vocal pacing. Team members must also be acutely aware that the singer may present in a heightened emotional state, and they must interact with the singer with compassion and understanding. The vocal health team must recognize that the singer may feel that he or she is in a crisis, as professional or academic success, livelihood, reputation, and future performing opportunities may all be jeopardized by their current voice problem. It is essential that the voice care team avoid use of the term "vocal abuse" as a concept and label. Voice injury is an occupational hazard and may reflect lack of education but is not "abuse." Use of such pejorative language may instill self-blame in the singer and may compromise the absolute trust that must be established between the singer and the voice care team.

The Singing Teacher's Role and Responsibilities

Review of the roles and responsibilities of the voice care team must begin with the patient's current singing teacher. The singing teacher is often on the front line for identifying a voice problem and is in the best position to ensure that appropriate referrals are made. The singing teacher is also most intimately acquainted with the singer's voice, voice history, and vocal habits, and can identify subtle changes in the voice.

In normal development of singing voice, the singing teacher is responsible for building technique in a healthy instrument. The singing teacher should be competent in a teaching technique that is style-appropriate to the singer. The singing teacher also teaches parameters of performance practice including diction, repertoire, stage deportment, and interpretation. The singing teacher should also teach appropriate practice protocol for the singer (American Speech-Language-Hearing Association, 2005; Roy et al., 2012)

Ideally, the singing teacher would work closely with the medical team managing the voice problem. In some cases, the singing teacher may work directly with the medical voice team, providing singing voice training or retraining under the supervision of the laryngologist, speech-language pathologist, and/or clinical singing voice rehabilitation specialist. In other cases, the singing teacher may function in a more auxiliary—but no less essential—role. This may include conferencing and consulting with the rehabilitation team to incorporate recommendations into ongoing voice training, or even attending singing voice therapy sessions so that he or she may ensure that strategies, techniques, and exercises are carried over into voice lessons and academic/professional singing activities while the singer is undergoing voice therapy and after discharge.

In some cases, the singing patient may not have any voice training background (this is often true for CCM singers) or may not currently be working with a singing teacher. In such cases, a singing teacher may become a part of the voice care team during the rehabilitation process, or the patient may be referred to an appropriate teacher in the community for ongoing voice training after completing the rehabilitation process (Benninger & Murry, 2006; Sataloff, 2006a, 2006b).

The Laryngologist's Role and Responsibilities

The laryngologist takes the patient's medical and voice history and conducts a full head and neck examination. This often includes laryngeal imaging as a means to diagnose laryngeal pathology via stroboscopy and in some cases, high-speed video. In some practices, the laryngeal imaging is conducted by the speech-language pathologist under the laryngologist's supervision. During image interpretation, the job of the speech-language pathologist is to interpret the impact of the injury on the vibratory characteristics of the vocal folds. Based on the laryngeal imaging results, the laryngologist makes a medical diagnosis of the voice problem (i.e., vocal fold lesions, paralysis or paresis, laryngitis, etc.). The laryngologist assesses and treats medical factors such as seasonal or chronic allergies, laryngopharyngeal reflux, and infections. The laryngologist provides surgical management of the voice problem when indicated and directs voice care with the speech-language pathologists and singing voice rehabilitation specialists. Voice re-evaluation with the laryngologist may be conducted at an interval appropriate to the diagnosis (Benninger & Murry, 2006; Sataloff, 2006a).

Steroids may be used as a diagnostic tool to get a clearer picture of underlying injury by temporarily resolving general edema. Steroids may also be necessary acutely to enable the singer to complete an important performance. It is important to avoid patient reliance on steroids, and stroboscopy should be conducted before prescribing steroids to ensure there is no contraindication and after treatment to ensure the injury has not been exacerbated (Sataloff, 2006b).

Allergy management may be provided by the laryngologist or through consultation with an allergy specialist. Singers should avoid systemically drying medications if at all possible (decongestants/antihistamines). The laryngologist may prescribe nasal treatment of allergies such as nasal steroid or antihistamine sprays instead. Sinus irrigation may be recommended as well as control of the patient's physical environment (bedding, floor covering, air filters, pets) (Sataloff, 2006b).

The laryngologist may prescribe medication for and provide information about behavioral management of laryngopharyngeal reflux. If reflux is determined to be inadequately managed through these interventions, the laryngologist may refer to a gastroenterologist for further assessment and recommendations (Benninger & Murry, 2006; Sataloff, 2006a).

Due to the complex nature of the voice, there are numerous medical problems that may be contributory. Any such factors, if present, will need to be addressed to achieve resolution of the voice problem. The laryngologist will make appropriate referrals to other physicians and practitioners as indicated. Examples may include referral to a neurologist for sleep disorders, dystonia, neck pain, and so on. A pulmonologist may be consulted for asthma, a rheumatologist for auto-immune dysfunction, or an endocrinologist for hormonal imbalance. A dentist, oral surgeon, or physical therapist may be helpful in managing temporomandibular joint dysfunction (TMJ). In some cases, referral to a psychiatrist or

psychologist may be indicated. (Benninger & Murry, 2006; Sataloff, 2006b).

The Speech-Language Pathologist's Role and Responsibilities

The speech-language pathologist who is ideally also a singing voice specialist, takes a detailed voice history. This should include onset and duration of the voice problem and any associated precipitating factors. Typical vocal demands should be reviewed, both for singing and speaking, including any phonotraumatic behaviors such as yelling or chronic throat clearing, as well as vocal hygiene habits such as hydration, caffeine, and alcohol intake and smoking history. While interviewing the patient, the speech-language pathologist will perceptually assess voice quality, coordination of breath to phonation, evident muscle tension, resonance, pitch, loudness, and vocal characteristics such as vocal fry, pitch, or phonation breaks (Benninger & Murry, 2006; Sataloff, 2006b).

In some clinics, the speech-language pathologist conducts the videostroboscopy and/or high-speed video examination. This may include use of flexible (distal chip) and/or rigid endoscope. Stroboscopy and high-speed video allow examination of the laryngeal structures, glottic closure, and vibratory patterns at various pitches. The examination provides information on vocal fold cover viscosity, vibration, and degree of closure (Hirano & Bless, 1993; Sataloff, 2006a).

The speech-language pathologist conducts and interprets acoustic and aerodynamic testing. Acoustic testing should include average fundamental frequency and pitch range. Measures of perturbation, noise-harmonic ratio, tremor, subharmonic noise, and soft phonation index have historically been included in acoustic testing, and are based on sustained vowel phonation (Benninger & Murry, 2006; Sataloff, 2006a). However, the results of some of these measures have not provided good correlation to perceptual ratings. New assessment programs have recently been developed that allow for acoustic assessment in continuous speech, such as the Analysis of Dysphonia and Speech and Voice (ADSV) from KayPentax, which performs cepstral-based measures. The ADSV is showing promising outcomes related to dysphonia severity and voice analysis measurement. This type of program is already being utilized at a number of clinics, and will likely soon become part of standard acoustic evaluation (Peterson, Roy, Awan, Merrill, & Tanner, 2013). Aerodynamic assessment typically includes measures of subglottic pressure, phonation threshold pressure, vital capacity, and characteristics of airflow and resistance (Benninger & Murry, 2006; Sataloff, 2006a).

The speech-language pathologist does not make a medical diagnosis, but describes vocal function though evaluation. Once he or she receives the medical diagnosis from the laryngologist, the speech-language pathologist makes recommendations for voice therapy related to speaking voice, develops a treatment plan with measurable goals, and provides rehabilitative voice therapy. In the case that the speech pathologist is also a singing voice rehabilitation specialist, the singing voice can also be addressed. Voice therapy includes training of maximal efficiency of vocal fold vibration via adequate breath support, appropriate balance of muscle activation in and around the larynx, and ideal configuration of the resonator/filter through a systematic, hierarchical training program. The voice therapy regimen will likely also include ongoing counseling regarding vocal hygiene, as well as regular review of voice use to optimize vocal pacing (Sataloff, 2006b).

The Singing Voice Rehabilitation Specialist's Roles and Responsibilities

As noted above, in some practices, the singing voice rehabilitation specialist is also a licensed, certified speech-language pathologist. If this is the case, speaking and singing voice evaluation and behavioral therapy can be conducted by the same person. This is an optimal arrangement, as it means fewer visits for the patient, and allows for a more holistic approach to the behavioral intervention, addressing the patient's speaking and singing voice simultaneously. A more unique setting would include both a speech-language pathologist who is also a singing voice specialist in addition to a vocal arts professional such as a voice teacher with expertise in vocal health. In this setting, the patient is receiving voice care from both the speech-language pathologist/singing voice specialist and the vocal arts professional, providing a truly multidisciplinary voice care experience (American Speech-Language-Hearing Association, 2005; Sataloff, 2006b).

The singing voice rehabilitation therapist will obtain additional details regarding the history of the problem relative to singing, including the specific singing symptoms they are experiencing, the style(s) the singer typically sings in, voice type, professional status, training background, typical performance activities, and any impending performances. The therapist will also review the singer's typical singing schedule, including individual practice time, rehearsals, performance, and recreational singing. If the therapist is conducting the evaluation with the laryngologist and/or speech-language pathologist, this information may be collected simultaneously with the medical history of the voice problem, resulting in a thorough and efficient voice history.

The singing voice rehabilitation therapist will conduct further perceptual assessment focusing on the singing voice. This may be accomplished by having the singer perform a series of vocalises and/or repertoire. As this can be a time consuming process, the singing voice evaluation may be conducted at a separate appointment. The therapist will assess the singer's pitch and dynamic range, voice quality, breath support, resonance, projection, pitch accuracy, ease of phonation, register negotiation, vibrato characteristics, appropriateness of declared voice part, posture, and body alignment. The therapist will also assess whether the singer's technique is appropriate and safe for the style(s) in which they sing. Ideally, the therapist will also review video and/or audio recordings of the singer, if available. This allows clearer assessment of the singer's function in real-world situations. If the singer has recordings that predate the injury, it can be very helpful to review them as part of the evaluation process to determine the patient's baseline and loss of function (Benninger & Murry, 2006; Sataloff, 2006a, 2006b).

Based on results of evaluation, the singing voice rehabilitation therapist determines guidelines for how high to sing, how long to sing, and what to sing. Whether voice therapy is conducted by a speech-language pathologist/singing voice specialist, or by collaboration between the speech-language pathologist and the singing teacher, voice rehabilitation therapy goals should encompass vocal pacing,

vocal hygiene, and vocal efficiency, permitting exercise of the voice in an amount and manner that supports healing. The singing voice specialist designs therapy exercises to unload maladaptive and nonproductive vocal behaviors, and develops an appropriate exercise regimen for rehabilitation and maintenance of vocal health. The exercises should be designed in such a fashion to promote healing and avoid further injury. This may include teaching basic vocal skills to untrained singers, or optimizing vocal function and technique in trained singers (Sataloff, 2006a, 2006b).

Collaborative Interaction and Decision Making

Clearly voice care for singers is complex and multifactorial in nature. There are numerous elements of voice evaluation and management that cannot be addressed or decided on by only one member of the team, or that require regular communication and collaboration to achieve optimal results. Obtaining a clear history of the voice problem can sometimes be hampered by communication breakdown, particularly if the singer uses technical singing language or abstract, imagery-based language to describe their vocal activities and what they are currently struggling with. Even the best-trained laryngologist may not be familiar with all the "singerese" that may arise in the discussion. A collaborative history-taking between the laryngologist and the clinical singing voice speech-language pathologist or singing teacher can be very beneficial in such a case, as the singing voice provider can function as interpreter (Benninger & Murry, 2006; Sataloff, 2006a, 2006b).

The speech-language pathologist and/or singing voice provider can also play an important role in follow-up education and ensuring the patient's adherence to medical recommendations, particularly as they will likely see the patient on a regular basis for multiple therapy sessions. The patient may be experiencing difficulty with a medication, may not have a clear understanding of the results of their evaluation or rationale for treatment recommendations, or may wish to explore options they had not previously wished to consider, such as surgery. In such cases, the therapist can facilitate communication with and/or reinforce the laryngologist's recommendations to ensure that all contributing factors are being addressed in an efficient and thorough manner.

The decision for how much to sing and whether to recommend voice rest is often a team-decision, and depends largely on professional status of the singer, style of singing, and degree of injury. Complete vocal rest is rarely indicated, as muscles need regular exercise. If maladaptive behavior is contributing to the voice injury, complete voice rest does not address the underlying behavioral problem. In addition, long-term voice rest can promote discouragement and fear of singing. The more important issue is determining how much to sing and when to "get back on the horse" and return to regular performing. This requires careful guidance of the laryngologist and clinical singing voice rehabilitation specialist to determine whether it is safe for the singer to sing. Conducting serial stroboscopy can be very beneficial in assessing progress and adjusting voice use recommendations. If the patient is currently working with a singing teacher, the singing voice rehabilitation therapist and laryngologist may also consult the singing teacher to determine the importance of any upcoming performances or other vocal activities. This type of collaboration is particularly critical when

deciding whether a singer should proceed with a performance in an injured state (Sataloff, 2006a, 2006b).

Indications for recommendation of "no singing" include vocal fold hemorrhage, vocal fold surgery, severe laryngitis/vocal fold ulceration, or whenever there is a danger of increasing the degree of injury by singing (Sataloff, 2006a, 2006b). Other considerations for recommending "no singing" include situations in which the performer's reputation will be damaged by a bad performance or when the performer cannot fulfill her performance obligations. When recommending "no singing," ramifications of cancellation or bad performance must be weighed by the team, possibly in consultation with the musical and production staff associated with the performance. Risk of further damage by continuing to sing must be assessed.

Many times singers may be concerned, whose decision is it to perform or not? The laryngologist provides information on medical risks for permanent injury; the speech-language pathologist/singing voice rehabilitation specialist advises the laryngologist and provides counseling to the patient; the patient's current voice teacher is best acquainted with the importance of the performance and the singer's vocal habits. All must advocate for the singer in communications with producers and directors, academic advisors, colleagues, and so forth. Ultimately, the singer decides whether to go ahead with the performance.

Discharge and Follow-Up

Team collaboration is essential in diagnosis and creation of the treatment plan and is no less so in determining discharge and an appropriate follow-up plan. Duration and intricacy of intervention will vary widely on a case-by-case basis, depending on the severity of injury, whether surgery was necessary, the nature and complexity of the contributing factors, and the degree of support that is likely needed to ensure that the patient can safely engage in singing activities. In some cases, medical management may be all that is needed. In others, the behavioral factors may be able to be addressed in only a few therapy sessions. Still other singers may require therapy over a period of months, and may need intermittent "brush-up" sessions after discharge. It is important to note that the patient may be discharged by one member of the team while continuing to work with another.

The most important consideration in determining when to discharge the patient is level of function. Through medical or surgical management and improvement of vocal pacing, vocal hygiene, and vocal efficiency, the singer may be able to return to a level of performance that meets his or her professional or avocational needs, even if some degree of physical injury, or vibration or closure impairment is still evident in laryngeal imaging results. Often, determining when to discharge from singing intervention can be the most challenging decision. As singing voice therapy inevitably and inherently addresses vocal technique, it is likely that the singer will continue to improve and make progress. The line between "singing therapy" and "singing lessons" can be quite blurry. The providing therapist must keep in mind that the goal of singing therapy is restoration of function that has been lost, and that of singing lessons is building technique in a healthy instrument. If the latter begins to be the case, it is likely time to discharge the patient. An excellent way to ensure continued improvement and help the singer stay on the path of vocal health is to encourage continued study with their current singing teacher, or refer them to a competent singing teacher in the community. Risk of reinjury is high if behaviors are not permanently changed and if necessary ongoing medical management is not continued. Periodic reexamination by all or part of the team is recommended for monitoring the singer's status and adjusting their maintenance plan.

Chapter Summary

Voice problems are almost always multifactorial, and the treatment for singers often involves multiple disciplines to address all facets of the problem. No single provider will have the education, training, experience, and qualifications to address all of these factors thoroughly, effectively, and efficiently. Therefore, singers should seek out a laryngologist physician who works collaboratively with a speech-language pathologist who is knowledgeable and skilled at working with singers and possibly other vocal arts professionals. Additionally, other physician specialties such as an allergist and pulmonologist may also play a vital role depending on the nature of the problem.

References

American Speech-Language Hearing Association. (2001). *Scope of practice in speech language pathology.* Rockville, MD: Author.

American Speech-Language Hearing Association. (2005). *The role of the speech language pathologist, the teacher of singing, and the speaking voice trainer in voice habilitation (Technical report).* Rockville, MD: American Speech and Hearing Association Ad Hoc Joint Committee with the National Association of Teachers of Singing and the Voice and Speech Trainers Association.

Benninger, M., & Murry, T. (2006). *The performer's voice.* San Diego, CA: Plural Publishing.

Hillman, R. (2013). *The way forward in clinical voice assessment.* The Voice Foundation 42nd Annual Symposium Care of the Professional Voice presentation. Philadelphia, PA.

Hirano, M., & Bless, D. (1993). *Stroboscopic examination of the larynx.* San Diego, CA: Plural Publishing.

Peterson, E., Roy, N., Awan, S., Merrill, R., & Tanner, K. (2013). *Performance of the Cepstral/Spectral Index of Dysphonia (CSID) as an objective treatment outcomes tool,* The Voice Foundation 42nd Annual Symposium Care of the Professional Voice presentation. philadelphia, PA.

Roy, N., Barkmeier-Kraemer, J., Eadie, T., Sivasankar, M. P., Mehta, D., Paul, D., & Hillman, R. (2012). Evidence-based clinical voice assessment: A systematic review. *American Journal of Speech-Language Pathology,* in press.

Sataloff, R. T. (2006a). *Vocal health and pedagogy, Volume I: Science and assessment* (2nd ed.). San Diego, CA: Plural Publishing.

Sataloff, R. T. (2006b). *Vocal health and pedagogy, Volume II: Advanced assessment and treatment* (2nd ed.). San Diego, CA: Plural Publishing.

SECTION III

Vocal Pedagogy for the 21st-Century Vocal Athlete

12

History of Classical Voice Pedagogy

If you want to understand today, you have to search yesterday.

PEARL BUCK

Overview

As a reader, you may ask, why does a book about contemporary vocal pedagogy contain a chapter on classical pedagogy? Understanding modern aspects of vocal pedagogy, results from having a basis and appreciation of how singers have been trained through the centuries. This knowledge provides the foundation for expansion of valid contemporary and future pedagogical development. Examination of historical training techniques provided early voice scientists a basis on which to investigate the validity of certain exercises and their physiological or acoustical manifestation. The purpose of this chapter is not to judge the validity of or to endorse any given pedagogical technique, but

rather to provide readers with a historical pedagogy overview with scientific validation where available. Because the majority of voice teachers training commercial music singers have personal training based in classical vocal pedagogy (as there are very few commercial music pedagogy training programs within the United States), this chapter also serves as a basis for incorporating historical pedagogical methodology into relevant commercial music pedagogy for themselves and their students.

Throughout the centuries, vocal pedagogues have attempted to train singers to emulate the aesthetically pleasing vocal sounds of a given vocal genre. A master-apprentice relationship of vocal training has provided the basis of today's commonly used pedagogical techniques. Within the last 50 years, technical advances have allowed us to look more accurately and objectively at aerodynamic, acoustic, and phonatory measurements of vocal output. Because of these advancements, scientists have had success in evaluating the soundness of respiratory, phonatory, and resonance training approaches for singers. By no accounts is the research complete. But the available literature provides both the singing teacher and the voice scientist evidence of specific training techniques that result in desired sound production. These scientific implications will continue to shape future directions of training for vocal athletes. It is therefore important to understand as singer, teacher, and scientist the historical roots of vocal pedagogy and the evolution and introduction of new pedagogical tools designed to meet changing the needs and high demands of the 21st century hybrid singer. A listing of available vocal pedagogy writings is included for the reader at the end of this chapter (Appendix 12–A).

Classical Vocal Pedagogy

As discussed in Chapter 2, the roots of modern day vocal pedagogy can be traced back to the first vocal pedagogy text, *Opinioni de' cantori antichi, e moderni o sieno osservazioni sopra il canto figurato* (Observations on the Florid Song), by Pier Francesco Tosi (1723) with many subsequent texts written on vocal training techniques. *Bel canto* vocal training is considered by many vocal pedagogues as the gold standard of classical voice (Blades-Zeller, 1994; Miller, 1986, 1996; Reid, 1982; Stark, 2003).

Today's training of the singing voice essentially remains the same as it was centuries ago, yet vocal demands on the commercial vocal athlete have changed (Cleveland, 1994; Deere, 2005). Pedagogical training is often based on techniques acquired by experience with previous voice teacher's (master-apprentice) and on the perceptual judgment (aesthetics) of a given teachers' ears. Research has established and documented important perceptual characteristics of the classically trained voice (Blades-Zeller, 1994; Ekholm, Papagiannis, & Chagnon, 1998; Robison, Bounous, & Bailey, 1994; Wapnick & Ekholm, 1997). Twelve perceptual parameters are considered to be essential for a perceived beautiful Western classical voice (Ekholm et al., 1998). These parameters include: appropriate vibrato, resonance/ring, color/warmth, clarity/focus, intensity, dynamic range, efficient breath management, evenness of registration, flexibility, freedom throughout vocal range, intonation accuracy, legato line, and diction (Ekholm et al., 1998, p. 183). The more proficient a singer is at producing these acoustic events, the more beautiful the voice is perceived.

A historical overview of vocal pedagogy provides readers with an understanding of the roots of vocal training methodology and common terminology. Without an understanding of the past, it becomes impossible to appropriately move forward in the training of the 21st-century vocal performer and the new demands encountered by the hybrid singer. This chapter aims to point out relevant and recurrent themes that have permeated both historical and contemporary vocal training.

Early Vocal Pedagogues

Pier Francesco Tosi and Giambasttisti Mancini provide early insight into vocal training, and some of their suggested vocal techniques offer a basis for the training of today's female voice. All of the early pedagogues had very strict standards on who they would accept as students. If aspiring singers lacked certain God-given talents and good looks, they were not considered for serious vocal training. In addition to a basic natural talent, ear training was essential. Recommendations made by both teachers included the strong conviction that all singers must be trained (and proficient) in solfeggio (textless exercise). Primarily focusing singing exercises on solfeggio allowed the singer to "unite articulation with vowel and establish good intonation" (Coffin, 2002). Even at that point in history, voice teachers were well aware of creating a solid vocal and musical foundation for future elite performance. Today's vocal teachers and studios often must train singers of various levels of skill and/or natural talent and often are not able to filter potential students with such rigor.

In addition to the training on solfeggio, Tosi professed that open vowels (/ɑ/, /ɛ/, /ɔ/) should dominate the training of scales, with no separation between notes using an /h/ or /g/. This alludes to the legato line which is the premise of *bel canto* singing. Fast passages were never to be sung on /i/ or /u/, perhaps because of the often-associated tongue and jaw tension created by many singers when these vowels are attempted. Another point of interest regarding Tosi's teaching includes the proposition that one should always "drag" the high notes to the low notes and never the other way around. No further exposition is provided by Tosi on this topic, but it leads one to believe that Tosi wanted the singer to approach the lower voice with a head voice dominant placement.

Training vocal agility and genre appropriate vocal ornamentation was imperative for historical vocal pedagogues. Specifically, Tosi required that all sopranos should be able to trill, although he offered no insight into how to teach the trill. The appoggiatura ("A dissonant pitch occurring in a strong musical position and resolving by ascending or descending a step to a consonance in a relatively weaker metrical position," Randel, 1986, p. 44) was considered the most important ornament to perfect as it pervaded the music of the day.

Mancini used many of the same underlying principles as Tosi. However, Mancini was the first to observe the effects of the mouth opening and its importance in tuning vowels. At the time his *Practical Reflections on the Figurative Art of Singing* was written (1912), little information on the physical acoustics of the singing voice was known, yet Mancini commented on the perceptual characteristics noted when singers performed with less than optimal formant tuning. He emphasized the relaxation and alignment of the throat, and that all vowels should be sung in a smile position, with /o/ and /u/ permitting slight lip rounding. If the mouth was perceived as too open, then the resultant tone was considered "crude," and a tone produced with too closed of a mouth position was considered "nasal." These statements by Mancini suggest that he was striving for his singers to attain optimum vowel placement. Mancini believed that for each note, there was an optimal voice placement that coordinated breath, phonation, and resonance. To achieve ideal vowel placement, he would have his students sustain whole notes crescendoing from piano to forte in order to find the perfect placement on each frequency and intensity. Once the impeccable note was achieved, the singer would move up or down one half-step at a time. The sheer discipline to move at such a slow pace would likely never happen in today's voice studio. Mancini goes on to comment that voices that are weak but have a good range and good high notes should sing in their chest voice every day to strengthen the voice.

He believed in teaching his students according to the basic talent and structure that they were given.

Keeping with the musical tradition of the time, the singer in Mancini's studio was required to master the artistic elements of the day, including, the portamento ("A continuous movement from one pitch to another through all of the intervening pitches, without, however, sounding them discretely," Randel, 1986, p. 649), the appogiatura, the *messa di voce*, and the trillo ("An ornament consisting of the more or less rapid alternation of a note with the one next above it in the prevailing key or harmony" (Randel, 1986, p. 869). When studying these techniques, Mancini maintained that the agility in the voice must be natural, breath must support the tones and the fauces should be "light." One might assume that when Mancini spoke of "light fauces" he was referring to the sense of openness in the back of the throat while attempting agility exercises.

Manuel Garcia I

Garcia I published *Exercises Pour La Voix,* which included 340 training exercises on: *messa di voce*, connection of tones with portamento, crescendi, diminuendi, trills, cadenzas, and agility. The agility exercises were designed to assist the singer with mastering the technical writings of the prominent *bel canto* composers of the day (Rossini, Bellini, and Donzetti). Progressively, the exercises in his book become more difficult in training both range and agility control.

The book of exercises includes "the secrets of the old Italian school divulged to him by Ansoni, and is the basis of the most rigid and through-going method by which he trained his students in Paris and London between 1816 and 1832" (Coffin, 2002, p. 14). One was not to undertake the 340 exercises without instruction. Instead, Garcia I advised that all singers study with a "master" who could help to alleviate any technical problems. If the student was unable to study with a master, then he provided a list of eight basic rules for the singer to follow as he practiced the exercises. In examining these rules, one encounters several aspects that may relate directly to methodology in teaching voice today.

Rule 1 suggests that the singer should always practice from the lowest note in the range to the highest note. Many voice teachers today believe that singers should begin vocalizing in the middle of their voice and work to both the frequency extremes of their pitch ranges in a systematic manner. Rule 2 begins teaching exercises on the most open vowel and progresses to the most closed vowel as the singer becomes more proficient at tuning the vowels without tension. Restating what Tosi and Mancini wrote about separation of notes with an /h/, Garcia felt the use of /h/ was in both poor taste and poor technique. Separation of notes was required, but Garcia advocated it be done with breath, not with glottal articulation. Rule 3 alludes to the inherent artistry the singer must master as he approaches cadences (i.e., the use of the appogiatura). Maintenance of correct posture was important for the singer in order to gain optimal chest expansion (Rule 4).

Garcia cautioned against facial and body contortions, suggesting that singing should require no abnormal tension in these areas. Deep, slow, quiet breathing was always employed by the singer prior to initiation of exercises or song, as not to engage in unnecessary laryngeal or respiratory tension (Rule 5). The singer was advised to keep an open throat, teeth, and lips as not to have tension in the laryngeal or articulatory space when singing (Rule 6). The perfection of *messa di voce* is described as Rule 7. Most importantly, the singer should never fluctuate in intonation when increasing intensity. Finally, Rule 8 focuses on maintaining portamento and its importance in the *bel canto* style throughout all exercises.

Manuel Garcia II— A Complete Treatise on The Art of Singing (1841)

From the rules and the training of his father, Garcia II further educated himself on the voice and voice production. The influence of his astute observations on the vocal mechanism has resulted in his title (Garcia II) as "the father of modern otolaryngology and pedagogy." During his lifetime, he was considered to be the premiere scholar and teacher of voice. Although Garcia II did not experience success of the singing career of his father, he brought far more to the pedagogical aspects of singing. For the first time in the history of the singing voice, Garcia II actually viewed the vocal folds during phonation, and was able to provide physiological explanations on voice production and to comment on the artistic expressions of song. Much of what Garcia II wrote has been debated through the years, and the language that he uses is often inconsistent. However, it is important to understand that he was attempting to describe things that had not yet been named, and it seems as if he struggled with terminology at times. Therefore, some of the discussion presented is based on these authors interpretation of Garcia II's writings

and what we know to be physiologically true today. An article by James Stark (1991) entitled *Garcia in Perspective: His Traite After 150 Years,* offers additional insight into the controversy surrounding Garcia's writings.

All singers were expected to be in good physical shape, and Garcia requested that they refrain from "excesses." The excesses that Garcia II warns against are some of the basic rules of good vocal hygiene that continue to be observed today. Some of his cautions include: watching the foods the singer consumes, not singing too high or too low for any length of time, not singing loudly for an extended period of time, not laughing, screaming, or crying loudly, or overexaggerating the "sombre" timbre. Garcia cautioned against singing too soon after eating, avoiding food that contained oil, certain fruits, and alcoholic beverages. Garcia II reported these things done in excess would result in damage to the voice, manifesting as hoarseness. If this hoarseness persisted over time, Garcia II believed that the singer would never regain the delicate control of the voice needed to perform in the professional arena. Although we now know that hoarseness or vocal pathology does not necessarily equate to the end of one's singing career, we continue to recommend many of these same truths to our singers today with now the scientific understanding of possible risks associated with phonotrauma and other vocal hygiene issues such as acid reflux.

Garcia also presented guidelines for practicing. First, the singer was advised to practice with a piano that was in tune as not to practice intervals with poor intonation. Second, Garcia felt that practicing in a small space with poor acoustics would fatigue the voice more quickly. The use of a mirror was recommended for personal reflection and correction of posture, facial expression, and any body tension. He set forth suggestions on how long to practice. Singers should begin with no more than 5 minutes of vocal exercise at one sitting for the first few days. They were permitted several 5-minute practice periods throughout the day. Once stamina had improved, the singer was then permitted to increase practice length 5 minutes at a time, until a half an hour was reached. Half-hour practice sessions, four times per day was the maximum time Garcia allowed his students to sing. Knowledge of current rehearsal and performance practices of today's singers indicate that total singing time is drastically greater in today's performance world.

Garcia trained breath as the necessary basis for production of optimal vocal quality (Chapter 2). Beyond respiration, to phonation, Garcia II is credited as the first man to view the vocal folds with a mirror during phonation and much of what he writes about the onset and maintenance of phonation is based on physical observations. His writings on phonation, specifically his avocation of the *coup de glotte*, are some of the most controversial points of his techniques (Stark, 1991). *Coup de glotte* literally means "stroke of the glottis," but *coup* also translates as "blow." This discrepancy in translation is the source of the much controversy surrounding Garcia's method of training vocal onset. It is the opinion of these authors, based on Garcia's writing and other writings on the subject (Stark, 1991), that Garcia was referring to the coordinated effort of expiration and the firm, not harsh, onset of phonation. A statement that supports this theory is one in which Garcia himself cautions against too abrupt a vocal onset: "One must guard against confusing the stroke of the glottis with the stroke of the chest (*coup de poitrine*), which resembles a cough, or the effort of

expelling something which is obstructing the throat" (Garcia, 1984, p. 42).

The *coup de glotte* was the basis in mastering Garcia's vocal technique, and it was advised to be taught in the first lesson (Stark, 1991). These authors interpret the *coup de glotte* to be the adductory movement of the vocal folds into a midline position, just slightly before the onset of breath. Therefore, when the force of exhalation begins, closure of the glottis results in a perfectly timed phonatory onset without prephonatory expiration noise. This phenomenon is the mark of any good voice onset for song or vocal exercise. Supported by the statements that guard against using an /h/ between each note, no aspirate noise was typically associated with optimal glottal closure. It is difficult to find an explanation of the phenomenon that occurs at the level of the vocal folds milliseconds before breath is initiated, and the accompanying sensation of maintaining all articulators and resonators in an optimal placement. Because of the poor description of Garcia's interpretation of this event, many people vehemently disagree with Garcia's *coup de glotte*, as a method for vocal onset. It is the assumption of these authors that these people envision the *coup de glotte* as a hard glottal attack (considered harmful to the voice) instead of a coordinated event involving expiration and vocal fold adduction.

Garcia recognized that the sound produced at the level of the glottis was not a beautiful musical tone. Rather the vocal folds generated a sound source, which the vocal tract was to shape and mold. In the writings of Garcia, resonation cannot be separated from registration, as they are interdependent, and an improper approach to resonation will directly affect the transition between registers. A discussion of Garcia's mention of both the "clear timbre" and the "sombre timbre" is addressed in conjunction with registration. Singers trained by Garcia were required to perform in both timbres and in all three registers (chest, head, and falsetto).

The clear timbre allows the voice to maintain a penetrating, piercing presence, but if taken to the extreme, it "makes the voice shrill, squalling, and yelping" (Garcia, 1984, p. 31). In the untrained voice utilizing the clear timbre, Garcia observed the larynx to rise as frequency increased. The rising larynx likely accounts for the shrillness of voice Garcia reported, as an increase in laryngeal height typically shortens the resonating tube and compresses the supraglottic structures. However, the sombre timbre offered a more round, full sound that was equated with a lowered larynx, thus creating a longer resonating tube. It was essential that the singer learn to sing with a balance of these two timbres in order to maintain a full round quality with a brightness and clarity to the tone (Garcia, 1984; Stark, 1991). The union and balancing of the two timbres resulted in a smooth transition between registers. Without the balance in timbres, a voice break or significant change in vocal quality was present. *Chiaroscuro*, an Italian word which means light-dark, best describes the quality of resonance that Garcia was attempting to achieve through the balancing of timbres.

Garcia believed that in order to prepare the oral and pharyngeal area for singing, a flattened tongue without tension, a raised velum, and separation of the faucial pillars at their base was required. In positioning the articulators as prescribed above, the oral and pharyngeal cavities were essentially "open" and prepared the vocal tract for open vowel sound productions. The shaping of the tone for various vowels and timbres required modification

of the pharynx, faucial pillars, tongue, and jaw. Tension in any of the articulators was reported to dampen the brilliance of the sound, as it could not adequately reflect the sound waves in such a way that is conducive to the recommended timbres.

Several timbres Garcia reported in the literature as "undesirable" for the singer and required immediate correction included: guttural timbre, nasal timbre, hollow timbre, and veiled tones. The guttural timbre was marked by a broad based of tongue which impinged on the epiglottis and constricted the pharyngeal resonating tube. This is consistent with excessive tongue tension/retraction and the resultant timbre. Nasal timbre is exactly what it implies, excessive undesired nasality in the tone. One of Garcia's students and future voice pedagogue, Matilde Marchesi, reported that all Americans presented with too much nasality in the tone. In contrast to nasal resonance is the hollow timbre. This can most likely be correlated with today's overly covered tone quality, or a "hooty" sound as Garcia reported hollow timbre to be caused by excessive tonsil swelling, lip constriction, or a tongue which is raised at the tip. A veiled tone is one in which the tone is clear but it lacks brilliance. Garcia reports this faulty veiled tone production resulted from a pinching of the glottis.

Garcia provided 314 vocal exercises to correct faults and train the most important elements of the singing voice. No reports on whether his students had to master all 314 exercises before they moved into singing vocal literature are given, but it is assumed to be true. These exercises focused on training the coordination of respiration, phonation, registration, and resonation. Portamento was used to help equalize registers, timbres, and power of the voice. Slurred vocalization (tones connected by a portamento) was the next step

Garcia proposed in training the voice. This parameter of voice training was likened to the violinist learning to connect tones consistently using his bow across the strings with a smooth, even tone. Maintaining adequate, consistent breath pressure as tones change frequency was the premise of these exercises. Because legato singing is the essence of *bel canto* singing Garcia reported it took at least a year and a half of vocal study to master this skill. In contrast to legato singing, Garcia also trained marked vocalization (marcato) in the singer. Marked vocalizations require the exact tuning of the vocal folds at discrete pitches, and are aimed at correcting the habit of sliding between pitches.

Garcia used specific training exercises to reflect the importance of the techniques discussed above and are organized in his text in such a manner. Exercises 5 through 10 and 32 through 37 become progressively more difficult in training portamento. The difficulty in these exercises comes from both increasing rhythmic difficulty and degree of the intervals used. Second, scales and roulades (an ornamental passage of melody in 18th-century music) were trained in exercises 11 through 31. These passages become increasingly longer in length, rhythmic complexity, and intervals. Exercises 38 through 189 are extensive, grueling vocal training tools, designed to train muscle memory for many possible interval and rhythmic patterns, while coordinating respiration, phonation, and resonation. Garcia requested that all exercises were produced on a pure Italian /ɑ/ before moving to /e/, /ɛ/, /o/, and /ɔ/. Also, /i/ and /u/ were considered the more difficult vowels and were postponed until later study.

Once the singer mastered the above exercises, students learned to vary vocal intensity on the vocalises and were then used for training inflection in the voice. Arpeggios (Exercises 190–206) aimed to facilitate a smooth passage from note to note regardless of the interval. One particular exercise of Garcia's requires the singer to ascend the scale stepwise to an interval of a 15th and then descend via arpeggio to a 5th below and then to a 12th below that. Ear training in coordination with precise intonation was considered a vital part of the vocal training process and was reflected in the difficulty of the exercises. Exercises 207 to 222 were devoted specifically to minor scales and chromatic scales for ear training purposes.

When the singer had progressed to this point in vocal training, they were then permitted to learn the *messa di voce*. Garcia's comments on the *messa di voce* include the recommendation that the singer was to use only air to increase intensity, and intonation must be maintained as intensity increased. Although Garcia did not have the acoustical knowledge Johann Sundberg or Ingo Titze would provide many years later, he recognized the fact that as subglottic pressure increased, the typical response was for the frequency to rise. The *messa di voce* became an extremely important task for the singer to master, as it allowed them to learn to control the muscles of phonation independent of breath pressure. Practiced on whole notes, Garcia's *messa di voce* exercise ascended by half steps throughout the singer's entire range.

Mastery of the above exercises prepared the singer to begin training specific ornaments that were characteristic of the day (Exercises 224–275). The ornaments that Garcia felt were the most important to train included: repeated tones (aspirated /h/), appoggiaturas, turns, trills, and little notes (grace notes). He ends his exercises on the major ninth chord and a variation thereof. It is not known how long it would take the singer to master the techniques presented by Garcia, but at the least, a year and a half could be expected.

Whether one agrees or disagrees with Garcia's method of training the voice, there is no dispute that he is considered the father of modern day vocal pedagogy. Those who studied under him modified his techniques and teaching methods and presented them as their own. Those who disagreed based their new techniques on the things they felt Garcia trained inappropriately. At the time, Garcia II was considered "the master," and his students were some of the best singers in the world. The pedagogues that followed him are discussed in terms of differences from the teachings of Garcia. The more contemporary voice pedagogues move toward a physiological approach to training the voice, using slightly different terminology, less imagery, and more definitive explanations. It is unclear whether this modern day physiological approach is more useful to the singer learning to master an artistic task. Chapter 14 provides insights for the teacher on how students plan and learn new motor tasks.

Mathilde Marchesi— Theoretical and Practical Vocal Method (1970) and Ten Singing Lessons (1901)

Marchesi studied under Garcia II for four years and was well-versed in his technique; so much so that Garcia asked her to teach for him when he was unable to do so himself. Because of Garcia's influence, Marchesi believed that her students had to possess physical and vocal talent and commit to at least 2 years of study. Marchesi refused to train male voices, but produced some of the most famous female voices of the time including: Caroline Dory, Gabrielle Krauss, Nellie Melba, and Ilma di Murska.

Much of Marchesi's technique is based on her time with Garcia; however, there are some fundamental differences about which she was quite adamant. Children were permitted to study voice by the age of seven and eight in a very limited range (from C–E, ten notes). The primary focus at that age was placed on piano (keyboard) skills and learning solfeggio. Between the ages of 12 and 18, singing was prohibited, as female voices during this time were considered "hoarse." Some of the most remarkable comments Marchesi makes are on the changes noted in the female voice during puberty and the guidelines she set forth. During puberty, female singers were advised to study vocal literature, music history, and three languages (French, German, and Italian). After the age of 18, a woman could truly begin to study voice with Marchesi. She felt that a minimum of 7 to 8 years of vocal training was necessary before any public performance.

Specific principles Marchesi professed regarding the singing technique included comments on posture, length of practice, phonation, diet and exercise, respiration, tongue placement, and the study of vocalises to blend registers. Strict vocal hygiene was of the utmost importance within Marchesi's studio. Posture was to be kept upright, with the head held erect, the shoulders back, and the chest free. She proposed all postural muscles were to be relaxed in order to maintain a free vocal sound. Marchesi's pedagogy regarding respiration is reviewed in Chapter 2. Her approach to vocal onsets was similar to the teachings of Garcia II. A firmly closed glottis was desired as not to allow any unwanted air escape. "The coup de glotte requires, then, a sudden and energetic approximation of the lips of the glottis, an instant before expiration commences" (Marchesi, 1970, p. ii). Marchesi likened her voice onset to that of a spontaneous action such as the cry at birth. Staccato was advised to be undertaken sparingly, as it was reported to be tiresome to the vocal mechanism.

Three registers acting and sounding as one was the goal of Marchesi's vocal exercises. In order to attain a balance between the chest, middle, and head voice, singers first had to achieve a correctly placed /ɑ/ vowel. Without the proper placement of the resonators, singers could not hope to attain a smooth register transition. Of the three registers, Marchesi considered the chest voice to be the most important, even for the soprano. Marchesi observed a correlation between the training of the chest voice and the security and solidity of the head register. In order for her singers to traverse their registers without a noticeable transition, the singer was advised to close/darken the tone as she made the ascending transition from chest to middle voice, and to open/brighten the tone as she descended from middle voice to chest voice. This process of navigating registers is consistent with the concept that if the chest voice relies too much on the "heavy mechanism" when ascending, the singer will present with a noticeable break into their middle or head voice.

All vocalizations were to be performed on pure Italian vowels beginning with /ɑ/. Contrary to previous pedagogues, Marchesi did not believe in the "smile position" of the lips as she felt it created a *voix blanche* (white voice), which may be interpreted as a bright, strident sound. The jaw was to be dropped and remain immobile during all vocalises, especially on fast passages. Also,

by engaging in immobility of the jaw, the singer was to learn to articulate with airflow/breath pressure, not with articulatory muscles. However, the image of a rigid jaw seems to present a problem in itself, creating undue jaw tension.

Once the vocal exercises were mastered on the vowel sounds, Marchesi introduced the following consonants (l, d, t, s, z, r, n, c, g, k, x), in order to train independence of the tongue and larynx. Mastery of the consonants allowed for transition to song, but only the Italian masters of song were allowed to be performed. The reasoning behind this is not addressed in her writings, but the Italian language does not contain stops at the ends of words and all vowel sounds are pure and are produced in a forward placement. Also, the Italian /l/ is much more forward in the mouth involving only the tip of the tongue as compared to its American counterpart (Adams, 1998).

Within her studio, Marchesi believed that a singer could only concentrate on one thing at a time, and her exercises reflected this concept. As with Garcia, the exercises became progressively more difficult, and no more than a half-hour lesson was allowed. The singers were advised to sing in 5- and 10-minute increments several times per day and were always to be done in full voice as if one were on stage, without forcing. In addition to private lessons, Marchesi believed in the benefit of group instruction. She found that singers learned a lot about their own technique from watching the mistakes of others. Marchesi was an extremely opinionated woman, with little slack for undedicated students. Marchesi wrote:

A singer who has learned how to breathe well, and who has equalized the voice, neatly blended the registers and developed the activity of the larynx and the elasticity of the glottis and resonant tube in a rational manner, so that all possible shades of tone, power, and expression can be produced by the vocal organs, would most assuredly be able to sing well, and without fatigue an effort the long and declaimed modern phrases. (Marchesi, 1901, viii)

Marchesi's vocal exercises were also presented and mastered in a specific order to achieve optimal voice production. The first exercise was to train the singer to initiate the tone with a *coup de glotte*, on a single pitch sustained for three beats. This exercise moved up by half steps throughout the singer's range. Next, the slur and portamento were introduced in a slow tempo and a stepwise fashion. Once intonation was secure, Marchesi believed that the singer should train intensity, power, and flexibility throughout the entire range. Exercises 9 to 36 work on scalewise passages with each tone produced with the identical intensity and duration as the other notes. Blending and equalization of registers was the focus of Exercises 37 to 73. Exercises 60 to 67 were specifically written for the high soprano, with an advanced degree of flexibility in the voice.

Additional exercises for register blending, using two, three, four, six, and eight note groupings encompass Exercises 74 to 125, with the latter exercises requiring exquisite control of intonation, respiration, and agility. Perfect intonation was essential for Marchesi's students, and Exercises 126 to 136 were devoted to training intonation using chromatic and minor scales. Scales were to be performed at varying dynamic levels (Exs. 138–151). Triplets and arpeggio were trained so that each note received the same intensity and dynamic level (Exs. 152–173).

Learning the *messa di voce* came along deep into Marchesi's vocal training process (Ex. 174). She advised, "The *messa di voce* should not be practiced until the voice has acquired a certain degree of suppleness and flexibility, and should never be attempted by beginners" (Marchesi, 1970, p. 39). Marchesi trained the *messa di voce* over 13 counts, ascending by half steps. At this point in the singer's training, the ornaments were added. Specific exercises aimed at training the appoggiatura, acciaccatura, mordente, turn, and the trill, complete the first portion of Marchesi's vocal method (Exs. 175–194).

Unlike previous voice pedagogues, the second portion of Marchesi's vocal method presented vocalises (song without words) to enhance and solidify optimal vocal technique. These 36 vocalises are complete with piano accompaniment and allow the singer a transition from vocal exercise (designed to train muscle memory), to songs without words (a transition from exercise to performance). Each of the technical voice exercises has a corresponding vocalise, so that the singer is able to transition into song more readily.

Franceso Lamperti—A Treatise on the Art of Singing (1877, revised 1890)

Lamperti was not a performer, but taught and wrote about vocal pedagogy. These writings emerged because of his disillusionment with the quality of the singer. He attributed the decline in singers due to several factors. The first problem was singers lacked the appropriate amount of time in training before public performances. Second, Lamperti felt composers were beginning to write syllables on every note, and it was disturbing the natural legato line of the voice. Finally, changes were being made in voice classifications, and from today's experience we know that singing out of range or in the inappropriate *fach*, a singer may at the very least, result in suboptimal voice production and at the very worst cause serious damage to his or her voice. Lamperti provides the example of one of the changes in classification involving the soprano being called upon to sing the highest roles, resulting in neglect of her chest voice. Thus, Lamperti felt a weakness in the strength of the soprano voice.

Much of Lamperti's pedagogical basis rests in appropriate training of respiration (Brown, 1968). Chapter 2 provides Lamperti's respiratory training guidelines. Lamperti believed each singer should learn to sing with full voice first, and gradually learn to diminuendo. When the singer produced a pianissimo intensity, the same amount of breath support should be felt by the singer as when singing forte. Following a mastery of the diminuendo, the singer was then trained in the entire *messa di voce*. Never was the singer to attempt to sing with more intensity than the breath could sustain. "The voice emitted should be less in force than the force of the breath which supports it" (Coffin, 2002, p. 60).

In training phonation, one great distinction between Lamperti and his predecessors is that each tone in agility exercises should be produced with a slight glottal "jerk." Possibly, the laryngeal sensation of glottal jerking was experienced by Lamperti, when in actuality it was the breath supporting the agility in the voice that was creating the sensation. Singers were advised never to sing the two highest or lowest notes in their range, but no basis was given for this training request. As with the other voice pedagogues, vocal exercises focused on training agility in the voice using portamento, legato, staccato, and marcato; with the most important of these being the legato voice.

One of the major concerns Lamperti (1905) expressed was the introduction of syllables on every note of a song in the vocal literature of the day. He recommended that all of his singers learn and train on solfeggio, sung with the pure Italian vowels and with different emotional contexts. This is the first example of a teacher promoting not simply muscle memory exercises, but muscle memory combined with an emotional component. Another reason for the singer training on solfeggio was to learn independence and freedom of the articulators from the vocal folds. Vocal literature for the singer was to include only the old Italian masters: Bellini, Donizetti, and Rossini. All other vocal literature was suspected to corrupt the voice.

William Shakespeare— The Art of Singing (1921)

Shakespeare (a student of Lamperti), trained his singers to incorporate speech into song. Likely because of Lamperti's influence, training of respiration in Shakespeare's students was essential (Chapter 2). Shakespeare believed that being aware of the minute action of the vocal folds during song was unnecessary. He did emphasize an understanding of the musculature and principles regarding the physiology of the vocal folds. But, he felt that the singer was not able to voluntarily control each minute movement. More important was finding the "natural place" of each individual note. The throat was to be free from tension and the voice feels as though it is floating on the breath in order to achieve this sensation. As with other voice pedagogues, Shakespeare emphasized the importance of maintaining independence of jaw, tongue, and throat.

The hard palate and teeth were considered the "soundboard," and correct placement and direction of the sound stream would result in a brilliant vocal quality. The pharyngeal area should feel open as it does the moment before swallowing. This may be the origin of the phrase "drinking in the tone." If the throat was open, there was no possibility for the singer to squeeze supraglottically during voice production. "The quality of a vowel has its origin in the freedom of the space behind and above the tongue, and in the freedom of the tongue itself" (Shakespeare, 1921, p. 42). One way in which Shakespeare taught his students the difference between an open throat and relaxed tongue and jaw, in contrast to the tight throat, tongue, and jaw, was to have them repeat "un italiano" six times (open) and then repeat "exactly" (closed) six times. In todays' clinical arena, speech pathologists sometimes use a similar technique referred to as negative practice to train a target voice production. This involves having the patient produce sound in the undesired way, and then in the desired way to increase learning of that particular skill.

Shakespeare wrote that several types of faulty singing were able to be assessed by the singing teacher through auditory cues alone. Four types of faulty production were addressed by Shakespeare including: throaty, frontal, nasal, and colorless. Throaty production could be recognized as an "aw" when the singer is attempting to produce an /ɑ/ vowel. Shakespeare reported that this flaw was a direct result of tongue and throat tension. Frontal singing was considered to be a result of excessive supraglottic squeeze in the middle voice as the singer ascends into head voice. Nasal singing was attributed to contraction of the soft palate. However, we know from speech science that nasality would actually

result from a relaxed, lowered soft palate, permitting the air to travel through the nasal cavity thus creating a hypernasality. Finally, colorless singing ("white voice") was said to be the result of the half smile that Garcia professed, but Marchesi cautioned against. In addition to the lips being pulled back and down, Shakespeare also felt that colorless singing was the result of lip, tongue, and jaw rigidity. Shakespeare also makes some inaccurate observations including reports such as "the vocal folds shorten as pitch increases" and "in middle voice the vocal folds don't vibrate their entire length."

Similar to his predecessors, Shakespeare subscribed to the three-register theory, with the chest voice being the most solid, serving as the anchor for the higher tones. Shakespeare warned that the chest voice should never be brought up too high and when forced up using muscular strength, resulted in poor production and technique. The medium voice (middle voice) could be brought up as high as one could take it and resulted in a brilliant quality when correctly produced. The singer was said to have felt both vibrations in the chest and the mouth with ideal production. Finally, the head voice, what we refer to today in singing terms as the falsetto or flute voice, was the highest of the tones produced, and sounded fluty and birdlike. Smooth register transition required the singer to know, through diligent exercise, where to "place" each note in terms of resonation. Shakespeare reported that forcing one register too high would always result in throat tightness and a tremolo.

Shakespeare also presented his vocal exercises from easiest to most difficult and offered exercises to train all of the vocal ornaments. Instead of beginning vocal exercises on the /ɑ/ vowel, Shakespeare had his singers learn all vowels (no diphthongs) on half step ascending dotted quarter notes. Once the singers could produce the vowels in isolation, he alternated different vowel sounds on sixteenth notes. He also added consonants, specifically /l, v, d, t, n, r, g, k, the/ at the very beginning of his exercise regimen attempting to achieve independence of jaw and tongue motion early in the training of his singers.

In addition to beginning the vocal exercises with a consonant, which was unprecedented until this time, Shakespeare also included two arias at the end of his text for singers to learn. "Una Voce Poco Fa" from *Il Barbiere di Siviglia* by Rossini is an aria which requires optimal agility in the voice as demonstrated through long, technically difficult runs. The second aria, "Oh Del Mio Dolce Ardor" by Gluck is a test in the legato line and demands a sense of artistry from the performer. Allowing singers to prepare arias at this early stage in their training may have been a reflection of the times. Singers were no longer satisfied with vocal exercises and vocalises alone. If they were paying for lessons, they wanted have a usable product. Therefore, Shakespeare may have condensed some of the basics in training and introduced song earlier than other pedagogues. It seems that this practice has continued, as recitals are expected within a singer's first six months of training.

William Vennard—Singing: The Mechanism and the Technic (1967)

Moving toward a physiological approach to pedagogy, William Vennard utilized science within his teaching. Understanding of basic anatomy and physiology of the vocal mechanism was required for his students as well as a basic understanding of acoustics.

Training respiration incorporated posture as well as breathing mechanics (Chapter 2).

Using high-speed photography, Vennard was able to print pictures of the vocal folds during various stages of vibration and used his high-speed photography to verify Garcia's *coup de glotte*. He was the first to comment on the sensory-motor integration needed for a coordinated onset of phonation. In order to train this type of attack, Vennard suggested moving from the panting exercise to a staccato exercise in which the singer would use a silent /h/ prior to initiation of the tone. The staccato exercises were to be followed by legato exercises while maintaining the same degree of glottal closure and breath pressure. Vennard emphasized the concept that separation and slurring of tones was not done at the glottal level, but rather by the muscles of the thorax and abdomen, in precise coordination with the onset of phonation. In addition to the physical onset of tone, the singer was trained to mentally prepare the respiratory and phonatory muscles prior to tonal onset. Vennard was the first to comment on the sensory-motor integration needed for a coordinated onset of phonation.

Vennard extensively examined the physiology of registration. He came to the conclusion that three distinct registers exist, and it is the job of the singer to train the muscles of the voice and resonators to sound as one register. Unfortunately, Vennard did not offer much insight into training the voice to sound as one register. Instead, he reported that as the voice ascends, the heavy mechanism should play less of a role in voice production, and the light mechanism should essentially take over.

With regards to resonance, Vennard described in detail the role of the pharyngeal, nasal, and oral resonating chambers and their effects on the quality of the singing tone. He advocated a low laryngeal placement, a loose jaw, a large throat (pharynx), a slightly grooved tongue, an arched soft palate, and slightly rounded lips in order to achieve the singer's formant. A large pharynx was encouraged because it tends to strengthen the lower partials of the voice and create a rich fullness to the sound. The oral cavity shape, as it is determined by the placement of the tongue, determines whether the pharynx-oral cavity acts as one large resonating tube or one large and one small tube. Tones that are produced with tongue tension were considered by Vennard to be "swallowed" or "throaty," while optimal tone placement was often said to be "in the mouth." Hypernasality in singing is never considered good vocal technique, and Vennard advocated the complete closure of the velopharyngeal port during singing. Vennard did not offer specific techniques for achieving these resonating positions, merely stating that singers who possess the "ring" in their voices possess these traits.

Chapter Summary

Vocal pedagogues of the past have set the foundation of much of today's vocal pedagogy for Western classical singing. Extensive study was expected with an apprentice-master model. Although there was not a strong anatomic and physiologic basis for much of what was taught, the pedagogical pioneers made inferences about the structure and function of classical singing based on sound and feel, and many of the landmark techniques are still prominent in today's teaching. Science and research over the past 50 years has helped to continue to shape vocal pedagogy, and many of the new pioneers in this field have

modified and evolved their approach as more information has emerged. However, there remains a gap in vocal pedagogy for the commercial vocal athlete. Unlike the centuries of tradition and information that exists on training the classical voice, there have been no texts based in scientific evidence of technique devoted solely to training the hybrid singing voice. Several teachers have published articles on exercises to train the contemporary commercial music (CCM) singer as well as recent research on this CCM voice production. A review of the existing literature related to CCM voice training and production is reviewed in Chapter 13.

References

Adams, D. (1998). *A handbook of diction for singers.* (In press).

Blades-Zeller, E. (1994). Vocal pedagogy in the United States: Interviews with exemplary teachers of applied voice. *Journal of Research in Singing, 17*(2), 1–87.

Brown, W. (1968). *Vocal wisdom: Maxims of G. B. Lamperti.* Reprint. New York, NY: Arno Press.

Cleveland, T. (1994). A clearer view of singing voice production: 25 years of progress. *Journal of Voice, 8*(1), 18–23.

Coffin, B. (2002). *Historical vocal pedagogy classics.* Metuchen, NJ: The Scarecrow Press.

Deere, J. (2005). *Singing in the 20th century: A recollection of performance and pedagogy.* Bloomington, IN: Author House.

Ekholm, E., Papagiannis, G., & Chagnon, F. (1998). Relating Objective measurements to expert evaluation of voice quality in western classical singing: Critical perceptual parameters. *Journal of Voice, 12*(2), 182–196.

Garcia, M. (1984). *A complete treatise on the art of singing: Part one*, Trans. and Ed.

D. V. Paschke. New York, NY: Da Capo Press (original work published 1841).

Lamperti, G. (1905). *The technics of bel canto*, trans. T. Baker. New York, NY: G. Schirmer.

Mancini, G. (1912). *Practical Reflections on the figurative art of singing.* Boston, MA: Gorham Press.

Marchesi, M. (1901). *Ten singing lessons.* New York, NY: Harper & Brothers.

Marchesi, M. (1970). *Vocal method* (2nd ed.). Milwaukee, WI: G. Schirmer.

Miller, R. (1986). *The structure of singing: System and art of vocal technique.* Los Angeles, CA: G. Schirmer Books.

Miller, R. (1996). *On the art of singing.* New York, NY: Oxford University Press.

Randel, D. (Ed.). (1986). *The new Harvard dictionary of music* (3rd ed.). Cambridge, MA: The Belknap Press of Harvard University Press.

Reid, C. (1982). *Bel canto principles and practices.* New York, NY: J. Patelson.

Robison, C., Bounous, B., & Bailey, R. (1994). Vocal beauty: A study proposing its acoustical definition and relevant causes in classical baritones and female belt singers. *The NATS Journal,* September/October, 19-30.

Shakespeare, W. (1921). *The art of singing.* Bryn Mawr, PA: Oliver Ditson Company.

Stark, J. (1991). Garcia in perspective: His traite after 150 years. *Journal of Research in Singing, 15*(1), 2-56.

Stark, J. (2003). *Bel canto: A history of vocal pedagogy.* Toronton, Canada: University of Toronto Press.

Tosi, P. (1723). *Observations on the florid song.* London, UK: J. Wilcox.

Vennard, W. (1967). *Singing: The mechanism and the technic.* New York, NY: Carl Fischer, Inc.

Wapnick, J., & Ekholm, E. (1997). Expert consensus in solo voice performance evaluation. *Journal of Voice, 11*(4), 429-336.

Appendix 12–A
Classical Vocal
Pedagogy Resources

Agricola, J., & Baird, J. (1995). *Introduction to the Art of Singing by Johann Friedrich Agricola (Cambridge Musical Texts and Monographs)*. Cambridge University Press.

Alderson, R. (1979). *Complete Handbook of Voice Training*. Prentice Hall Trade.

Andrews, D., & Dik, D. (2009). *How a Voice Teacher Shapes the Performance of His Students: A Study of the Pedagogy and Life of Giuseppe De Lucca*. Edwin Mellen Press.

Appleman, D. (1986). *The Science of Vocal Pedagogy*. Bloomington, IN: Indiana University Press.

Benninger, M., & Murry, T. (2006). *The Performers Voice*. San Diego, CA: Plural Publishing.

Boytim, J. (2003). *The Private Voice Studio Handbook: A Practical Guide to All Aspects of Teaching*. Hal Leonard Corporation.

Brown, W. (1968). *Vocal Wisdom: Maxims of G. B. Lamperti*. Reprint. New York, NY: Arno Press.

Bunch, M. (1982). *Dynamics of the Singing Voice*. New York, NY: Springer-Verlag.

Burtis, H. (2011). *Case Studies in Vocal Pedagogy*. Alberti Publications.

Bybee, A., & Ford, J. (Eds.). (2002). *The Modern Singing Master: Essays in Honor of Cornelius L. Reid*. Lanham, MD: Scarecrow Press.

Callaghan, J. (2000). *Singing and Voice Science*. San Diego, CA: Singular Publishing.

Caruso, E., & Luisa, T. (1979). *Caruso and Tetrazzini on the Art of Singing*. New York, NY: Dover Publications (Reprint of 1909 ed.).

Chapman, J. (2005). *Singing and Teaching Singing: A Holistic Approach to Classical Voice*. San Diego, CA: Plural Publishing.

Coffin, B. (2002). *Historical Vocal Pedagogy Classics*. Metuchen, NJ: Scarecrow Press.

David, M. (2008). *The New Voice Pedagogy*. Scarecrow Press.

Dayme, M., & Besterman, A. (2009). *Dynamics of the Singing Voice*. Springer.

Deere, J. (2005). *Singing in the 20th Century: A Recollection of Performance and Pedagogy*. AuthorHouse.

Doscher, B. (1994). *The Functional Unity of the Singing Voice* (2nd ed.). Lanham, MD: Scarecrow Press.

Downing, W. (1927). *Vocal Pedagogy for Student, Singer, and Teacher*. Carl Fischer.

Duey, P. (2007). *Bel Canto in Its Golden Age*. Duey Press.

Fields, A. (1947). *Training the Singing Voice.* DaCapo Press.

Garcia, M. (1984). *A Complete Treatise on the Art of Singing: Part One*, Trans. & Ed. D. V. Paschke. New York, NY: Da Capo Press (original work published 1841).

Hampton, M., & Acker, B. (2000). *The Vocal Vision: Views on Voice by 24 Leading Teachers, Coaches and Directors.* Applause.

Henderson, L. (1991). *How to Train Singers.* West Nyack, NY: Parker Publishing.

Joiner, J. (1998). *Charles Amable Battaille: Pioneer in Vocal Science and the Teaching of Singing.* Lanham, MD: Scarecrow Press.

Kagen, S. (1960). *On Studying Singing.* New York, NY: Dover Publications.

Klingstedt, P. (1941). *Common Sense in Vocal Pedagogy as Prescribed by the Early Italian Masters.* Stillwater, OK: Self Published.

Koster, R. (1990). *The Commonsense of Singing: Some Reflections on Technique, Performing and Repertoire.* New York, NY: Leyerle Publications.

Lamperti, G. (1905). *The Technics of Bel Canto*, trans. T. Baker. New York, NY: G. Schirmer.

Lehmann, L. (1952). *How to Sing.* New York, NY: Macmillan.

Leyerle, W. (1986). *Vocal Development through Organic Imagery* (2nd ed.). Mt. Morris, NY: Leyerle Publications.

Manén, L. (1974). *The Art of Singing.* London, UK: Faber Music.

Marafioti, M. (1981). *Caruso's Method of Voice Production.* New York, NY: Dover Publications.

Marchesi, B. (1978). *Singer's Pilgrimage.* New York, NY: Da Capo Press.

Marchesi, M. (1901). *Ten Singing Lessons.* New York, NY: Harper & Brothers.

Marchesi, M. (1967). *Vocal Method* (2nd ed.). Milwaukee, WI: G. Schirmer.

Marchesi, M. (1970). *Bel Canto: A Theoretical and Practical Vocal Method.* Dover Press.

McCoy, S. (2004). *Your Voice: An Inside View. Multimedia Voice Science and Pedagogy.* Princeton, NJ: Inside View Press.

McKinney, J. (1982). *The Diagnosis & Correction of Vocal Faults.* Nashville, TN: Genevox Music Group.

Miller, R. (1986). *The Structure of Singing: System and Art of Vocal Technique.* G. Schirmer Books.

Miller, R. (1993). *Training Tenor Voices.* New York, NY: G. Schirmer Books.

Miller, R. (1996). *On the Art of Singing.* New York, NY: Oxford University Press.

Miller, R. (1997). *English, French, German, and Italian Schools of Singing.* New York, NY: Scarecrow Press.

Miller, R. (2000). *Training Soprano Voices.* Oxford, UK: Oxford University Press.

Miller, R. (2004). *Solutions for Singers: Tools for Performers and Teachers.* Oxford, UK: University Press.

Monahan, B. (1978). *The Art of Singing.* Metuchen, NJ: Scarecrow Press.

Pesenti, S. (2011). *Basic Elements of Vocal Artistry for Young Singers.* AuthorHouse.

Potter, J. (2006). *Vocal Authority: Singing Style and Ideology.* Cambridge University Press.

Regal, R. (2005). *With a Voice of Singing (Vocal Pedagogy).* Ideal Sacred Music.

Reid, C. (1971). *The Free Voice.* New York, NY: J. Patelson.

Reid, C. (1975). *Psyche and Soma.* New York, NY: J. Patelson.

Reid, C. (1982). *Bel Canto Principles and Practices.* New York, NY: J. Patelson.

Ristad, E. (1982). *A Soprano on Her Head.* Moab, UT: Real People Press.

Samuelsen, R. (2010). *With a Song in My Heart: Reflections on 50 Years of Teaching and Performing.* Norlightspress.com.

Sataloff, R. (1998). *Vocal Health and Pedagogy.* San Diego, CA: Plural Publishing.

Schmidt, J., & Schmidt, H. (2007). *Basics of Singing.* G. Schirmer Books.

Sell, K. (2005). *The Discipline of Vocal Pedagogy: Towards a Holistic Approach.* Ashgate Publishing Company.

Shakespeare, W. (1921). *The Art of Singing.* Bryn Mawr, PA: Oliver Ditson Company.

Stanley, D. (1929). *The Science of the Voice*. New York, NY: Carl Fischer.

Stark, J. (2003). *Bel Canto: A History of Vocal Pedagogy*. University of Toronto Press.

Stockhausen, J. (1884). *Method of Singing*. London, UK: Novello.

Sundberg, J. (1987). *The Science of the Singing Voice*. Dekalb, IL: Northen Illinois University Press.

Tosi, P. (1743). *Observations on the Florid Song*. London, UK: J. Wilcox.

Vennard, W. (1967). *Singing: the Mechanism and the Technic*. New York, NY: Carl Fischer.

Ware, C. (1997). *Basics of Vocal Pedagogy*. McGraw-Hill.

Whitelock, W. (1975). *Profiles in Vocal Pedagogy: A Textbook for Singing Teachers*. Clifton Press.

13

Belting Pedagogy: An Overview of Perspectives

Introduction

Semantics regarding the term belting have historically resulted in much debate regarding both its definition and production. For the purposes of this text, belting will be considered as a vocal style commonly found and used in contemporary commercial music (CCM). Unlike the multitude of classical vocal pedagogy writings and degree programs designed to prepare the next generation of teachers, there are very few pedagogical training programs at the collegiate level that offer education and training specifically in teaching CCM vocal pedagogy. However, the demand to train commercial artists in a nonclassical aesthetic is growing rapidly.

Voice teachers of the 21st century will likely encounter requests from students to learn and perform styles other than Western classical singing. As part of commercial music training, the ability to train belting will inevitably need to be addressed by the teacher. This chapter provides the reader with a brief overview of the origin of belting and its presence in various styles of music. Summaries of commercial music pedagogical approaches from some of the current well-known and successful teachers are described. The intent of these authors is to neither dispel or endorse a specific pedagogical method; rather, it is to provide the reader with an overview of some of the prominent CCM pedagogues who have pioneered and contributed to this field by formalizing, publishing, and presenting their methods for others to learn.

Readers should keep in mind that most of the pedagogical approaches and methods for both classical and CCM styles described have not necessarily undergone rigorous scientific investigation demonstrating efficacy. However, the CCM pedagogues presented in this chapter have refined their methods over years of teaching or research with an understanding that CCM styles require a unique pedagogical approach that is different from traditional classical pedagogy.

Many of these teachers have been generous with their methods, presenting at conferences, contributing papers and books, leading workshops, intensive seminars, and master classes.

Increasing Demand for Commercial Pedagogy and Belting

There is a rich musical history and transformation of the very early or "common styles" of singing from minstrel shows, to vaudeville, through today's contemporary styles of jazz, pop, rock, gospel, and music theater. Elaborating on the historical development of each of these genres is beyond the scope of this book, but commercial vocal styles continue to evolve and reflect society. The popularization of musicals into conventional media (e.g., *Glee*, *Smash*, *Nine*, *Chicago*, *Les Miserablés*, *The Sound of Music*) has resulted in cross-pollinated singing within popular vocal music. This popularization has now seemingly made singing more approachable and accessible to both the technically skilled and novice vocalist. Additionally, the emergence and popularity of televised singing talent shows such as *The Voice*, *American Idol*, and *America's Got Talent*, further brings CCM styles of vocal music into mainstream culture.

As a consequence, there has been an influx of singers of all ages and stages of life and skill wanting to sing in CCM styles. In the best of scenarios, the singer has sought out a skilled voice teacher who is willing and able to guide the singer. For the classical teacher, development of their own pedagogy to meet the demands of their students may have evolved out of necessity. Interestingly, it has been reported that

approximately 34% of university level teachers who train nonclassical singers have neither performance or pedagogy training in commercial music (Weekly & LoVetri, 2009). Certainly, many have been successful out of experience and have learned to adapt to the needs of the student's various demands. Others, however, perhaps maintain a traditional classical approach asserting that a solid classical technique is sufficient to sing many styles of music, although not all pedagogues endorse this thinking.

In a less desirable scenario, the singer performs CCM styles without proper vocal training or with no vocal training at all. This could result in an inefficient or potentially harmful singing approach, increasing the risk of vocal injury. Today, more than ever, there is a need for voice pedagogues to understand how to guide students seeking to sing in commercial music styles. The field of vocal pedagogy has evolved over the past 20 years, and there is now added consensus acknowledging commercial styles of singing, including belting, as a valid genre requiring sound vocal technique.

Overview of History and Pedagogical Approaches for Belting

Unlike the plethora of information that exists on training the classical voice, there are few if any formalized texts devoted solely to training the belt voice. Several teachers have published articles and books (primarily based in their own teaching experience) on approaches and exercises to train the musical theater singer (Boardman, 1992; Edwin, 1998a, 1998b; Estill, 1988; LeBorgne, Lee, Stemple, & Bush, 2009; Sullivan, 1989).

The vocal style of belting has been around hundreds of years and can be traced in part back to the Negro settlements and plantation life in North America where slaves would engage in sacred shouting, ballads, and moans. This form of vocal expression was characterized by wails, high pitches, glides, and voice breaks and was a far cry from Baroque and Classical styles of music that originated from royalty and high society.

Within the last 30 years, an emergence of specific vocal pedagogy regarding training of belting and the commercial music singer has begun to develop. An overview of these pioneers in training belters is presented below. The teachers and pedagogues included in this chapter vary in their contribution to training belting. Some of the teachers have published detailed methodology, while others have published educated opinions based on their years of teaching experience. Overviews of works are presented below in order of their first date of publication.

through various exercises and sounds. Singers who are able to learn and master her 13 Figures for Voice™ should result in optimal vocal flexibility for multiple styles without strain or effort. Her method targets mastery of six-voice characteristics including twang, sob, belt, opera, falsetto, and speech. The utility of Estill's vocal training effects improved flexibility of the laryngeal mechanism by attempting to define for the singer/speaker many different vocal qualities. Perceptual feedback regarding sound quality is emphasized using technical software programs, which record and analyze the acoustic signal of the voice. Estill Voice International proposes both theory and motor acquisition as part of the training. Similar to the classical pedagogues, Ms. Estill initially used a master-apprentice relationship to train her future teachers, and today there are at least two levels of teachers: course instructor and master teacher. In-depth discussion of Estill's training methodology can be found at the Estill Voice International website.

Jo Estill—Estill Voicetraining™

Jo Estill was the founder of Estill Voice Training™ and Figures for Voice™ in 1988. She was known for contributions to voice research on physiology of belting and has collaborated with voice scientists exploring elements of voice physiology during singing and speaking. Considered as one of the pioneers of belting research, Jo Estill studied laryngeal movement during belting via laryngeal imaging and videostroboscopy. Additional research included EMG in conjunction with acoustic measurements of voice. This research led to development of her methodology to train nonclassical singers, which emphasizes mastering volitional control of the laryngeal structures

Jan Sullivan—How to Teach the Belt/Pop Voice (1989)

Jan Sullivan's text attempts to clarify what perceptually constitutes the belt voice, and how to produce the belt sound. This article uses terms such as belt, quasi-belt, legitimate (classical), chest, nasal, pop (soft belt), pop legitimate, middle gospel, and soul. Different physiological mechanisms are described as needed to produce each of the voice types, and musical excerpts are provided as examples. No scientific research to date has been conducted to determine whether or not the "different mechanisms" theory she described is true for belters and whether the terminology used is consistent.

The most important distinction among voice types Sullivan makes is that she does not consider belting the same as chest voice. She states that chest voice is trained as the lowest part of a classical singer's range. Belting is considered an entirely different production than the classical mezzo, soprano, or coloratura chest voice. Belting as described by Jan Sullivan:

A sound produced by a vocal mechanism in which the larynx is slightly higher than in the classical voice, and the vocal cords come together firmly and cleanly. The shape of the word and how it is spoken is intrinsic to the sound. The sound seems forward in comparison to classical even to the point of sometimes seeming nasal, but it is not nasal. The amount of energy in the support areas is immense. The lips, teeth, tongue, and jaw are shaped and positioned in a specific way for consistent projection of the word so that the word stays between the teeth and the sound formed is not destroyed by an ever-changing projection as it leaves the mouth. The space inside the mouth is not as large as in the classical technique. (p. 42)

Four specific training techniques are addressed by Sullivan in order that a singer may be able to achieve the belt sound if they can successful do all four things. First, mouth positioning is extremely important in the belt voice. Second, good posture, respiration, breath support, and vocal onset is essential (further discussed in Chapter 2). Third, ideal vowel placement is indicated so that the singer may not only be intelligible, but maintain the strength and consistency of the vowel throughout the range. Finally, she considered diction to be the utmost importance, as the belter must be understood in order to move the plot of the story forward through song.

Ms. Sullivan's discussion on breath support and attack are limited to a few sentences in her writings. She alludes to the *lutte vocale* (vocal struggle) when she addresses breath support. No information regarding training of phonation is addressed in Sullivan's article. The only mention of the larynx is with respect to its relative height during belting, suggesting that the laryngeal positioning is higher than that of the classical voice. She goes on to state that training appropriate resonance in belters as the essence of good technique. Specifically, articulation and appropriate mouth position must be trained differently from the classical singer. Sullivan suggested the proper mouth position resembles the bell of a trumpet because both the upper and lower teeth are visible with this mouth position.

Articulation resulting in excellent diction must be achieved by the belter. Sullivan suggests a complex system of coding the text using shapes, colors, arrows, and symbols. This coding system is designed to help the singer know exactly where vowel modification, glottal attacks, and diphthongs are to occur and alert them to certain vocal pitfalls. Consonants, especially in the word-final position, should be clearly and distinctly articulated without shortening the previous vowel. Also, Sullivan suggested that tongue placement maintains a forward position throughout the entire song and rests with the tip touching the bottom front teeth. The only instance when the tongue is permitted to move is during specific consonant production.

Following text coding, Sullivan provides information on training a singer in how to produce a belt sound. She uses the words "bay," "may," and "pay" as the starting point for belters. Production (spoken) of these words is initially to be as nasal as possible. The highest degree of nasality is given a rating of "one." Students are then asked to produce these same three words with a forward placement without nasality and that sound is given a rating of a "two." The process continues moving the placement of these words further back until the words become "deep and throaty." The placement that is perceived as furthest back is given a rating of "ten." For each of the ten ratings, Sullivan provides a definition of what type of singing is produced by that vocal tract configuration. The next step of the process is the spoken production of the song lyrics. Ultimately, the lyrics are put to music. Finally, she suggests pairing the belt style and with classical singing style on vocalises, so that the singer learns to differentiate between them (Sullivan, 1989).

Larra Henderson—How to Train Singers (1991)

Within Henderson's chapter on performance technique in her book *How to Train Singers* (1991), she addressed the belting voice. She defined belting as a mix of chest and head voice requiring a frontal focused tone, with more active engagement of the abdominal muscles than with classical singing. The belt tone was never to be considered nasal; rather the singer should feel the sympathetic nasal vibrations when belting. Belting, as interpreted by Henderson, is a color/timbre of the voice that all singers should be able to access.

Henderson advocated a solid basis for appropriate breath support based in the classical diaphragmatic breathing technique.

Her text includes an entire chapter devoted to postural alignment and breathing technique. Similar to the classical pedagogues in her techniques, no significantly new information regarding respiratory training is offered in this text. However, Henderson is a strong believer in the Alexander Technique™ with respect to postural alignment.

Henderson wrote that the primary perceptual difference between belting and classical singing is achieved through vowel placement and tone color. Tone production was not specifically addressed as it relates to belting, with the exception of loudness. However, she discouraged increased intensity in the beginner and required a solid foundation in classical technique prior to teaching a singer to belt.

Forward placement of vowels and a sensation that they vibrate off of the hard palate she reported as the primary differences noted between the classical and belt tone quality. She provided ten vocalises designed to promote this frontal focus in singers, designed to reprogram a muscle memory task. Henderson reported training singers is similar to training athletes; one must train muscle memories in order to perform certain tasks vocally and physically (Henderson, 1991).

Jeannette LoVetri— Somatic Voicework™ The LoVetri Method

For over four decades, Ms. LoVetri has been a strong proponent of the belief that CCM requires distinct technical training, aimed at the sounds vocalists make in the various styles, which are frequently different than those that classical singers make. She published her first article in 1993 regarding the differences in voice production between classical and musical theater singing (Sundberg, Gramming, & LoVetri, 1993). Credited for coining the term CCM (for contemporary commercial music), formerly called "nonclassical." Jeanie LoVetri is the creator of Somatic Voicework™ (SVW) The LoVetri Method (Lovetri, 2008), a body-based system of training for CCM incorporating techniques derived from the disciplines of speech pathology, acting, movement, yoga, Alexander Technique™, and Feldenkrais®. Her training methodology strongly advocates for vocal health and collaboration with otolaryngologists and speech pathologists. Somatic Voicework™ The Lovetri Method emphasizes developing a fully balanced vocal mechanism while cultivating increased aural discernment. It focuses on hearing subtle differences in vocal qualities such as registration (head, chest, mix) and vowel sound accuracy, while also observing external postural and physical behavior as contributors to overall vocal production. Success in this method is based on the teacher's ability to apply vocal exercise to promote change in the student's vocal response, and to hold in mind the desired musical goals of the student while so doing.

Certification in her method is offered in three levels. Level I introduces an organized pedagogical approach based on vocal function and the principles of voice science medicine. Level II delves deeper into her method, teaching participants how to troubleshoot common technical problems seen in singers. Ms. LoVetri has created the Solution Sequence®, which is taught in Level II and is a grid of common problems observed in singers, causes for those problems, and exercises to remediate the problem. Level III delves deeper into troubleshooting technical issues, and applying Somatic Voicework™ principles

to CCM repertoire. Somatic Voicework™ is the chosen pedagogical method at the CCM Vocal Pedagogy Institute at Shenandoah Conservatory (LoVetri, 2013). Further understanding on the background and development of Somatic Voicework™ training, methodology, and certification can be found at the Somatic Voicework™ website.

Robert Edwin— Belting 101 (Part 1 & 2)

Singing teacher Robert Edwin provides another perspective to training the belt voice. Edwin's recurring article series in the *NATS Journal* (The Bach to Rock Connection) are based primarily in his experience with teaching (Edwin, 1998a, 1998b). His two-article series on belting provides his interpretation of the definition of the belt voice and its pedagogical methods. Edwin defined belting as "A term describing a chest voice dominant vocal quality used in many styles of nonclassical singing" (p. 53). His definition of belting is based in registration terminology. He hypothesized that in belt voice production, the thyroarytenoid muscle demonstrates more activity resulting in the heavy mechanism (which would include the chest voice), while the cricothyroid muscle predominates in the light mechanism (head voice). Edwin stated that belting is a result of thyroarytenoid dominant phonation, but resolved that it is not the same as chest voice. EMG evidence suggests that register changes are based on the activity of the vocalis muscle. Heavy registration resulted in increased activity of the vocalis while light registration noted decreased EMG activity of the vocalis (Hirano, Vennard, & Ohala, 1970).

Edwin also reported that not all singers voices may be able to sustain a belting tone, just as all classical singers may not be able to perform Wagner. The classical literature concurs with Edwin's statement as singers have always been cautioned not to sing for long periods of time outside of their appropriate *fach*. Advocating breath as the foundation for good singing technique, Edwin further suggested training efficient breath management. He did not provide any explanation of what constitutes efficient breath management in the belter, nor did he provide insight as to whether breath management strategies used in training the classical singer are appropriate for the belter. One would assume that if belting is produced with intensity demands different from that of the classical singer, it may require a different breathing strategy.

No specific mention of training vocal onset, glottal attacks, or other commercial stylistic elements is addressed by Edwin. Rather he provided specific vocalises with which to train students in the belt technique. The recommendations to begin vocalizing include beginning in the low-frequency range of the singer's voice. He reported sound productions should be a "chest-mix," not an exclusively chest voice production but does not offer perceptual or physiologic cues that would differentiate "chest mix" and pure chest voice productions. He goes on to say the sound quality should be "brassy," "twangy," and "nasal-tinged." In order to achieve the correct placement, he advocates using alternating /nɑ/-/ni/ in a five-note ascending and descending diatonic scale. A fast tempo is recommended to avoid vocal strain on the higher notes. This exercise was advised not to be taken into head voice (beyond the first passaggio).

Other than the terminology mentioned above, no mention of training resonance is given. Edwin proposed that belting, like classical singing, should not permit jaw or tongue tension, nor the observation of neck veins or muscles protruding during song (Edwin, 1998a, 1998b).

Seth Riggs

Seth Riggs, a voice coach based in Hollywood, is the creator of Speech Level Singing™. His work states that one must always use a speech-level tone when singing across their entire frequency range regardless of the style of music. He emphasizes stable posture advocating an open rib cage. Mr. Riggs' Speech Level Singing™ does not focus solely on resonance or breathing stating, "good resonance and breathing are the by-product of good technique." Although, he does not necessarily endorse use of imagery, he does detail specific exercises to achieve a desired outcome. Mr. Riggs offers several levels of certification in his methodology that can be located on his website (Riggs, 2007).

Lisa Popeil

Lisa Popeil is a Los Angeles-based voice teacher and creator of Voiceworks® Method. The Voiceworks® Method is based on over 50 years of voice study and almost 40 years of professional teaching. It promotes the idea that there are certain skills that all singers should have: posture; five jobs of support; breathing; knowing one's absolute vocal range; how to control vocal fold closure; vertical laryngeal positioning; the ability to control resonance with ring, brightness, and nasality; pharyngeal width and constriction; registration mastery for all styles; and skill in vibrato types and speeds. For more advanced singers interested in vocal styles such as pop, rock, country, jazz,

R&B, musical theater legit, musical theater belting, opera, and operetta, Ms. Popeil's method provides detailed analysis.

Her published article, The Multiplicity of Belting (2007), defines belting as speech-like or yell-like in character. She subcategorizes different types of belting based on sound. These include heavy belt, ringy belt, nasal belt, brassy belt, and speech-like belt. Her method places strong emphasis on proper posture and precise abdominal support to minimize or eliminate vocal fold pressing. She further discusses some of the physiologic differences of vocal fold activity based on her research. Discussion of registration and emphasis on a tactile awareness of laryngeal activity associated with various pitches is important in her pedagogy. She offers a variety of DVDs, CDs, books, classes, and workshops, which teach her method (Popeil, 2007, 2010). More information can be found on her website Lisa Popeil's Voiceworks®.

Mary Saunders-Barton— Bel Canto/Can Belto: Learning to Teach and Sing for Musical Theatre

Mary Saunders (Professor of Music at Penn State University, where she serves as Head of Voice Instruction for the Bachelor of Fine Arts in Musical Theater at Penn State University and as Head of the MFA in Vocal Pedagogy for Musical Theatre), has developed and published on her Bel Canto/Can Belto pedagogy techniques and implemented a new terminal degree program in Musical Theatre Pedagogy.

The pedagogical basis for her teaching of both the male and female musical theater performers is to produce healthy, versatile singers with necessary endurance to support an eight-show week. Specifically,

her technique works on "balancing classical vocal technique with the techniques specific to musical theater singing and contemporary commercial music." All students are exposed to and expected to master with some degree of proficiency appropriate "breath management, legato, vibrancy, clean onset and release, and ease of production" (Saunders-Barton, 2013). Control of palatal elevation and flexibility of laryngeal height allow the singer to alter resonance spaces in an infinite number of possible combinations for both speech and song providing them with an available vocal and resonance "palette" necessary to manipulate for the demands of musical theatre performance (Saunders-Barton, 2005).

The aesthetic priorities which drive the pedagogy for Saunders-Barton Bel Canto/Can Belto are strongly based in the elements and mastery of the speaking voice. Saunders-Barton states, "Musical theatre is a speech-based, vernacular form anchored in drama. We are teaching actors to sing. Our primary allegiance is to character and story. This does not negate the concept of aesthetic beauty but it certainly broadens the definition!" As a result, she embodies the pedagogy that you must "train the speech, train the singer" (Saunders-Barton, 2013). Speaking voice placement, inflection, flexibility, and range are also essential voice components to master within her musical theater pedagogy training. One cannot build the necessary stamina for musical theater performance, if the speaking voice is inappropriately functioning or lacks flexibility. Therefore, students are exposed to text-based exercises designed to incorporate both the speaking and singing aspects of coordinated sound production in one task. Cross-conditioning, incorporating both fully classical sounds and chest voice, are essential components of the Bel Canto/Can Belto pedagogy. Saunders-Barton advocates that a balance of both vocal qualities and muscle group activity (thyroarytenoid and crico-thyroid) results in a balanced middle voice with the ability to increase intensity without vocal strain (Saunders-Barton, 2013). Information on Mary Barton-Saunders pedagogy can be found on her Bel Canto Can Belto website.

Chapter Summary

The Black Crook, first performed in 1866, is considered by most to be the first American Musical. However, the first musical theater degree program was not established until about 100 years later (1968, Cincinnati College-Conservatory of Music). As of this writing, over 140 musical theater preprofessional training programs exist: three offer an Associates of Arts in Musical Theater (MT); 46 offer a Bachelor of Arts in MT; 81 offer a Bachelor of Fine Arts; 5 offer a Bachelor of Music in Interdisciplinary Musical Theater; 5 offer a Bachelor of Music in MT; 2 offer an Masters of Arts in Music Theater; and 2 offer an Masters of Fine Arts in Musical Theater. But there are currently only two universities who offer advanced degrees specifically in nonclassical pedagogy (Pennsylvania State University and Shenandoah University). This disparity between pedagogy training programs and performance programs has likely left many teachers to devise their own nonclassical pedagogy to meet the demands of their students.

Although limited formal pedagogy programs focus on CCM styles, there are many teachers who have dedicated themselves to teaching this vocal style. The above chapter provided a general overview of some of these pedagogues. Fortunately, several have published their methods or made them accessible with workshops and seminars. These authors reiterate that it would be impossible to claim one approach as superior or inferior to another; however, the same would be true for classical pedagogical approaches as none of them have been rigorously, scientifically studied. The field of vocal pedagogy in general, continues to rely on conventional wisdom and empirical observation combined with the research that does exist to further refine our approach and methods for teaching. These CCM pedagogues have made valuable contributions to our field. Many of them have collaborated with voice scientists and even served as subjects in research to help further our knowledge in this pedagogical area. Additionally, most have been vocal proponents for decades, highlighting the need for an approach to CCM that is distinct from traditional classical pedagogy in order to better serve the needs of these singers.

References

Boardman, S. (1992). Vocal training for a career in music theater: A pedagogy. *The NATS Journal, 49*, 8–15, 47.

Edwin, R. (1998a). Belting 101. *Journal of Singing, 55*(1), 53–55.

Edwin, R. (1998b). Belting 101, Part two. *Journal of Singing, 55*(2), 61–62.

Estill, J. (1988). Belting and classic voice quality: Some physiological differences. *Medical Problems of Performing Artists*, 37–43.

Henderson, L. (1991). *How to train singers*. West Nyack, NY: Parker Publishing.

Hirano, M., Vennard, W., & Ohala, J. (1970). Regulation of register, pitch, and intensity of voice. *Folia Phoniatric, 22*, 1–20.

LeBorgne, W., Lee, L., Stemple, J., & Bush, H. (2009). Perceptual findings on the

Broadway belt voice. *Journal of Voice, 24*(6), 678-689.

LoVetri, J. (2008). Contemporary commercial music. *Journal of Voice, 22*, 260-262.

LoVetri, J. (2013). *Somatic voicework. The LoVetri method.* Retrieved from http://www.somaticvoicework.com.

Popeil, L. (2007). The multiplicity of belting. *Journal of Singing, 64*, 77-80.

Popeil, L. (2010). *Lisa Popeil's Voiceworks.* Retrieved from http://www.popeil.com.

Riggs, S. (2007). *The Seth Riggs Vocal Studio.* Retrieved from http://www.sethriggs.com.

Saunders-Barton, M. (2005). *The well spoken singer. Essays on voice and speech.* Voice and Teachers Association, August.

Saunders-Barton, M. (2013). Broadway bound: Teaching young musical theater singers in a college training program. *NYSTA VOICE Prints,* March-April.

Sullivan, J. (1989). How to teach the belt/pop voice. *Journal of Research in Singing and Applied Vocal Pedagogy, 13*(1), 41-56.

Sundberg, J., Gramming, P., & Lovetri, J. (1993). Comparison of pharynx, source, formant, and pressure characteristics in operatic and music theater singing. *Journal of Voice, 7*(4), 301-310.

Weekly, E., & LoVetri, J. (2009). Follow-up contemporary commercial music (CCM) survey: Who's teaching what in nonclassical music. *Journal of Voice, 23*(3), 367-375.

14

Belting:
Theory and Research

Introduction

Although we know more today than we ever have about the science of the singing voice, there is much to be learned about the nuances of the singing voice for both classical and CCM vocal styles. Fortunately, classical singing, belting, and some of the other CCM vocal styles have been the focus of voice science research in the last 40 years. Results of these studies provide useful information for the teacher, scientist, and student about laryngeal and acoustic function. Study results should be regarded with caution, because, like much of the research we have on singing voice, many of the studies for CCM styles are limited by small subject pools. This chapter serves to highlight some of the peer-reviewed seminal and current physiological research on belting and other CCM singing styles. Perceptual and objective data are presented. Readers are encouraged to familiarize themselves with

the concepts and terminology discussed in Chapter 5 before reading this chapter.

Belting—Perceptual Research

Prior to objective investigation of the belt voice, one must first make an attempt to define it perceptually. Terminology used to define the nature and production of the belt voice is almost as controversial as the style itself. At a 2001 NATS Winter Workshop conference specifically designated to better understand and train the belt voice, the terminology and use of various training techniques was diverse. Sixteen different printed opinions on the definition of belting were presented at that conference. Although presenters used inconsistent terminology, there was little dispute about the quality of sound they desired to achieve. Semantic confusion permeates the literature with a plethora of terminology used to describe the acoustic events related to commercial voice sound production. There are multiple papers on terminology and descriptions about commercial voice production (Bourne, Garnier, & Kenny, 2011; Lovetri, 2006; Popeil, 2007; Spivey, 2008; Sundberg, 1994). Presentation of literature in this segment is limited to articles published in scientific journals. Without an accepted definition, objective evaluation of a given vocal quality is difficult.

Early attempts to define the perceptual attributes of belting were conducted by Miles and Hollien (1990). They reviewed the limited literature on defining perceptual characteristics of belting as well as surveying voice teachers and other voice professionals. The results of their study concluded with four perceptual judgments of belting (loud, heavy phonation, little-to-no vibrato, high degree of nasality) that reoccurred in both the literature and survey. The conclusion of their paper challenged others to further investigate perceptual findings and objectify the acoustic parameters.

LeBorgne, Lee, Stemple, and Bush (2009) evaluated perceptual and objective measures of pre-professional belters. Casting directors were asked to evaluate the belt voice quality of 20 musical theater majors who were proficient in the singing style referred to as belting. The raters (casting directors) were asked to judge the belters on a set of seven perceptual parameters (loudness, vibrato, ring, timbre, focus, nasality, and registration breaks), and then report an overall score for these student belters. The four highest and lowest average scores were used to establish the elite and average student belters. A correlation analysis and linear regression analysis provided insight regarding which perceptual judgments correlated most highly with the elite and average scores. The LeBorgne et al. (2009) study found the perceptual ratings of vibrato and ring to be most highly correlated to the elite student belter. In addition, vibrato and ring were found to highly correlate with perceived loudness. Findings related to the objective measures conducted in this study are presented later in this chapter.

Sundberg, Thalen, and Popeil (2012) sought to further examine different subtypes of belt qualities that they describe as heavy belt, brassy, ringy, nasal, and speechlike. One of the coauthors on this investigation also served as the single subject for all vocal tasks. A classical sample of the same musical phrase was also recorded by the same subject for comparison. A panel of eight listeners had good agreement (61%–100% accuracy) with identifying the appropriate category of vocal production. Objective measure of these vocal productions were completed and are discussed further in the segments below.

Laryngeal Muscle Activity and Action during CCM Singing

Some of the earliest research on laryngeal muscle activity during belting was presented at one of the first scientific assemblies of multiple disciplines from the worlds of vocal pedagogy and vocal arts medicine in 1988 (now referred to as The Voice Foundation Annual Symposium). Jo Estill (1988) presented a pilot study using bipolar electrodes on a single subject. She looked at muscle activity of the vocal folds along with seven other extrinsic laryngeal muscles including pharyngeal constrictors and muscles of the tongue. Estill concluded that the primary difference in muscle activity between belting and classical style singing involved the relative position and angle of the thyroid and cricoid cartilage. She concluded that their positioning was opposite for classical style and belting.

Further research into the investigation of vocal registers used hooked wire EMG electrodes to monitor activity of thyroarytenoid and cricothyroid muscles in seven female singers (Kochis-Jennings, Finnegan, Hoffman, & Jaiswal, 2012). Two subjects were professional classical singers, two sang both classical and nonclassical and one was nonclassical. All subjects were deemed able to produce the four distinct registers by a voice teacher prior to the study. Chest voice demonstrated greater TA activity and greater vocal process adduction compared to head voice. Chestmix showed greater TA activity compared to headmix on the same pitch on the high frequencies. TA activity for chestmix and headmix on the low frequencies was comparable. Muscle activity patterns appeared to be consistent with the style of vocal training. For example, classically trained subjects showed less range of TA activity across registers (25%-38%) compared to CCM singers (5%-75%) particularly at higher pitches. Cricothyroid activity did not appear to be tied to changes in registration compared to TA activity (Kochis-Jennings et al., 2012).

Although the next study does not relate to laryngeal muscle activity directly, it does provide insight into possible supraglottic muscle activity in CCM singing styles. This study aimed to compare laryngeal behavior during different singing styles used transnasal fiberoptic laryngoscopy to examine muscle tension patterns of 100 healthy singers representing different styles of singing including art song, choral, opera, musical theater, pop/jazz, blue grass/country western, and rock/gospel. After looking at these singers during varied singing tasks, the authors rated muscle tension patterns based on: (1) level of glottal adduction, (2) supraglottic constriction, and (3) anterior to posterior constriction of the laryngeal vestibule during singing. Overall, choral, art song, and opera had the lowest percentage of muscular tension (41%-58%) music theater in the middle with (74%) and rock/gospel and blue grass/country western having the highest muscle tension scores (87%-94%). Incidentally, 15% of the singer subjects had asymptomatic laryngeal pathology (nodular swelling) identified at the time of the study (Kouffman, Radomski, Jojarji, & Pillsbury, 1996). This finding illustrates the point that singers (regardless of genre) can be free of voice complaints and present with asymptomatic vocal pathology. This presents an interesting issue for the CCM singer as to what constitutes a vocal complaint, as we do not know what a CCM singer's threshold might be for variations in vocal functioning compared to classical singers. Another consideration with this study is that the different laryngeal configurations identified as muscle tension patterns may be simply related to vocal tract adjustments which have acoustic implications for varied styles of singing rather than aberrant muscular tension.

In an attempt to quantify the glottic closure, supraglottic, and laryngeal height patterns during belting, both rigid and fiberoptic evaluation of seven professional belters was conducted (LoVetri, Lesh, & Woo, 1999). Findings of their study indicated that individual singers utilized a variety of glottic and supraglottic configurations to produce an acceptable belt sound. Two of the seven female belters used a lowered laryngeal position on their belting. This is in contrast to much of the literature which reports the need for a high larynx position.

Voice Source Information on Belting

In addition to using needle electrodes into the intrinsic and extrinsic laryngeal muscles and direct observation (nasendoscopy) to determine muscle activity, multiple studies have used less invasive measures (Electroglottograpy [EGG] and inverse filtering). EGG provides information about how long the vocal folds are open and closed and how quickly they come together, which will ultimately impact the vocal spectrum output. Similarly, inverse filtering uses technology to "decouple" the effects of the vocal tract from the vocal folds (i.e., what are the vocal folds doing separately from how the vocal tract modifies and enhances the sound).

Open Quotients, Closed Quotients, and Subglottal Pressure Measures

The belt voice has been identified as having a longer closed quotient (CQ) with higher subglottal pressures than classical singing (Bestebreurtje & Schutte, 2000; Bjorkner, 2008; Bjorkner, Sundberg, Cleveland, &

> **Open Quotient (OQ)** refers to the ratio of the time vocal folds are open during a full cycle of vocal fold vibration. **Closed Quotient (CQ)** refers to the ratio of how long the vocal fold are closed during a full cycle of vocal fold vibration. **Subglottal Pressure** refers to the amount of air needed to set the vocal folds into vibratory motion.

Stone, 2005; Bourne & Garnier, 2012; Kochis-Jennings, Finnegan, Hoffman, & Jaiswal, 2012; Lebowitz & Baken, 2011; Schutte & Miller, 1993; Stone, Cleveland, Sundberg, & Prokop, 2003; Sundberg, Cleveland, Stone, & Iwarsson, 1999). Relevant research studies in a variety of styles and contexts are presented. Schutte and Miller (1993) defined belting as having over a 50% closed phase. Other researchers have used the parameters set forth by Schutte and Miller as a basis for further investigation. Vowel variations were not observed to impact changes in CQ when belting, but degree of CQ has been noted to increase with increased frequency (Bestebreurtje & Schutte, 2000). Specifically, an increase of 3% or greater in CQ percentage for belt compared to speech was observed in 10 of the 18 trials conducted. The authors surmised that in addition to CQ playing a role in belting there are likely individual vocal tract modifications based on singer physiology and style/aesthetic goals for the tone (Bestebreurtje & Schutte, 2000).

Bjorkner et al. (2005) examined voice source differences in chest register versus head register for seven professional music theater singers who reported having classical training. These authors looked at subglottal pressures, closed quotient, and several other parameters to explore how the vocal folds behave in different vocal registers. In general, chest voice demonstrated increased closed quotient compared to head register. Higher overtones were stronger and perceived phonatory pressedness was greater for chest voice production (Bjorkner et al., 2005).

Belting in several defined qualities (heavy chest, brassy, ringy, and head) resulted in CQ patterns noted in previous studies within a single subject design (Sundberg et al., 2012). Within the Sundberg et al. study, heavy belt and brassy belt showed the longest closed quotient, nearing 50%. Bourne and Garnier (2012) published findings using a larger sample size (six subjects) in the qualities of chesty belt mix, twangy belt and legit. Legit voice quality had the longest open quotient (OQ), with twangy belt and chesty belt showing a similar amount of CQ. Mix voice production found that the six subjects all demonstrated various strategies somewhere in-between legit and belt for resonance and glottic behavior (Bourne & Garnier, 2012).

On the other hand, Lebowitz and Baken's (2011) findings on CQ conflicted with that of most previous studies. The authors compared closed quotient (CQ); how long vocal folds stay closed during the open/closed phased of vibration, speed quotient (SQ); how quickly vocal folds close, in 20 professional belters (who were asked to sing in both a belt and classical style). Their findings indicated that belting consistently yielded a higher SQ compared to classical style. Interestingly, there was little difference in CQ during belting, with only a small (12%) increase in CQ. The mean CQ for belting and classical was equal to or below 50% in this group of singers.

Another component that has yielded investigation on belting is subglottal pressure measures. Subglottal pressure is the amount of pressure needed to set the vocal folds into vibration. Theoretically, the more firmly the vocal folds are closed, the more subglottic pressure is required to set the vocals into vibration. The increase of subglottic pressure as a means to increase vocal intensity is well-documented in the literature (Sundberg, 1990; Titze, 1994). As belters are generally perceived to be loud, measures of and comparisons of subglottic pressure measures should be quantifiable. Studies are consistent with respect to subglottic pressure measures (Bjorkner, 2008; Bjorkner et al., 2005; Stone et al., 2003; Sundberg et al., 1999). Specifically,

musical theater voice production has demonstrated generally increased subglottal pressure in comparison with classical singing (Bjorkner, 2008; Sundberg et al., 2012). Brassy and ringy qualities were in the mid-range of pressure, with ringy trending slightly more toward lower subglottal pressures (Sundberg et al., 2012).

Formants and Harmonic Findings/Singers Formant/Formant Tuning

Recall from Chapter 5 that location of formants (resonances of the vocal tract) are determined by vocal tract shape, and the harmonics are integer multiples of the fundamental frequency. Changes in vocal tract configuration (i.e., raising or lowering the larynx, changing jaw opening, altering lip position) alter the location of the formants, and ultimately how the vowel is perceived by the listener (recall that vowel identification is determined by F1 and F2). Additionally, when a formant is located near a harmonic, that harmonic is amplified. As commercial music singers learn to alter the shape and size of their resonators, they mold the sound source (produced by the vocal folds) into infinite possible timbres.

Some of the more interesting research on belting has focused on the interaction of the formants and harmonics as qualitative markers of belting and other nonclassical singing. The literature has looked at country

> Timbre is in part determined by the strength of the harmonic. Harmonics become strengthened when they are near formants.

singers, musical theater singers, pop singers, and some folk singers. Formant frequencies of five professional country singers were examined for both speaking and singing voice (Sundberg et al., 1999). The authors concluded that the formant structure for these five high-level professional country performers was similar between singing and speech formants. This, is in contrast with what we know about classical style singing where the formant structure is very different from speech (Singer's Formant). It makes sense that country style singing has a comparable formant structure to speech because much of this style of singing occurs in the speech range with speech-like vowel shaping. Additionally, given that country music singing is almost always amplified, these singers do not necessarily need to modify the vocal tract in order to increase amplification of higher formant frequencies in order to project over an orchestra, as is the case with classical singing (Sundberg et al., 1999).

The lyrics of musical theater songs are required to be understood on the first hearing, because they are essential for plot advancement and emotional content, so speech-like quality is imperative. Therefore, it has been postulated that the singer's format is eliminated in belting, as the formants that define vowels (F1–F2) are paramount for text comprehension (Schutte & Miller, 1993). The reported lack of a singer's formant in belting may be a result of the consistent use of body microphones. It is generally accepted that the singer's formant was developed so that professional classical singers could be heard over an orchestra without amplification. One study found that professional opera singers had difficulty being heard and understood when singing musical theater literature (Stone, 1994).

Consistent general findings (with some subject and semantic variability) have been confirmed in multiple studies within the last 20 years. The following studies report findings related to formants and harmonics of belting. Sundberg, Gramming, and LoVetri (1993) examined four voice qualities within a single subject (chest, chest-mix, headmix, and head) and reported that female mix voice production had qualities from both classical and belting. The first two formants were higher in belting compared to the classical singing, but subglottic pressure levels were not significantly different. Stone, Cleveland, Sundberg, and Prokop (2003) compared aerodynamic and acoustic data for Broadway compared to classical singing. Their single subject was a female professional singer with a background in both vocal styles. The result demonstrated lower F1 and F2 in general for opera compared to Broadway.

As single-subject designs tend to populate this literature, Bestebreurtje and Schutte (2000) evaluated the resonance strategies used for belting in a single subject. Specifically, a singer would "formant tune" by adjusting their vocal tract configuration, thereby altering formant locations, in order to boost the amplification of certain harmonics of the sound source. For this subject, there was a tuning of her lower formants (F1 and F2) to the second and fourth harmonics. The authors also described different tuning behaviors for different vowels. For example, there was no adjustment of the formants for the /a/ vowel, and this vowel was considered a "belt friendly" vowel. This is likely because F1 and F2 for /a/ are already higher, compared to other vowels, therefore insuring that there is a boost in amplification of some of the higher harmonics, without having to modify vocal tract shape in order to tune formants to harmonics. Conversely, the /u/ vowel appeared to be the least "belt friendly." This is because the /u/ vowel inherently has lower formants because of the lengthened vocal tract due to the lip rounding. As a result, the /u/ vowel required modification of the vocal tract to raise the formant Hz in order to amplify higher harmonics for this subject. The optimal formant to harmonic tuning pair was

> *The Singer's Formant.* The acoustic phenomenon known as the singer's formant is well-documented in the literature with respect to its physiological basis and expected frequency values (Schutte & Miller, 1993; Sundberg, 1990; Titze, 1994). Research has established the physiological and mathematical calculations for the singer's formant (Titze & Story, 1996). From this research, one expects to find the singer's formant located in the 3000 Hz frequency range. This finding is fairly consistent among men, but there is a question as to whether sopranos possess a singer's formant (Sundberg, 1990). No specific reference to the singer's formant was made with regard to belting in the research completed by Sundberg et al. (1993) or Schutte and Miller (1993). LeBorgne (2001) reported an increase in spectral energy in elite belters around 4000 Hz on /i/ and /u/ vowels. In theory, if the literature is correct with respect that belters elevate the larynx (Miles & Hollien, 1990; Schutte & Miller, 1993; Sundberg et al., 1993) thus shortening the vocal tract, an increase of the singer's formant may be noted based on mathematical principle (Fn = 35,000 cm/sec/(4 × 2.2 cm) = 3977 Hz).

F1 tuned to the second harmonic as was observed for the spoken /eh/ vowel. The authors hypothesized that for belting, it is ideal to boost the amplitude of the higher harmonics because it facilitates the bright, loud quality associated with belting.

Three recent studies (Bourne & Garnier, 2012; Kochis-Jennings et al., 2012; Lebowitz & Baken, 2011) have focused on the F1/H2 interaction. Results demonstrated that chest and chestmix had the greatest acoustic energy in the mid and upper harmonics compared to head register, which had less energy in the upper harmonics (Kochis-Jennings et al., 2012). In the Lebowitz and Baken study (2011) of 20 professional singers, classical style singing consistently yielded higher H1 amplitudes compared to H2. However, for belting, H1 was greater in amplitude than H2 70% of the time, and H2 has higher amplitude than H1 30% of the time. Finally, within the Bourne and Garnier study (2012), the first formant had little variation for the classical/legit style, meaning there was no "tuning" of the first formant to the second harmonic, which was observed in the belt productions. Additionally, the second format was significantly higher, tuned toward the H2 for belt compared to legit singing. This conflicts with the previously described study, where there was not an F1/H2 tuning. It should be noted that higher pitches were measured in this current study with measurements going up to B4, C5, and D5.

Intensity Findings

Despite indications that elite belters are perceived as louder than average belters, LeBorgne (2001) did not find significant intensity differences between elite and average belters. The average vocal intensity ranged from 62.7 dB to 74.5 dB within the elite and average groups. Overall intensity had not previously been reported in the literature for belters. Reported maximum intensities produced by trained vocalists across their frequency range (with a comparable microphone to mouth distance as the LeBorgne study) ranged from 63.1 dB (at low frequencies) to 102.7 dB (at high frequencies).

Although loudness did not correlate highly with overall score in the LeBorgne (2001) investigation, the interaction of vibrato and ring with loudness may indirectly account for the perceived increase of intensity. Specific differences between elite and average belters with respect to vibrato and ring may result from influences of vibrato rate and extent as well as formant tuning (creating a "ring") increasing the overall perceived intensity of a tone (Dejonckere, Hirano, & Sundberg, 1995; Horii, 1989; Schutte & Miller, 1993). Similar studies on measurements of intensity on sustained voices found increased rates of vibrato as the intensity of sustained tones increased (Michel & Myers, 1991; Titze et al., 1999).

Many belters are perceived to include both straight tone and vibrato on belted, sustained notes. Differences in the intensity of the head, middle, and tail portions of several vowels were noted by LeBorgne (2001). Either the head or middle portion of the vowel presented with the greatest intensity. The tail portion of the vowel always presented with the lowest intensity. This finding suggests one of two possibilities. The first is that the singer essentially performs a modified *messa di voce* on sustained tones; the second is that the singer may use an increased rate of vocal vibrato at the tail of the sustained tone to give listeners the perception of increased vocal intensity. The second theory also speaks to

the fact that belters may intuitively utilize vibrato to decrease the amount of time increased intensity is sustained.

One other note on intensity relates to the use of personal amplification by belters. The majority of belters, even at the amateur level, use personal amplification. Therefore, belters may not employ increased vocal intensity especially when compared to classical singing, but may only be perceived as doing so.

Vibrato Findings

The classical voice literature reports a high correlation of a consistent, even vibrato with overall vocal beauty in the classical singer (Ekholm, Papagiannis, & Chagnon, 1998). However, early literature on belting reports that little-to-no vibrato was an essential characteristic of belting, but more recent studies indicate that vibrato (delay of onset, amplitude, and magnitude) is used as a stylistic choice and was highly correlated with elite belters (Miles & Hollien, 1990; LeBorgne, 2001; Stone et al., 2003). Jazz singing is reported to mix straight tones with vibrato by altering the rate and amplitude of the vibrato (Titze, 1994). Readers are referred back to Chapter 3 for further discussion on vibrato.

Timbre/Spectral Slope Findings

Perceptually, the literature reports belting to be associated with a bright timbre (Miles & Hollien, 1990; Schutte & Miller, 1993). The degree of brightness in the singing voice is an aesthetic choice in most cases. Typically, the operatic voice is considered darker and rounder in comparison to the belting quality in musical theater (Schutte & Miller, 1993). It is also noted in the literature that in order to traverse the passaggio, male singers in the Western classical tradition "cover" (slight darkening of tone) as they ascend in frequency (Hertegard, Gauffin, & Sundberg, 1990). Without "covering" a noticeable passaggio is heard. Belters do not seem to employ this strategy as they ascend in frequency.

Bloothooft and Plomp (1988) noted the vast vocabulary used to describe vocal timbre, yet found little literature to support the perceptual use of the various terms. Their article, "The Timbre of Sung Vowels" looked at spectral attributes of the perceived vocal qualities. "Sharpness" of voice was found to correlate with the slope of the spectrum. Baken and Orlikoff (2000) also report that as the slope of the spectrum becomes more shallow, the voice or instrument is perceived as brighter than if the slope is steeper. The typical spectral slope of the voice shows a rolloff of approximately -12 dB per octave (Baken & Orlikoff, 2000).

Trends examining spectral slope of elite student belters reveled a likely perceptually brighter voice based on the degree of spectral sloping (LeBorgne, 2001). Not surprisingly, /i/ vowel, which is typically perceived as brighter than /ɑ/ and /u/, showed a consistently shallower spectral slope than the /ɑ/ or /u/ vowels across all subjects with the steepness or shallowness of the spectral slope directly related to the amplitudes of the higher harmonics. Specifically, increased amplitudes of the higher harmonics will result in a more shallow spectral slope. The author speculated that perhaps it is this increase in the higher harmonics that gives the elite belters not only the brightness in timbre, but also the richness of tone (LeBorgne, 2001). Further investigation of the amplitude differences of the high-frequency harmonics in these singers is warranted.

Nasality Findings

The literature reports that one of the characteristic perceived parameters of belting is a high degree of nasality in the tone, yet classical voice considers nasality a vocal flaw (Estill, 1988; Miles & Hollien, 1990; Schutte & Miller, 1993; Zraick & Liss, 2000). Several studies have examined the velopharyngeal port (where the velum closes off the nasal cavity from the oral and pharyngeal cavities) in classical singing (Sundberg, Birch, Gümoes, Stavad, Prytz, & Karle, 2007; Tanner, Roy, Merrill, & Power, 2005). Findings indicate that many classical singers have some degree of velopharyngeal port opening during certain vowels. The addition of the nasal resonance changes the interaction of the resonance tubes resulting in some degree of formant tuning, which ultimately attenuates the first formant and enhances the higher partials (i.e., give more brilliance—not nasality to the voice; Sundberg et al., 2007). LeBorgne (2001) examined the nasalance scores between elite and average belters. Significant differences between groups were not observed. Because of the limited data on nasalance scores, further research on normative ranges for both classical singers and belters needs to be completed in order to determine if belters display a higher degree of nasality in singing than their classical counterparts.

Registration Findings

It has been hypothesized that belters employ laryngeal elevation placing stress on the thyroarytenoid muscle, and maximal strain will eventually result in a registration break (Estill, 1988; Miles & Hollien, 1990; Titze, 1994). Registration breaks were noted to occur in both elite and average belters, primarily during scalewise movement (Le-Borgne, 2001). However, elite belters were more proficient in traversing the passaggio area without perceptual notice. LeBorgne (2001) reported that all of the average singers except one demonstrated a registration break on at least one vowel on the scale passage.

The Science Behind the Singing: Inertance and Compliance Theories

We know from studies described earlier in this chapter that there appear to be general differences between how classical and CCM singers produce the sounds associated with their genre. These differences occur in various combinations at all levels of voice production including the power source (respiration), sound source (phonation), filter function (vocal tract), and articulation (shaping sound). As a result, acoustic, aerodynamic, and muscular measurements differ not only from classical to CCM, but even within various CCM styles. The synergy of the nuanced adjustments between these subsystems, particularly the vocal tract and the sound source are what make a truly great singer regardless of style; however, the results of studies have demonstrated some variability in how these interactions actually occur.

Ingo Titze, in his theory of nonlinear source-filter coupling (Titze, 2008), postulated that the vocal tract can interact with the sound source in a way that can either enhance or inhibit output and that there are a variety of factors that determine how this interaction occurs and whether or not it is constructive. In 2009, Titze and Worley expanded on Titze's original theory and compared acoustic measures in both high-pitched operatic singing and belting in a male singer (Titze & Worley, 2009). The authors described stylized shapes of a singer's vocal tract for different styles of singing. For example, they hypothesized that the inverted megaphone vocal tract configuration commonly used in Western classical singing and the noninverted megaphone configuration commonly seen in belting (i.e., trumpet shaped lips) result in different voice source and filter (vocal tract) interactions, which, in turn, change the acoustic components and perceived sound.

Titze and Worley proposed the two following hypotheses:

1. Laryngeal posture of Western classical style of singing employs the inverted megaphone (i.e., narrow toward lips, wide at pharynx) allowing for reinforcement of the harmonics above the first formant (F1) because the formants are all lowered due to lengthening of the vocal tract. From a pedagogical standpoint, this vocal tract alteration could be a method necessary for managing passaggio transitions in order to avoid or reduce sound source/vocal fold instabilities. These instabilities could include transient changes in vocal fold vibration patterns, pitch jumps, and subharmonics, all of which can occur during changes in pitch where harmonics pass through formant regions. If a classical singer is ascending in pitch on the same vowel, the harmonics will eventually pass though the formants, which have remained steady in order to preserve that vowel. Modification of the vocal tract might be warranted to lower formant locations, keeping them below the H1 thus avoiding the undesired, abrupt intersecting of F1 through the first harmonic. This could be more problematic

for a vowel such as /a/ where the first formant is already higher compared to other vowels.

2. In contrast, the authors speculate that in belting, a megaphone, or trumpet shape to the lips serves to reinforce the fundamental pitch and second harmonic (H2) below the first formant. Spreading the lips to create a trumpet-like posture raises all formants when no other vocal tract modification is occurring.

The authors go on to further to describe the interaction potentials between vocal fold vibration (sound source) and the vocal tract. There is the possibility of a constructive interaction between the two if they have comparable impedance. The concept of impedance as it relates to voice production is complex and readers wanting in-depth information are encouraged to read Titze and Verdolini-Abbott (2012), where comprehensive explanations are provided. Figure 14–1 provides a schematic of impedance and impact on voice. Generally speaking, impedance refers to a lack of response to an applied stimulus and is a ratio of acoustic pressure to glottal flow. If there is a delayed response, it is considered an inertive reactance, and this is desirable because this configuration facilitates more efficient vocal fold vibration. The goal for optimal voice production is to get as many areas in the vocal tract to have an inertive reactance as possible (Titze & Verdolini-Abbott, 2012). Various modifications of the vocal tract by a skilled singer can facilitate these interactions to reinforce harmonics.

The three primary ways to alter the inertive areas of the vocal tract are: (1) modify vocal tract length (altering laryngeal height, and/or jaw/lip/tongue position), (2) modify vocal tract shape (megaphone versus inverted megaphone), and (3) facilitate epilaryngeal narrowing (Titze & Verdolini-Abbott, 2012). Figure 14–2 provides a schematic of ways to alter the vocal tract in order to increase inertive areas in the vocal tract. Titze and Worley (2009) propose that this interaction between the sound source and vocal tract reinforces vocal fold vibration and promotes stability of vocal fold vibration during changes in pitch and/or vowel. If a singer is not successful, than a deconstructive interaction can occur resulting in impact on vocal fold vibration possibly resulting in transient pitch instability or aperiodic vocal fold vibration. These authors are not the first to describe changes in vocal tract configuration causing abrupt disturbances of vocal fold vibration (Hatzikirou, Fitch, & Herzel, 2006).

Titze and Worley (2009) go on further to discuss that physiologic differences in biomechanics of the vocal folds can also come into play with regard to stability of vocal fold vibration and ability of the vocal folds to self sustain vocal fold oscillation. For example, if a singer has thick, pliable, and responsive mucosal layer of the vocal folds, they are more able to sustain oscillation. Therefore, the sound source does not rely on or require as much reinforcement from the vocal tract to help sustain vocal fold vibration. In this case, the harmonics are more stable and, theoretically, this singer is at less risk for instability of vocal fold vibration when harmonics intersect with formants during pitch and/or vowel change. The downside is that, although vocal fold oscillation is more stable, the output power is not as robust. Conversely, if a singer does not inherently have thick, pliable mucosal covering of the vocal folds, he may need to rely more on the nonlinear interaction of the sound source with the vocal tract. In this scenario, the singer has greater efficiency and output power, but is also at greater risk for experiencing harmonic instability.

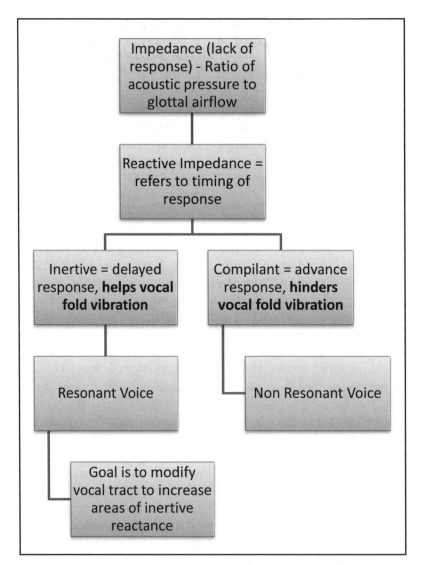

Figure 14–1. Schematic of impedance. *Source*: Titze and Verdolini Abbott, 2012.

Titze and Worley (2009) expand on this idea by presenting a scenario in which the H2, attributed to the female belt or male chest register, must be managed carefully by the singer in order to avoid destabilizing vocal fold oscillation. If there is an abrupt change in how the H2 is reinforced, the vibratory pattern of the vocal folds can potentially destabilize. Additionally, according to this theory, the chest register can involuntarily flip into head or falsetto if the H2 is not reinforced. For example, elevating the larynx and lowering the jaw will raise the F1 above the H2 up to a certain point. However, when the pitch becomes high enough that the singer can no longer modify the vocal tract to raise the F1 above the H2, a break into the head or falsetto regis-

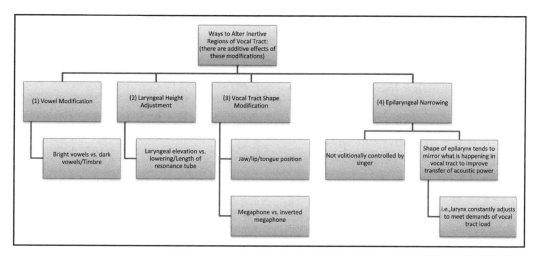

Figure 14–2. Ways to alter the inertive regions of vocal tract.

ter occurs. According to Titze and Worley (2009), blended transition through registers occurs when the interaction of F1 and H2 is smooth. For belt, /ae/ and /a/ have the highest F1 region compared to other vowels; therefore, it is easiest to maintain F1 above H2 for higher pitches without as much vocal tract modification (i.e., laryngeal elevation), and these vowels are typically easier to belt. Conversely, classical singers modify toward a more covered or longer versions of vowels in order to lower the formants and keep F1 below the H2. This helps to maintain even timber during change in pitch for classical singing.

Titze and Worley (2009) provide a very thorough discussion about the interaction between the sound source and the filter, and how singers might need to modify the vocal tract to stabilize the voice during changes in pitch. They discuss the difference in the relationship between the F1 and H2 and offer a theoretical basis for why singers choose different vocal tract modification to achieve stability when singing. Additionally, the authors discuss some physiologic differences in the thickness and responsiveness of the vocal fold

mucosal covering also playing a possible role in how dependent the sound source is on vocal tract interaction for that singer. The authors do not go into discussion about the roles of the ratio of open to closed quotient during vocal fold vibration and how this factors into changes in registration.

Chapter Summary

During the 19th century, the emergence of voice science came to light evoking a need to investigate voice production from a perspective of mechanics and function. Over the past 150 years, our knowledge of voice science has evolved. The merging of vocal arts and voice science has brought us far in our knowledge of vocal acoustics and physiology, but there is still much to be learned. This chapter has provided a chronologic overview of the research on belting regarding current thinking on the acoustic and laryngeal differences of this style of singing. As with much research on singing science, most of the studies reviewed in this chapter are limited because of low subject numbers.

Information provided by the aforementioned studies may appear to ask more questions than they answer. Quantifying art rarely provides clear-cut results, and perhaps it is for that reason many choose not to delve into such research. Consensus on a perceptual definition of the belt voice is closer to being a reality, but semantic differences continue to present a stumbling block to the scientist.

The new millennium provides opportunities for singers, teachers, and scientists to bridge the gaps in knowledge previously unexplored; with these answers will come more questions. Current technological advances in the areas of voice science should enable the voice community to answer questions related to the nature and production of voice with greater accuracy and understanding. This increased understanding of the voice will supplement and enhance previous research and provide teachers of voice a rationale for methodology in the voice studio, and we must continue to seek out information to better understand pedagogical implications for managing these vocal athletes.

References

Baken, R., & Orlikoff, R. (2000). *Clinical measurement of speech and voice* (2nd ed.). San Diego, CA: Singular Publishing.

Bestebreurtje, M., & Schutte, H. (2000). Resonance strategies for the belting style: Results of a single female subject study. *Journal of Voice, 14*(2), 194–204.

Bjorkner, E. (2008). Musical theater and opera singing—Why so different? A study of subglottal pressure, voice source, and formant frequency characteristics. *Journal of Voice, 22*(5), 533–540.

Bjorkner, E., Sundberg, J., Cleveland, T., & Stone, R. (2005). Voice source differences between registers in female musical theater singers. *Journal of Voice, 20*(2), 187–197.

Bloothooft, G., & Plomp, R. (1988). The timbre of sung vowels. *Journal of the Acoustical Society of America, 84*(3), 847–860.

Bourne, T., & Garnier, M. (2012). Physiological and acoustic considerations of the female music theater voice. *Journal of Acoustical Society of America, 131*(2), 1586–1594.

Dejonckere, P., Hirano, M., & Sundberg, J. (1995). *Vibrato.* San Diego, CA: Singular Publishing.

Bourne, T., Garnier, M., & Kenny, D. (2011). Music theater voice: Production, physiology and pedagogy. *Journal of Singing, 67*(4), 437–444.

Ekholm, E., Papagiannis, G., & Chagnon, F. (1998). Relating objective measurements to expert evaluation of voice quality in Western classical singing: Critical perceptual parameters. *Journal of Voice, 12*(2), 182–196.

Estill, J. (1988). Belting and classic voice quality: Some physiological differences. *Medical Problems of Performing Artists*, 37–43.

Hatzikirou, H., Fitch, W., & Herzel, H. (2006). Voice instabilities due to source-tract interactions. *Acta Acustica united with Acustica, 92*, 468–475.

Hertegard, S., Gauffin, J., & Sundberg, J. (1990). Open and covered singing as studied by means of fiber optics, inverse filtering, and spectral analysis. *Journal of Voice, 4*(3), 220–230.

Horii, Y. (1989). Acoustic analysis of vocal vibrato: A theoretical interpretation of data. *Journal of Voice, 3*(1), 36–43.

Kochis-Jennings, K., Finnegan, E., Hoffman, H., & Jaiswal, S. (2012). Laryngeal muscle activity and vocal fold adduction during chest, chestmix, headmix, and head registers in females. *Journal of Voice, 26*(2), 182–193.

Kouffman, J., Radomski, T., Jojarji, G., & Pillsburry, D. (1996). Laryngeal biomechanics of singing. *Otolaryngology-Head and Neck Surgery, 115*(6), 527–537.

LeBorgne, W. (2001). *Defining the belt voice: Perceptual judgements and objective measures* (PhD dissertation). University of Cincinnati, Pro Quest, UMI Dissertations Publishing.

LeBorgne, W., Lee, L., Stemple, J., & Bush, H. (2009). Perceptual findings on the broadway belt voice. *Journal of Voice, 24*(6), 678–689.

Lebowitz, A., & Baken, R. (2011). Correlates of the belt voice: A broader examination. *Journal Voice, 25*(2), 159–165.

LoVetri, J. (2006). Contemporary commercial music: Editorial. *Journal of Voice, 22*(3), 260–262.

LoVetri, J., Lesh, S., & Woo, P. (1999). Preliminary study on the ability of trained singers to control the intrinsic and extrinsic laryngeal musculature. *Journal of Voice, 13*(2), 219–226.

Michel, J., & Myers, D. (1991). The effects of crescendo on vocal vibrato. *Journal of Voice, 5*(4), 292–298.

Miles, B., & Hollien, H. (1990). Whither belting? *Journal of Voice, 4*(1), 64–70.

Popeil, L. (2007). The multiplicity of belting. *Journal of Singing, 64*(1), 77–80.

Schutte, H., & Miller, D. (1993). Belting and pop, nonclassical approaches to the female middle voice: Some preliminary considerations. *Journal of Voice, 7*(2), 142–150.

Spivey, N. (2008). Music theater singing . . . Let's talk. Part 2: Examining the debate on belting. *Journal of Singing, 64*(5), 607–614.

Stone, E. (1994). The emperor's new voice (Can opera singers sing Broadway?), *Opera Monthly,* November/December, 2–5.

Stone, E., Cleveland, T., Sundberg, J., & Prokop, J. (2003). Aerodynamic and acoustical measures of speech, operatic, and broadway vocal styles in a professional female singer. *Journal of Voice, 17*, 283–297.

Sundberg, J. (1990). What's so special about singers? *Journal of Voice, 4*(2), 107–119.

Sundberg, J. (1994). Perceptual aspects of singing. *Journal of Voice, 8*(2), 106–122.

Sundberg, J., Birch, P., Gümoes, B., Stavad, H., Prytz, S., & Karle, A. (2007). Experimental findings on the nasal tract resonator in singing. *Journal of Voice, 21*(2), 127–137.

Sundberg, J., Cleveland, T., Stone, E., & Iwarsson, J. (1999). Voice source characteristics in six premier country singers. *Journal of Voice, 13*(2), 168–183.

Sundberg, J., Gramming, P., & Lovetri, J. (1993). Comparisons of pharynx, source, formant, and pressure characteristics in operatic and musical theatre singing. *Journal of Voice, 7*(4), 301–310.

Sundberg, J., Thalen, M., & Popeil, L. (2012). Substyles of belting: Phonatory and resonatory characteristics. *Journal of Voice, 26*, 44–50.

Tanner, K., Roy, N., Merrill, R., & Power, D. (2005). Velopharyngeal port status during classical singing. *JSLHR, 48*(6), 1311–1324.

Titze, I. (1994). *Principles of voice production.* Englewood Cliffs, NJ: Prentice Hall.

Titze, I. (2008). Nonlinear source-filter coupling in phonation: Theory. *Journal of the Acoustical Society of America, 123*, 2733–2749.

Titze, I., Long, R., Shirley, G., Stathopoulos, E., Ramig, L., Carroll, L., & Riley, W. (1999). *Messa di voce*: An investigation of the symmetry of crescendo and decrescendo in a singing exercise. *Journal of the Acoustical Society of America, 105*(5), 2933–2940.

Titze, I., & Story, B. (1996). Acoustic interactions of the voice source with the lower vocal tract. *Journal of the Acoustical Society of America, 101*(4), 2234–2243.

Titze, I., & Verdolini-Abbott, K. (2012). *Vocology: The science and practice of voice habiliation.* Salt Lake City, UT: NCVS.

Titze, I., & Worley, A. (2009). Modeling source-filter interaction in belting and high-pitched operatic male singing. *Journal of Acoustical Society of America, 126*(3), 1530.

Zraick, R., & Liss, J. (2000). A comparison of equal-appearing interval scaling and direct magnitude estimation of nasal voice quality. *JSLHR, 43*, 979–988.

15

Exercise Physiology Principles for Training the Vocal Athlete

Introduction

As with all physical actions, voice production requires a combination of muscular strength and coordination of multiple body systems even for the most basic phonatory tasks. Consider the complex mental, physical, and vocal actions necessary for high-level singing regardless of style. Although there are physiologic differences in how these styles are produced, all genres of singing require stable, strong musculature functioning in a balanced, efficient manner for optimal output. The concept of applying the principles of motor learning and exercise physiology to voice training is not new for the speech-language pathologist specializing in rehabilitation of the voice. These concepts and principles have also been adopted by some vocal pedagogues who use a physiologic approach to voice training in their studios.

The following chapter highlights some of the key principles of how muscles work, the exercise science behind movement, and how these philosophies might be applied when training high-level singers. The subsequent chapter (Chapter 16) provides an overview of basic motor learning principles with emphasis on how the teacher/clinician/singer can maximize practice patterns, cueing, and modeling to facilitate permanent carryover of new vocal skill sets. For further reading on these topics, the reader is encouraged to explore the references provided in this chapter for books and papers on exercise science and motor learning.

Muscle Fibers and Laryngeal Function

A basic knowledge of what a muscle is and how it works provides the voice pedagogue and singer with the building blocks for functional understanding. There are three types of muscle in the human body: (1) smooth muscle, (2) cardiac muscle, and (3) striated muscle. Smooth muscle is regulated by the autonomic nervous system. Examples of smooth muscle structures include: the uterus, stomach, and esophagus. For these structures, involuntary peristalsis (propelling contraction), is the primary pattern of muscle contraction. Cardiac muscle is a striated muscle that is also involuntary. The heart is composed of cardiac muscle. Skeletal limb muscles and muscles of the larynx are striated muscles under voluntary motor control and will be the focus of this section.

Skeletal (Limb) Muscles

The human body contains about 400 skeletal muscles making up about 40% to 50% of human body weight (Powers & Howley, 2009; Suzuki et al., 2002). These muscles allow for movement, postural stability, and generation of heat. Skeletal muscle can be grouped by fiber type with two primary categories: type I-slow twitch fibers or type II-fast twitch fibers. Slow twitch fibers have certain characteristics that make them more resistant to fatigue compared to fast twitch fibers. Two reasons slow twitch fibers are fatigue-resistant are because: (1) they have a higher number of capillaries surrounding them compared to other fiber types, providing increased blood supply and (2) they have numerous oxidative enzymes (which help slow down the way a muscle gets energy). Fast twitch fibers can further be subcategorized into type IIa and type IIx. Type IIx fibers are now thought to be the fastest but least efficient because

the characteristics of this fiber type lead it to expend a significant amount of energy per unit of work (Powers & Howley, 2009). Type IIa fibers fall between type I and type IIx. IIa fibers have some degree of fatigue resistance, though they are not as fatigue-resistant as type I fibers. Type IIa are adaptable with training and can further arm them against fatigue by increasing their oxidative capacity with training (Powers & Howley, 2009).

Research on human laryngeal muscles and rat models indicates that human laryngeal skeletal muscles have similar characteristics to skeletal limb muscles with regard to fiber type, capillary density, and metabolic features (Hoh, 2005; Suzuki et al., 2002). Studies on fiber typing have been conducted for the thyroarytenoid muscle, posterior cricoarytenoid muscle, and interarytenoid muscles (Tellis, 2004; Tellis, Rosen, Thekdi, & Sciote, 2004). The thyroarytenoid muscle (TA) and lateral cricoarytenoid muscle (LCA) are composed of about 80% type II fibers and 20% type I fibers. In contrast, the posterior cricoarytenoid muscle (PCA) is composed primarily of type I fibers (65%; Happak, Zrunek, Pechmann, & Streinzer, 1989; Tellis, 2004). Type I fibers also appear to be abundant in the cricothyroid muscle (CT) (Li, Lehar, Nakagawa, Hoh, & Flint, 2004). Interestingly, the metabolic characteristics of the interarytenoid (IA) muscle fibers make them susceptible to quick fatigue. Based on studies that have differentiated muscle fiber types for the laryngeal muscles, the fast twitch fiber density of the TA, IA, and LCA allow for rapid valving and closure for airway protection. In contrast, the slow twitch fibers that predominate the PCA make the muscle very fatigue-resistant, allowing for repetitive opening of the airway for respiration 24 hours per day.

Basic Training Principles for Exercise Science

There is ample research on impact of exercise and strength training on general skeletal muscles, such as limb muscles; however, adequate research on impact of exercise on laryngeal muscles is inherently more challenging because of the locations and sizes of these muscles. Findings from research done on limb muscles cannot necessarily be transferred to laryngeal muscles. There is research to suggest that there are reasonable similarities between limb muscles and intrinsic laryngeal muscles (Hoh, 2005; Sciote, Morris, Horton, Brandon, & Rosen, 2002; Tellis et al., 2004). Specific similarities that have been described include muscle fiber type, metabolic attributes, changes in neuromuscular junction, and capillary density changes associated with aging (Kersing & Jennekins, 2001; McMullen & Andrade, 2006; Suzuki et al., 2002).

There are five primary principles described in exercise science literature to maximize strength, function, endurance, and longevity. The overriding tenet of these principles is that muscles, if trained in the appropriate manner, will undergo muscle fiber changes in addition to neural and metabolic changes, resulting in an adaptation to the new demand imposed upon them. This concept is referred to as Specific Adaptation to Imposed Demand (SAID). There is evidence in exercise physiology literature that if training is done with the following principles in mind, the above described physiologic changes will occur. The five principles of exercise training are: intensity, frequency, overload, specificity, and reversibility.

Intensity, frequency, and overload are best described inclusively. In order for the target muscle to undergo the desired physiologic adaptations, there must be adequate frequency, and an appropriate amount of intensity. These two factors will help ensure that the third (overload) principle is realized. Both frequency and intensity must surpass the target muscle's comfort zone; otherwise, the target muscle will persist in a state of homeostasis (maintenance) and adaptation will not occur. Demanding muscular exertion beyond its maintenance level will overload the muscle, leading to adaptation and change.

There are a number of changes that occur during this process. Of particular interest are the changes in the muscle fibers, neural adaptations, and metabolic changes. These changes are not in tandem, however. In fact, the neural and metabolic adaptations typically precede the muscle fiber hypertrophy (Lieber, 2010; Sale, 1988). Initial gains in strength are due to the neural adaptations, which occur over a period of four to five weeks. These changes can be seen after about two weeks of training before any measurable increase in actual muscle bulk (Lieber, 2010).

Metabolic changes are also an important contributor to improved muscular strength. When the appropriate frequency and intensity levels are implemented for the target muscle, there is increased efficiency in the delivery of adenosine triphosphate (ATP), which provides energy to the muscle for contraction. In turn, muscle fatigue is reduced. Over time an increase in capillary density around the muscle occurs.

> The neuromuscular junction is the place where the nerve meets the muscle.

Real-life physical example of intensity, frequency, overload, specificity, and reversibility principles: If you wanted to improve leg muscle strength by using squats (specificity), the frequency (how many times you performed the exercise), the intensity (how challenging you make the squat influenced by how low you go or by adding weight), and overload (challenging the muscle via heavier weight and/or lower bend beyond its maintenance level to the point of muscle failure) will over time result in progressive muscle change. If you stop doing squats, the muscle fibers will revert (reversibility) back to their pre-exercise state.

especially when employing different registers or vocal genres.

The final exercise principle is reversibility or detraining. Put very simply, if you stop going to the gym, you lose previously attained gains in strength and endurance. Recall that the muscle adapts to increased demands. Therefore, if the demand decreases or stops, there will be a detraining effect, and the muscle will return to its pre-training level of function, as all of the physiologic gains will have reversed. Detraining happens very quickly. Further, the longer the hiatus from training, the longer it will take to regain the strength. For example, if you stop strength training for two weeks, exercise science research suggests that it could take up to four weeks to reacquire post-training gains (Sandage & Pascoe, 2010). If this applies to voice training, there are implications to consider regarding complete vocal rest.

This ensures that there is better oxygen transmission from the blood to the target muscle (MacIntosh, Gardiner, & McComas, 2006). This is an important benefit because capillary density has been shown to decrease with age (Russell, Nagai, & Connor, 2008).

Specificity refers to the concept that strength training must be designed to appropriately target the specific muscle or muscle group with the intended skill or task. Research in exercise science suggests that while some generalization exists across muscles, there is not full carryover to the muscles if the training task differs from the demanded task. As an example, consider the two activities of running and cycling. Both tasks require the use the majority of the muscles in the leg, but training specifically for one task (running) does not automatically make one skilled in the other (cycling). This concept likely has implications regarding different styles of singing

Research on Exercise Science for Voice

Historically, there is an association between exercise physiology and kinesiology with physical fitness, athletics, and physical therapy. Speech pathologists have also applied these principles to voice therapy and rehabilitation (Patel, Bless, & Thibeault, 2010; Sandage & Pascoe, 2010; Saxon & Schneider, 1995; Stathopoulos & Duncan, 2006; Stemple, Lee, D'Amico, & Pickup, 1994; Thibeault, Zelazny, & Cohen, 2009). Vocal pedagogy has also moved toward a physiologic and functional approach to voice training.

Physiologic studies regarding specifically exercise physiology principles and voice provide the basis for consideration of possible modalities to improve the muscle strength of both the respiratory and the laryngeal muscles as well as detraining effects (Baker, Davenport, & Sapienza, 2005; Illi, Held, Frank, & Spengler, 2012; Sabol, Lee, & Stemple, 1995; Sapienza, 2008; Sapienza, Davenport, & Marti, 2002; Sapienza, Troche, Pitts, & Davenport, 2011; Stemple, Lee, D'Amico, & Pickup, 1994; Tay, Phyland, & Oates, 2011; Wingate, Brown, Shrivastav, Davenport, & Sapienza, 2007).

Respiratory Muscle Strength Training

Respiratory muscle is skeletal muscle and therefore can be trained and conditioned (Illi et al., 2012; Sapienza, 2008). Depending on the needs of an individual, either an expiratory muscle trainer (EMT) or inspiratory muscle trainer (IMT) may be appropriate. Research has indicated respiratory

muscles can be strengthened and trained via a paradigm of daily practice (with a specified number of repetitions at specified resistance level) using a handheld resistance device (which contains an adjustable valve) to provide increased load on the respiratory muscles. Figure 15–1 shows an example of a respiratory muscle trainer. If a singer with high physical and vocal demands can increase respiratory muscle strength, it should decrease laryngeal load. For those interested in a detailed description of respiratory strength training, readers are referred to Respiratory Muscle Strength Training: Theory and Practice (Sapienza & Troche, 2011).

Laryngeal Exercise

Vocal Function Exercises (VFEs) are a systematic approach to improving glottal efficiency

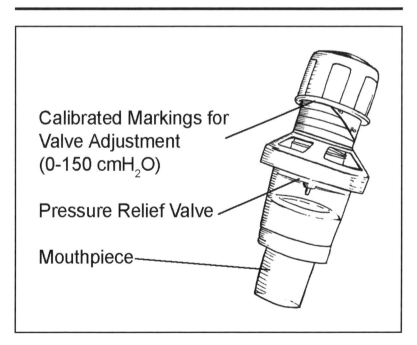

Figure 15–1. Schematic of expiratory muscle strength trainer. Courtesy of Dr. Christine Sapienza.

and function through a series of specific isometric exercises. Initial research on Joseph Stemple's VFEs was published in 1994, with over 15 research articles to date documenting effects of this exercise program. The exercises are a series of four voice tasks to be completed twice per day designed to optimize balance of laryngeal musculature and airflow. These exercises were piloted on 35 vocally healthy, non-singer graduate students for a period of 4 weeks (Stemple et al., 1994). The group that completed VFEs demonstrated improved post-program measurements with respect to increased frequency range and decreased airflow rates. Since the introduction of VFEs, they have commonly been used in voice therapy for a variety of disorders (Stemple et al., 1994).

Sabol and colleagues further assessed the impact of Stemple's Vocal Function Exercises on 20 graduate level voice majors. The test group of singers in this study added VFEs to their current vocal training routine for 4 weeks. The control group continued their vocal training regime but did not add VFEs to their vocal training program. At the end of the 4-week period, the singers who added VFEs to their regular training regimen demonstrated improved phonation times and aerodynamic measures compared to the singers who did not add VFEs. The authors surmised that the isometric nature of the VFEs resulted in increased glottal efficiency over the 4-week period. These exercises have also been adapted and modified by voice teachers and are used as part of vocal training. Additional studies have looked at impact of VFE training program on older voices with similar results to previously mentioned studies (Gorman, Weinrich, Lee, & Stemple, 2008; Tay et al., 2011). Finally, the use of VFEs as part of pop singers' warm up demonstrated improved spectral output immediately following the exercises (Guzman, Angulo, Muñoz, & Mayerhoff, 2013).

For those interested in a detailed description of VFEs, readers are referred to Vocal Function Exercises DVD (Stemple, 2006).

Application of Exercise Physiology Principles for Training Vocal Athletes

In the exercise physiology and kinesiology literature, recommendations of frequency and duration for muscle training for flexibility are 3 to 7 days per week with emphasis on holding a given stretch for 15 to 60 seconds. Muscle training for strength and endurance involves 2 to 3 days per week with emphasis on muscle overload completing 8 to 12 repetitions for 1 to 3 sets (Powers & Howley, 2009). It is clear that some of these parameters do not easily translate into voice training. For example, it might be very challenging for a singer to engage in a stretch of a muscle, for example a slow ascending glide for 60 seconds. However, these general principles can be used by the teacher and singer to establish guidelines with baseline skill levels for that student. Progress can be measured by comparing current skill to baseline skill levels. Studies in exercise physiology have indicated there needs to be a minimum of 3 days per week of appropriate training for gains to be made (Saxon & Schneider, 1995). Because voice lessons typically occur weekly, the student needs to maintain a scheduled practice regimen in order to achieve goals in vocal improvement, muscle memory, and vocal fitness.

Translation of strength and endurance into voice involves the overload principle. As with general fitness, progression to muscle overload must be slow and thoughtful. This comes into play when singers train their chest register up into the belting range (above the first break) at loud volumes. Re-

> A slow, targeted approach will often get results faster and more efficiently.

call the concept of SAID described earlier. Muscles over time will adapt to increased demands of higher pitch and louder volumes; however, a slow deliberate approach will minimize risk of injury and allow for development of balance and strength. Singers most likely get into trouble when they impose physical demands on the voice that they have not yet trained and adapted to. This could lead to pressed, hyperfunctional singing and would also lead to increased risk of injury because of laryngeal compensation, resulting in increased medial compression and sheering stresses. Another consideration when overloading a muscle is to alternate muscle groups to allow for recovery. This will help build strength and endurance while minimizing risk of injury.

The principle of specificity stipulates that when training for a task you must target the appropriate muscle group and that there will not necessarily be carryover to a different skill. For singers, this applies to registration. The previous paragraph discussed a slow approach to training the chest voice toward a belt as one example of the overload principle. This is also a good example of application of the specificity principle in singing. The only way to train a singer to belt is to target and train the appropriate muscles to produce that sound. Multiple years of sound classical training will likely not enable a singer to safely sing in a belt because a different set of muscular activation is targeted and required for classical singing compared to belting, particularly for women. Conversely, if a singer is working on a high, melismatic role, then voice exercises must target those skills.

That is not to say that a singer should only train for one vocal default setting. Recall from the chapter on The Singer's Body that muscles exist in agonist/antagonist pairs and problems can occur from long-term, aberrant tension/length relationships between muscle pairs. With this in mind, it makes sense to cross-train registers to avoid imbalance between head register (CT dominant) and chest register (TA dominant), as this could ultimately lead to technical problems and decreased vocal flexibility. In fact, for music theater singing, the performer's voice has to be a hybrid mix, requiring use of multiple vocal styles depending on the role. Therefore, cross-training the body and voice is an important component not only to vocal fitness, but also for marketability as a performer.

The final principle is reversibility (or detraining). In other words, use it or lose it. If we train our voice to adapt to the demands of a specific role or song and then stop, we will lose those gains fairly quickly. Additionally, the longer you refrain from training, the longer it takes to re-establish gains. In musical theater singing, a performer prepares for a role and then maintains gains by performing the role multiple times per week even if specific exercises are no longer targeting the desired tasks. A similar scenario could be true for a country

> In order to have functional legs, one must have strength and stability in both the quadriceps and hamstrings. An imbalance of these agonist/antagonist muscle pairs could lead to problems with gait and balance. Similarly, singers also need strength and coordination across the vocal mechanism to achieve balance and flexibility.

or pop singer on tour with multiple shows per week. The trap here is to avoid getting into a dominant vocal mode because that could lead to imbalance in the vocal mechanism over time. The goal for the singer is to find the balance between safely training up to meet a specific vocal demand, for example, a heavy belt role, while still maintaining some balance between the agonist/antagonist muscle pairs (in this case, head voice). In the physical therapy spectrum, the therapist uses exercises to focus on the weak antagonistic muscle group in order to rebalance the mechanism (Saxon & Schneider, 1995). In vocal terms, that would mean if the voice has become too heavy from consistent frequent use of chest voice (TA dominant), exercises focusing on balancing the antagonist muscle (the CT) to re-establish equilibrium in the voice should be considered.

> Vocal warm-ups, like physical warm-ups, should be designed as a gentle exercise to "get things moving." Vocal warm-ups should be differentiated from a vocalize. A vocalize should be used to target specific vocal technical issues.

Vocal Warm-Ups

Exercise physiology literature describes the importance of warming up muscles before active physical exercise for multiple reasons: (1) it increases blood flow and oxygen delivery to skeletal muscles, (2) it increases musculature temperature thereby increasing activity of muscle enzyme, and (3) it gently increases flexibility and range of motion of muscles and joints (Powers & Howley, 2009). Athletes typically incorporate a physical warm-up into their fitness regimen. Similarly, vocal warm-up is typically part of conventional practice for singers but how may singers truly incorporate a functional warm-up before active singing and what does a "vocal warm-up" consist of? A survey of vocal warm-up and cool-down practices of 117 classical singers indicated

that 54% of these singers regularly warmed their voices up before singing. Length of vocal warm-up ranged from 5 to 10 minutes, and female singers reported more frequent use of vocal warm-up and for longer periods of time compared with males (Gish, Kunduk, Sims, & McWhorter, 2012). The results of this survey might be viewed as surprising given that almost one-half of the classical singers polled did not report using vocal warm-up as part of their standard practice. Reasons for this are not known. However, a 10-year retrospective study of 188 musical theater singers in a pre-professional conservatory program found that approximately 90% of incoming freshman used vocal warm-ups before engaging in singing activity (Donahue, LeBorgne, Brehm, & Weinrich, in press). Yet, only approximately 15% of the singers in this study reported using vocal cool-downs. Both the Gish et al. (2012) study and the Donahue et al. (2013) study indicated that the singers who warmed-up ranged from 5 to 20 minutes in duration, but types of exercises used for warm-up were not specified.

Research on Warm-Ups and Cool-Downs

Studies looking at physiological impact of vocal warm-ups and cool-downs in both singers and non-singers have yielded varied

> Phonation threshold pressure (PTP) refers to the least amount of subglottal air pressure needed to set the vocal folds into vibration.

results. Researchers have looked at impact of vocal warm-up on the viscosity of the vocal folds and phonatory effort reflected in phonation threshold pressure (PTP) (Elliot, Sundberg, & Gramming, 1995).

This research was based on sports medicine data postulating that warm-up heats skeletal muscle resulting in reduced mucus viscosity (Safran, Seaber, & Garrett, 1989). The authors postulated that if vocal warm-up reduced viscosity of the vocal folds, then PTP would decrease resulting in less effortful phonation. The subject pool consisted of 10 trained, non-professional singers who all reported benefit from the vocal warm-up. Following vocal warm-up tasks, the PTP measurements across subjects was varied despite the report that all subjects stated they felt well warmed-up. This suggested that lowered PTP is not the only factor contributing to the singer's sense of feeling vocally warmed up. Additionally, differences among subjects with regard to biomechanical properties of the vocal folds likely impact an occurrence of a shift of PTP after vocal warm-up (Elliot, Sundberg, & Gramming, 1995).

Another study examined impact of vocal warm-up on PTP measurements of 10 sopranos after extensive vocal warm-up. Post warm-up PTP measurements actually increased in the higher pitch ranges indicating that increased air pressure was required to maintain vocal fold vibration at higher pitches after warm-up. This was inconsistent with many singers' perceptions

that higher range is more accessible and less effortful after vocal warm-up. The authors speculated that the increased PTP was due to increased viscosity of the mucosal layer of the vocal fold that may actually have served as a stabilization mechanism of the vocal fold for higher pitches (Motel, Fisher, & Leydon, 2003).

Other studies have looked at different vocal parameters such as perturbation, noise-to-harmonic ratio, and amplitude of the singer's formant following vocal warm-up. Twenty singers completed their own vocal warm-up time (averaging 7 to 23 minutes). Results showed improved measurements for both amplitude perturbation and frequency perturbation in addition to improved noise-to-harmonic ratios. Mezzo-sopranos had improvements in the frequency perturbation values post vocal warm-up that were nearly three times that of sopranos. The most significant post warm-up effect was found for lower pitches compared with higher pitches (Amir, Amir, & Michaeli, 2005).

Physical body warm-up has also been considered in terms of impact on vocal function. Ten male and ten female actors were given two physical warm-up conditions completed 1 week apart. The first condition consisted of a general body relaxation and vocal warm-up, and the second condition consisted of aerobic activity prior to completing the same vocal warm-up. Measurements of phonatory threshold pressures (PTP) were taken following both conditions. The results demonstrated that males and females both perceived reduced vocal effort after both aerobic and nonaerobic conditions, but females benefited more (decreased PTP) from adding aerobic exercise to their vocal warm-up regimen compared to the males (McHenry, Johnson, & Foshea, 2009).

Moorcroft and Kenny (2012) looked at differences between a singer's perception of vocal changes and improvement after vocal warm-up and listener's perceptions. Both listeners and singers reported improvement in voice post warm-up; however, there was not agreement as to what vocal aspects demonstrated improvement (Moorcroft & Kenny, 2012). These same authors also investigated the impact of vocal warm-up on vibrato rate and found that vibrato rates stabilized and moderated after vocal warm-up (Moorcroft & Kenny, 2013).

The use and understanding of vocal cool-downs as a part of the daily practice regimen appears less common in singers. However, physical athletes rely on some degree of cool-down following a race or intense practice session. A recent study looked specifically at the benefits of vocal cool-downs in elite choral singers and found that singers who used a vocal cool-down had decreased effort (PTP) to produce voice the following day (Gottliebson, 2011).

Although empirical data on the impact that vocal warm-up has on objective measures is variable, almost all singers who participated in the above-mentioned studies reported a better sense of tone placement, ease of voice production, and improved vocal quality following vocal warm-up (De-Fatta & Sataloff, 2012). The majority of studies to date have used classically oriented singers, and results cannot necessarily be transferred to CCM singers who have different physical and vocal performance demands. The variability of results may speak to the individuality principle in exercise physiology advocating that each individual singer likely requires a very specific set of exercises suited for his or her voice. The prudent teacher and student understand the need for flexibility and adaptability of the singer. Vocal warm-ups and cool-downs should be tailored to meet these demands.

Voice Fatigue

Voice fatigue can be experienced not only by singers but also by other professional voice users such as teachers who place high demands on their voices. The actual mechanism of voice fatigue is a complex physiologic phenomenon that is not completely understood with regard to voice use. Exercise physiology literature defines two primary types of fatigue: (1) neuromuscular fatigue, which refers to the decrease in maximal force production of the muscle resulting in a reduced ability to perform work, and (2) central fatigue, which occurs in the central nervous system when either the frequency of motor unit firing is reduced or the amount of motor units is reduced. There is no consensus on whether central fatigue is a viable theory (Powers & Howley, 2009).

Voice fatigue can be described as an awareness or sensation of increased effort after a period of voice use. Voice fatigue can occur either with or without perceived and measurable change in vocal quality. The de-

Using an exercise analogy: If you run for 4 hours (marathon), you will experience muscular fatigue. Depending on your level of training and current level of physical fitness, the degree and longevity of the fatigue will vary. Singing and speaking are no different. If you sing for 4 or 5 hours, depending on your level of training and muscle strength, you will experience normal vocal fatigue. However, if after only 30 minutes of voice use, you experience vocal fatigue (in a well-conditioned singer), that may indicate an abnormal vocal fatigue.

gree of vocal fatigue will vary in terms of both duration and recovery of symptoms.

Ongoing episodes of voice fatigue should not be ignored by the singer as it can indicate a vocal pathology. However, voice fatigue can occur without presence of a vocal fold lesion or other organic pathology. The most common symptoms of voice fatigue include: (1) decline in vocal quality (hoarse, husky, breathy), (2) loss of voice, (3) decreased ability to sustain pitch, (4) loss of endurance and/or intensity, (5) increased vocal effort, and (6) throat discomfort/fatigue/pain (Kostyk & Rochet, 1998).

Titze (1994) discusses vocal fatigue as neuromuscular fatigue resulting in a diminished capacity for a muscle to sustain the same degree of tension with repetitive stimulation. In singing, this means that either the laryngeal intrinsic and extrinsic musculature can no longer sustain the vocal task. This theory only takes into account the muscular aspect and does not include the impact and sheering stresses of repeated impact that may also contribute to vocal fatigue. With respect to minimizing muscular aspects of vocal fatigue, thoughtful and methodical training to strengthen and balance respiratory and laryngeal musculature would potentially help increase vocal endurance and stability during high voice demands.

An additional component to vocal fatigue that strength training cannot combat is mucosal fatigue. Recall that the vocal folds are multilayered with the outermost mucosal layer encompassing the vocal fold. Increased viscosity of the vocal folds results in increased vocal fold stiffness. This in turn, requires more lung pressure to sustain vocal fold vibration as well as increased effort to start phonation (PTP), which results in inefficient laryngeal mechanism. Increased viscosity of the vocal fold mucosa results in generation of more friction

during vocal fold vibration, creating more heat dissipating over the vocal fold resulting in vocal fatigue, vocal fold edema, and erythema.

If a vocally healthy singer is experiencing new onset of fatigue, consider whether or not the fatigue may be muscular or mucosal in nature. This distinction may not be apparent to the singer, and it may not be possible to easily discern the difference, but some thoughtful reflection of recent events may help clarify possible contributing factors. Mucosal fatigue can sometimes respond to both systemic and environmental hydration. Systemic hydration occurs by consuming hydrating liquids such as water. Additionally, "wet snacks" such as plums, watermelon, applesauce, and other water infused foods can also help to some degree with systemic hydration. Environmental hydration refers to humidifiers and steamers. Nasal breathing can also help reduce immediate desiccation of vocal fold mucosa, although during live performance this is often difficult for a CCM performer especially if they are also dancing (see Chapter 10 for a detailed explanation of hydration).

Muscular fatigue, on the other hand, can be managed by altering voice intensity and use. "Vocal naps" (where the singer does not use the voice) in 5- to 30-minute increments may help recovery from voice fatigue after heavy vocal load. Additionally, vocal cool-down can also help bring the voice back to a "neutral" setting after very active or extreme use. For daily voice use, variation of pitch, rate, and volume with adequate use of airflow during conversational speech can help reduce vocal load. Consider the analogy of carrying a heavy backpack using only your left arm. The arm would fatigue fairly quickly because it is carrying the entire workload. This can be likened to speaking in the very narrow pitch range with reduced intonation and prosody during connected speech. Now consider you are carrying the same backpack, but you are distributing the workload more evenly by alternating arms and also carrying it on your back. You will be able to carry the same weight for a much longer period of time because the weight of the backpack is distributed more evenly. This can be equated to speaking with a greater range of motion in pitch volume and loudness, thereby more evenly distributing the vocal load across the entire mechanism. There is also application of this concept to some CCM styles of music, which use grace notes and riffs as these can sometimes be less fatiguing then sustained straight tones.

Recently, a survey of professional music theater singers was undertaken, investigating how their heavy vocal load impacted their perceptions of their voice functioning. These singers all considered themselves to be vocally healthy and were in current productions performing eight shows per week. Results of the survey and a series of focus interviews were interesting in that, singers reported not only negative descriptors such as soreness in the throat, weakness, phlegm, dryness, and irritation, but some also reported positive descriptors such as warm, strong, energized, free, activated, and moves easily. There was variation across singers as to whether or not the negative descriptors were cause for concern, or just part of the job. In fact, more than one half considered this to be just normal variation in their voice over the course of a performance week. This study provides a basis of information about possible trends in perceived vocal stability/durability during an eight-show week, but rationale for the stability or instability is not included (Phyland, Thibeault, Benninger, Vallance, & Greenwood, 2013). This study implies the need for singers to know when they have merely "worked their voice out"

and when they have fatigued their instrument. Despite the ability of a voice dosimeter to track amount and intensity of actual vocal use, an internal vocal calibration may be important for maintaining longevity in vocal health given the high demands in CCM singing.

Monitoring Vocal Effort

All professional voice users are at risk for experiencing voice fatigue. The important distinction to make is when fatigue is transient and when it could be an indication of emergence of a vocal problem. It is critical for singers to establish an internal scale of vocal effort to use as a comparator and gauge. For example, maximal vocal effort would be rated as a 10, and 0 would represent no vocal effort. Normal conversational speaking vocal effort may be around a 1 to 2 on the 10-point scale, and maximal vocal effort (10/10) may represent a maximal muscular and vocal strain and intensity. The singer should not confuse intensity (soft and loud) with effort, as speaking softly often takes more effort than speaking at a moderate intensity. Because this is a self-perception scale, the goal is to get maximum output with the least amount of effort on the scale. Using this scale (or something similar) will allow both the teacher and the singer to gauge whether a given exercise or song is decreasing (or increasing) in effort level with time and practice.

The scale also allows a quantitative measurement for effort level as singers are adept at masking technical problems and even masking vocal pathology by producing pleasing sounds, even if they are very effortful. This method helps the singer and teacher to monitor physical and vocal limitations, which can help guide vocal choices and future training. A vocal effort scale can also help monitor for gains in strength and endurance, keeping in mind that there will always be slight variations in perceived effort for a variety of reasons. Singers should always have a general idea of how quickly they rebound from transient fatigue, so that if fatigue becomes persistent, it is clear that a medical assessment is warranted. The key concept is to know your own instrument and to seek guidance and medical intervention from a laryngologist if you suspect onset of vocal fatigue is reflective of possible underlying pathology.

Chapter Summary

The focus of this chapter has been to introduce the principles of exercise physiology as they relate to voice training. Different types of muscle fibers were described relative to resistance and fatigue. Literature regarding muscle fiber typing for the human larynx was also discussed. The principles of exercise physiology were described with emphasis on how these might be incorporated into a vocal training regimen with respect to both respiration and phonation. Current literature on vocal warm-ups, cool-downs, and voice fatigue were also reviewed with emphasis on how current practice of voice training might be altered to maximize training and voice efficiency. Chapter 16 continues with motor learning principles and how they apply to voice training and skill acquisition.

References

Amir, O., Amir, N., & Michaeli, O. (2005). Evaluating the influence of vocal warm-up on singing voice quality using acoustic measures. *Journal of Voice, 19*(2), 252–260.

Baker, S., Davenport, P., & Sapienza, C. (2005). Examination of strength training and detraining effects in expiratory muscles. *Journal of Speech Language and Hearing Research, 48*(6), 1325–1333.

DeFatta, R., & Sataloff, R. (2012). The value of vocal warm up and cool down exercises: Questions and controversies. *Journal of Singing, 69*(2).

Donahue, E., LeBorgne, W., Brehm, S., & Weinrich, B. (in press). Reported vocal habits of first-year undergraduate musical theatre majors in a pre-professional training program: A ten-year retrospective study. *Journal of Voice.*

Elliot, N., Sundberg, J., & Gramming, P. (1995). What happens during vocal warm-up? *Journal of Voice, 9*(1), 37–44.

Gish, A., Kunduk, M., Sims, L., & McWhorter, A. (2012). Vocal warm-up practices and perceptions in vocalists: A pilot survey. *Journal of Voice, 26*(1), 1–10.

Gorman, S., Weinrich, B., Lee, L., & Stemple, J. (2008). Aerodynamic changes as a result of vocal function exercises in ederly men. *Laryngoscope, 118*(10), 1900–1903.

Gottliebson, R. O. (2011). *The efficacy of cool-down exercises in the practice regimen of elite singers* (Dissertation). University of Cincinnati.

Guzman, M., Angulo, M., Muñoz, D., & Mayerhoff, R. (2013). Effect on long-term average spectrum of pop singers' vocal warm-up with vocal function exercises. *International Journal of Speech Language Pathology, 15*(2), 127–135.

Happak, W., Zrunek, M., Pechmann, P., & Streinzer, W. (1989). Comparative histochemistry of human and sheep laryngeal muscles. *Acta Otolaryngologica, 107*(3–4), 283–288.

Hoh, J. (2005). Laryngeal muscle fiber types. *Acta Physiologica Scandinavica, 183*, 133–149.

Illi, S., Held, U., Frank, I., & Spengler, C. (2012). Effect of respiratory muscle training on exercise performance in healthy individuals: A systematic review and meta-analysis. *Sports Medicine, 42*(8), 707-724.

Kersing, W., & Jennekins, F. (2001). Age-related changes in the human thyroarytenoid muscles: A histological and histochemical study. *European Archives of Oto-Rhinology-Laryngology, 261*(7), 386-392.

Kostyk, B., & Rochet, A. (1998). Laryngeal airway resistance in teachers with vocal fatigue: A preliminary study. *Journal of Voice, 12,* 287-299.

Li, Z., Lehar, M., Nakagawa, H., Hoh, J., & Flint, P. (2004). Differential expression of myosin heavy chain isoforms between abductor and adductor muscles in the human larynx. *Otolaryngology-Head and Neck Surgery, 130*(2), 217-222.

Lieber, R. (2010). *Skeletal muscle structure, function, and plasticity: The physiological basis of rehabilitation* (3rd ed.). Baltimore, MD: Lippincott, Williams & Wilkins.

MacIntosh, B., Gardiner, P., & McComas, A. (2006). *Skeletal muscle: Form and function* (2nd ed.). Champaign, IL: Human Kinetics.

McHenry, M., Johnson, J., & Foshea, B. (2009). The effect of specific versus combined warm-up strategies on the voice. *Journal of Voice, 23*(5), 572-576.

McMullen, C., & Andrade, F. (2006). Contractile dysfunction and altered metabolic profile of the aging rat thyroarytenoid muscle. *Journal of Applied Physiology, 100,* 602-608.

Moorcroft, L., & Kenny, D. (2012). Vocal warm-up produces acoustic change in singers' vibrato rate. *Journal of Voice, 26*(5), 667-e613.

Moorcroft, L., & Kenny, D. (2013). Singer and listener perception of vocal warm up. *Journal of Voice, 27*(2), 258-e251.

Motel, T., Fisher, K., & Leydon, C. (2003). Vocal warm-up increases phonation threshold pressure in soprano singers at high pitch. *Journal of Voice, 17,* 160-167.

Patel, R., Bless, D., & Thibeault, S. (2010). Boot camp: A novel intensive approach to voice therapy. *Journal of Voice, 25,* 562-569.

Phyland, D., Thibeault, S., Benninger, M., Vallance, N., & Greenwood, K. (2013). Perspectives on the impact on vocal function of heavy vocal load among working professional music theater performers. *Journal of Voice, 27*(3), 32-39.

Powers, S., & Howley, E. (2009). *Exercise physiology: Theory and application to fitness and performance*. Boston, MA: McGraw Hill.

Russell, J., Nagai, H., & Connor, N. (2008). Effect of ageing on blood flow in rat larynx. *The Laryngoscope, 118,* 559-563.

Sabol, J., Lee, L., & Stemple, J. (1995). The value of vocal function exercises in the practice regimen of singers. *Journal of Voice, 9,* 27-36.

Safran, M., Seaber, A., & Garrett, W. (1989). Warm-up and muscular injury prevention. An update. *Sports Medicine, 8*(4), 239-249.

Sale, D. (1988). Neural adaptation to resistance training. *Medicine and Science in Sports and Exercise, 20,* 135-145.

Sandage, M., & Pascoe, D. (2010). Translating exercise science into voice care. *Perspectives on Voice and Voice Disorders, 20*(3), 84-89.

Sapienza, C. (2008). Respiratory muscle strength training applications. *Current Opinion in Otolaryngology & Head and Neck Surgery, 16,* 216-220.

Sapienza, C., Davenport, P., & Marti, A. (2002). Expiratory muscle training increases pressure support in high school band students. *Journal of Voice, 16*(4), 495-501.

Sapienza, C., & Troche, M. (2011). *Respiratory muscle strength training: Theory and practice*. San Diego, CA: Plural Publishing.

Sapienza, C., Troche, M., Pitts, T., & Davenport, P. (2011). Respiratory strength training: concept and intervention outcomes. *Seminars in Speech and Language, 32*(1), 21-30.

Saxon, K., & Schneider, C. (1995). *Vocal exercise physiology*. San Diego, CA: Singular Publishing.

Sciote, J., Morris, T., Horton, M., Brandon, C., & Rosen, C. (2002). Unloaded shortening velocity and myosin heavy chain variations in human laryngeal muscle fibers. *Annals of Otology, Rhinology, and Laryngology, 111*, 120–127.

Stathopoulos, E., & Duncan, J. (2006). History and principles of exercise-based therapy: How they inform our current treatment. *Seminars in Speech & Language, 27*(4), 227–235.

Stemple, J. (2006). *Vocal function exercises: DVD*. San Diego, CA: Plural Publishing.

Stemple, J., Lee, L., D'Amico, B., & Pickup, B. (1994). Efficacy of vocal function exercises as a method of improving voice production. *Journal of Voice, 8*, 271–278.

Suzuki, T., Bless, D., Connor, N., Ford, C., Kyungah, L., & Inagi, K. (2002). Age-related alterations in myosin heavy chain isoformsin rat intrinsic laryngeal muscles. *Annals of Otology, Rhinology, and Laryngology, 111*, 962–967.

Tay, E., Phyland, D., & Oates, J. (2011). The effect of vocal funciton exercises on the voices of aging community choral singers. *Journal of Voice, 26*(5), 19–27.

Tellis, C. (2004). *A review of human skeletal muscle histology, physiology, and metabolic properties: Relationship to the intrinsic laryngeal muscles, muscle fatigue, and instrumentation* (Doctoral comprehensive examination paper). University of Pittsburgh. Pittsburgh, PA.

Tellis, C., Rosen, C., Thekdi, A., & Sciote, J. (2004). Anatomy and fiber type composition of human interarytenoid muscle. *Annals of Otology, Rhinology, and Laryngology, 113*(2), 97–107.

Thibeault, S., Zelazny, S., & Cohen, S. (2009). Voice bootcamp: Intensive treatment success. *The ASHA Leader, 14*, 26–27.

Titze, I. (1994). *Principles of voice production*. Englewood Cliffs, NJ: Prentice Hall.

Wingate, J., Brown, W., Shrivastav, R., Davenport, P., & Sapienza, C. (2007). Treatment outcomes for professional voice users. *Journal of Voice, 21*(4), 433–449.

16

Application of Motor Learning Principles to Voice Training

Introduction

Motor learning is defined by Schmidt and Lee (2010) as "a set of processes associated with practice or experience leading to relatively permanent changes in the capability for movement." Motor learning is not something we can always see or observe. More importantly, level of performance during skill acquisition does not necessarily reflect degree of learning that has taken place. While there are studies demonstrating neural adaptive changes (i.e., changes in the brain) over time for motor skills during physical tasks, studies on morphologic changes in the brain as a result of vocal training are scarce. There has been one study demonstrating that elite opera singers exhibited increased cortical networks for both sensorimotor, and kinesthetic motor control with accumulated practice compared with unstrained nonsingers

with additional increased involvement in the motor memory areas at subcortical and cerebellar areas of the brain (Kleber, Veit, Birbaumer, Gruzelier, & Lotze, 2010).

This chapter provides an overview of motor learning principles and the application of these techniques for voice training. Concepts will be introduced highlighting rehearsal and practice techniques that can facilitate motor learning. A discussion on how different teaching styles including feedback, verbal and physical cueing can help or hinder students' learning and skill acquisition is included. Basic exercise physiology concepts can be applied to voice training to maximize motor learning. Readers seeking further detail are encouraged to read *Motor Learning and Performance: A Situation-Based Learning Approach* by Schmidt and Wrisberg (2008), and *Motor Control and Learning: A Behavioral Emphasis* by Schmidt and Lee (2010).

Motor Performance Versus Motor Learning

Before introducing the stages of motor learning, it is important to understand the difference between motor learning and motor performance. Although seemingly similar, there are some key differences between the two. Motor performance is the result of the performer completing an acquired motor skill (i.e., singing a scale, hitting a ball). Motor performance fluctuates and can be impacted by fatigue, motivation, and illness. Motor learning is different from motor performance and refers to actual physical and neurologic changes that occur as a result of practice or experience giving an indication of the performer's level of skill in executing a particular motor task. Motor learning is stable with a rule system that has been internalized as a result of practice, whereas motor performance could be executed in a suboptimal manner because of a variety of factors, but that does not necessarily indicate that particular skill has not been well learned. For example, a tennis player may miss his serve because the strings on the racket need to be tightened, or because his shoulder is injured. This does not actually mean that he has not internalized the movement pattern for serving a ball. It simply means in this instance, he did not hit it accurately for external reasons. Conversely, another tennis player may hit the ball exactly in the right place in one instance, but then miss it on subsequent tries. On his successful try, he demonstrated good motor performance, but his subsequent misses indicate that motor learning of that skill has not fully taken place yet.

The important thing to keep in mind about motor learning and motor performance is that as teachers, we cannot assess the student's level of skill based on one performance of that skill. Rather, we must observe multiple performances before we can determine if motor learning has occurred and motor rules in the form of neuromuscular patterns have actually been internalized. Further, though it may seem counterintuitive, a student's achieving a high level of performance during acquisition of a new skill does not automatically equate to permanent learning of that skill. In order to determine if actual motor learning has occurred, observation of multiple successful performances of that skill under various conditions and challenges are necessary. The task of the singing teacher is to distinguish between the two to determine if further learning needs must occur before the given skill is stable and internalized. For example, a student's ability to glide with smooth transition from chest register to head mix at the same volume with no audible registration shift must be observed multiple times in order to feel confident that the skill has been internalized, and the proper coordination of musculature adjustments has been well established for that task. As discussed in Chapter 15, in addition to coordination of various muscular adjustments for movement patterns, gradually

> *Motor performance* is the result of the performer completing an acquired motor skill (i.e., singing a song, hitting a ball).
> *Motor learning* refers to physical and neurologic changes that occur as a result of practice or experience giving an indication of the performer's level of skill in executing a particular motor task.

building muscular strength and coordination also plays a significant part in development of these skills.

Stages of Motor Learning

During any new skill acquisition, there are considered three primary stages in motor learning: (1) verbal/cognitive stage, (2) motor learning stage, and (3) automatic stage (Schmidt & Wrisbreg, 2008). Importance in understanding these stages and where the student falls within the motor learning continuum will determine for the teacher how and when to provide cueing and feedback in order for the student to fully acquire a certain skill.

Verbal/Cognitive Stage

During the early stages of the motor learning process is where the student is getting the "feel" of the movement through verbal, tactile, and other sensory cues. Cognitive processing at this stage is generally slow, requiring a lot of attention and increased repetition as the learner establishes newly acquired movement patterns. Multiple errors are made during this part of the skill acquisition process, and there is substantial teacher cueing and guidance regarding positive and negative attempts at a given task. The way we structure practice and provide feedback in the lesson in this stage is different compared with later stages of motor learning, and this will be further discussed in this chapter. The teacher and student will see the most noticeable gains within the early stage of motor learning compared with the latter stages.

Motor Learning Stage

The second stage is referred to as the motor learning stage. This is the longest stage in acquiring a skill and can last years. During this stage, the student has an understanding of the basic movement pattern and has become more consistent and efficient in producing that skill. Emphasis is now focused on refining the movement patterns for that skill. The important development in this stage is the learner's ability to internally recognize and detect errors within their movement patterns/skill. Feedback and cueing required of the teacher become less necessary compared with the early stage as the learner becomes less dependent on teacher guidance.

Automatic Stage

The final stage in the motor learning process is the automatic stage. Processing and appropriate execution of the skill is fast with fluid and efficient movements. The learner has quick error detection and self-correction. Very little active processing occurs at this stage. External cueing and feedback are not needed by the teacher as learner provides their own feedback. An athletic example is the Olympic gymnast who merely thinks about the very first step in her floor routine and the rest of her performance is completely automatic because all of the movement patterns are internalized and stable. On the rare occasion that we see an abrupt disruption in a performance of Olympic caliber, the performer likely was abruptly pulled out of the automatic processing mode and into more conscious mode processing of movement, which temporarily impedes performance.

This is likely what is happening when an athlete or performer chokes up during a performance. Similarly, the vocal athlete executes singing tasks at an automatic level often combined with other physical motor tasks such as dancing.

Practical Application in the Studio

When working with a student, the teacher should be aware of where the student falls in terms of the stage of motor learning for that various skills, keeping in mind that they will have mastered different levels for various motor tasks. When meeting with a new voice student, the teacher likely will assess areas of strength and coordination versus areas of weakness and reduced coordination. For example, a student may have a strong head register but no chest voice or vice versa. Furthermore, a student may exhibit reduced coordination of registration evidenced by difficulty transition from chest to head efficiently. Certain vowels may be easy and free while others are stuck and poorly produced in certain ranges of the voice. Another important consideration is what motor skills have been learned and internalized by the student that are inefficient and need to be unlearned and re-trained. Often a new student will present with tension resulting in inefficient voice production, and this can present in a multitude of ways. The student's default setting, though suboptimal, is often firmly established in the motor plan of that singer. Early work would likely involve establishing new, more efficient movement patterns. Time and patience are often required as a new internal template for voice production is established. In this scenario, emphasis might not focus as much on strengthening and coordination; rather, early lessons may incorporate exercises to reduce extraneous muscle activity. These observations can help the teacher and student establish appropriate goals for training.

Establishing Training Goals

Goals should be realistic for the singer but challenging. The teacher should structure learning to be productive for the student rather than leaving them overwhelmed and frustrated. If the student appears overwhelmed, a reassessment of the vocal goals should be made to ensure that goals are consistent with the student's capabilities and level of motivation. The teacher must balance choosing challenging goals with choosing goals that will enable the student to experience some success early on. Motivation is a critical factor in acquiring new skills. If the teacher can create some early goals that will enable the singer to achieve some gains quickly, then they are paving the way for success when more challenging goals are then approached.

These considerations are important for the teacher not only with repertoire choices, but also with technical work. Goals should also be specific, meaning the exercise is chosen to work on a specific skill (e.g., onsets, respiratory patterns, navigating the passagio). These goals must also be attainable for the student. A goal for a graduate level student or a preprofessional singer will be different from that of a novice singer. If a student is just beginning to explore belting as a vocal style, choose songs that are challenging but not impossible, given that the vocal mechanism is still gaining strength. Choosing attainable goals must of course be balanced with the need to impose higher demands on the musculature in order to overload the muscle and build strength. This is discussed in Chapter 15.

A methodical approach utilizing observation of baseline and skill acquisition development is critical to minimize vocal strain and possible injury especially when building vocal strength, stamina, flexibility, and agility. The teacher and student must carefully monitor this process to ensure that the mechanism is being challenged, but not strained. The overload principle, an exercise physiology principle, was discussed in Chapter 15. As a reminder, this principle states that in order to gain strength and endurance, one must "overload" the muscle beyond its current level of functioning in order to see gains in strength. Challenge the healthy instrument just a bit beyond the student's comfort zone to gauge readiness to move on. If necessary, simplify the task and then build up the level of complexity when the student is ready.

As singers and performers, a significant amount of time is spent rehearsing to minimize mistakes. Therefore, it stands to reason that we should set up voice lessons to minimize mistakes. However, this thinking can actually hinder learning of new motor skills. Although it seems counterintuitive, errors (and the recognition of these errors) are critical for long-term, permanent learning. We certainly don't learn to walk without falling down once or twice. It is the falling down and learning from that fall that ultimately allows us to walk.

The caveat is that as teachers, we are inclined to guide the student toward the best performance possible, by modeling, cueing, and manipulating, but with too many of these examples, we may actually be reducing their independent learning. This idea that reduced performance of a motor skill during early stages of acquisition leads to better learning is well-documented in exercise physiology literature (Schmidt & Bjork, 1992). Another potential negative outcome of only allowing a mistake-free performance is that it gives the student a false sense of security only to be let down at the next lesson or during home practice when they are unable to duplicate their initial transient success. Teachers need to be aware of this potential problem, so that student motivation is not impacted by thinking they have failed to perform the skill. If the student understands that errors are not only OK but can enhance learning, they will learn quickly to take advantage or their errors to maximize skill acquisition. Similarly, if you encounter a student who has an inefficient vocal pattern, the "undoing" of the pattern and new skill acquisition will certainly result in a vocal setback before moving forward. Students should be forewarned of this as they are paying to sound better, not worse.

> As a general rule of thumb, within a lesson, take the student just to the point in the difficulty of the skill where they begin to break down. Then, take it back one or two steps in the process and that is the level they should be practicing at home (80% of their maximum). Next session, that 80% level will have moved the bar higher, and a new 80% level will be reached.

Structuring a Lesson

With the knowledge of motor learning and skill acquisition, a discussion on how to structure a lesson or practice session in order to maximize learning and generalization of motor skills by actually creating opportunities for errors will be addressed. There are several types of practice styles discussed in exercise physiology literature. Blocked practice style emphasizes only one skill during practice (i.e., vocal agility exercises only) versus random practice style in which multiple skills are rehearsed (i.e., resonant voice + vocal agility + register blending). Additionally, each skill can be addressed and rehearsed in multiple ways. A good teacher will have knowledge of each individual student and their learning style to provide the appropriate exercises and implementation of those exercises for maximal gain.

How a given skill is rehearsed is another consideration for the teacher. Constant practice means there is no variation in how the skill is rehearsed. For example, if practicing agility in a constant format, the student would be singing on the same vowel, in the same pattern, at the same volume each time. Varied practice refers to a format in which the skill is rehearsed in multiple ways. Skills can also be practiced in a blocked format where only one skill is practiced over and over, or a random format where multiple skills are practiced. Going back to a tennis analogy, an example of constant practice would be practicing forehand swing to the same spot at the same speed over and over. Varied practice would involve practicing forehand to different spots at varied speeds. If the teacher is using a blocked format, the student would only be practicing forehand during that session. If a random format is used, the student would practice forehand, backhand, and serves within one session. During a voice lesson, a student could be guided to work only vocal agility on the same vowel and the same volume with the same scale pattern (constant practice), or the student could work on agility with varied vowels at different volumes, legato, staccato (varied practice).

These practice styles can be combined, and the type of practice style used would depend on what motor learning stage the student is in for that skill. For example, if the student is still in the early verbal/cognitive stage, the teacher may elect to use a blocked constant pattern initially. This allows the learner to experience multiple repetitions of the target skill in order to establish an internal reference for correct movement relative to sound and feel. For example, if the student has no reference at all for what head register sounds or feels like in her own voice, early lessons may incorporate simple stepwise vocal exercises designed to elicit and access that movement pattern while allowing the student to establish a reference for the sound and sensory experience of that particular motor task (head voice).

The student's performance of this particular skill will likely improve simply as a result of multiple uninterrupted repetitions of the same skill within one voice lesson. However, as soon as the student has a reference for the goal, and begins to hit the target even some of the time, the teacher could elect to transition toward a random/varied paradigm (varied pitch, volume, scale). In this case, that might include switching from exercises in head register to exercises in chest register. What will likely follow are increased errors because the teacher has just increased the complexity of the practice. However, though perhaps counterintuitive, the random varied model has demonstrated the greatest gains in motor learning compared with other practice styles (Lee, Magill, & Weeks, 1985). Additionally, this practice model is relevant to voice because singing and acting involves and requires numerous simultaneous motor skills. This model promotes flexibility and adaptability, two very necessary skill sets for a performer (Catalano & Kleiner, 1984).

The Forgetting Hypothesis

Let's return to the concept that we want to set up our students to make errors in order to maximize motor learning. The "Forgetting Hypothesis" endorses the notion that by producing nonsequential, random repetitions of various motor skills, the learner is forced to generate and/or retrieve a new motor paradigm for each new skill. For example, skipping from Skill A to B to C back to Skill A keeps the brain from going on autopilot by repeating one skill over and over in a closed loop. Performance will indeed improve with uninterrupted repetition, but only by virtue of the repetition not because of learning. Therefore, carryover will not occur (Shea & Morgan, 1979). To further clarify, let's return to the tennis lesson analogy. Student A is being taught in a blocked/constant format, and student B is being taught in a random/varied format. Student A has only practiced forehand from the same area of the court and the same speed. Performance of that skill for student A becomes quite good by the end of the lesson. In contrast, student B running up and down the court hitting forehand and backhand presented at varied speeds. Student B makes significantly more errors during the lesson, and performance is not as good compared with student A. The following week however, when both students return for their lesson, student B will actually perform better than student A. The reason for this is because student A demonstrated improved performance only as a result of rote repetition but did not actually internalize or learn any of the new movement patterns. Student B, although poor in performance initially, actually internalized more of the movement patterns and demonstrated some learning of the new skills. This concept is well-described in the exercise physiology literature for athletic performance.

Once the student has established a reference for the target motor skill and can produce it at least sometimes, we want to create a practice environment where the learner generates errors by constantly having them switch from one task to another. This may reduce performance in the short-term but will facilitate learning and long-term carryover of new skills. How might we view this within the context of the vocal athlete? We could apply this concept not only to acquisition of vocal skill sets, but also to actual learning of music. Let's take the former scenario into consideration. As an example, one of the distinguishing features of many music theater performers is they often need to be skilled in many vocal styles including facility with both a belt and "legit" sound in order to be more hirable. Therefore, vocal training might be designed to vary registration across these parameters within the lesson. For example, exercises might vary from head register, to chest, to belting, back to head and so on. In addition to varying the use of registration, there are other parameters to be varied such as timbre, vowels, intensity, and pitch range. In order for this to be effective, the teacher must have a clear intention of how they structure technical work during a lesson. Careful listening for subtle changes in response to the exercise is important to maximize efficiency. This has the benefit of helping to internalize these different vocal default settings fairly easily. Additionally, as was discussed in Chapter 15, this type of vocal cross training also has the added benefit of muscular strengthening and conditioning for multiple vocal styles.

Feedback and Cueing

Take a moment to consider your teaching style. What strategies do you use to convey a concept? Do you verbalize a lot of concepts in your lessons? Do you have a hands-on approach? Do you stop and correct often? Do you provide a vocal model each time? Do you use poetic or anatomic imagery? How often do you provide feedback? The next section discusses how teaching style can either promote or hinder motor learning.

Cueing and feedback refers to the manner in which we communicate to the student whether or not they hit the target skill. There are two primary types of feedback: intrinsic and extrinsic. Intrinsic feedback provides the learner with sensory information about what is going on with their body during skill production. It is learner-driven by what the learner sees, feels, and hears. Extrinsic, or augmented feedback, is sensory information provided by an outside source. It is controlled by the teacher or observer (or perhaps a recording). Information derived from extrinsic feedback gives the learner information about how he or she did while performing the task. The primary difference between these two types of feedback is that one is teacher or observer controlled, and one is learner controlled.

The two primary modes of cueing are knowledge of performance (KP) and knowledge of results (KR). KP provides the singer with some sort of information about the quality of the movement they produced. For example, telling a student that

they didn't drop their jaw wide enough is an example of KP, or telling a student you noticed nice rib expansion during inhalation is another example of KP. This type of feedback is common; however, it does not allow the student to assess their own performance. Instead, the teacher is doing the thinking for the student. It is important to pause and let the student first process what she did before the teacher provides KP (Wulf & Schmidt, 1988).

In contrast, KR does not provide the student with information regarding the quality of the movement rather, it simply tells the student how close they came to the target. Telling a singer she was sharp on a given note is an example of KR. It tells the student she didn't hit the target, but gives her no information about the quality or correctness of her movements during her attempt. To use a golf analogy, KP provides the golfer with information about his swing, and KR tells him how close he came to getting the ball into the hole. KR feedback is only useful if the student understands what the target actually is because the singer needs to be able to assess whether there is a mismatch between the desired production and the actual production. Therefore, telling a student you would like her to sing in head register is not helpful for her if she has no auditory or tactile reference for what head register sounds and feels like in her voice. This is why blocked, constant practice becomes important earlier in skill acquisition. It allows the singer to establish a reference for correctness, which is critical for error detection. Otherwise the learner will become dependent on the teacher to always provide feedback (Bilodeau, Bilodeau, & Shumsky, 1959).

The leaner's reference for correctness can help the teacher determine what type of feedback to provide. For example, early in the motor learning process when

> Describing the activity of the CT muscle relative to the TA muscle during head register won't likely help the student better understand how to produce the sound correctly.

reference for correctness is not firmly established, KR along with blocked/constant practice might help to more firmly establish the learner's reference for correctness for that skill by associating a certain movement pattern to a resulting action. If a singer has never really sung in chest voice, the teacher should structure the lesson to elicit that sound through modeling and appropriately chosen exercises. This will increase learner confidence and motivation; however, the teacher must then transition to intrinsic feedback as soon as the learner demonstrates they can approximate the target at least some of the time and are aware of whether they did or did not produce the target skill. Keep in mind that extrinsic feedback artificially inflates performance, so the teacher and student should expect a temporary reduction in performance when you transfer to intrinsic feedback. Verbal instruction on mechanics of movement is much less productive than simply experiencing the movement. This has been demonstrated in both kinesiology and voice literature (Wulf & Weigelt, 1997; Yiu, Verdolini, & Chow, 2005).

Reducing Learner Dependency

The above section discussed how structuring cueing and feedback can impact learning. There are some additional guidelines that may further facilitate or hinder motor learning. The overarching goal during instruction is to reduce learner dependency on teacher feedback, so that the learner ultimately can self-monitor. Delayed imitation is a key component that was touched upon earlier. Having the student wait several seconds before repeating a sound allows them to process and evaluate what they have done. It increases their ability to provide intrinsic feedback. This has been demonstrated in kinesiology studies that indicate that immediate KR after completion of a skill impedes performance, whereas a short delay with learner evaluation of a completed task can enhance learning of that skill (Swinnen, Schmidt, Nicholson, & Shapiro, 1990). It also provides a "desirable difficulty" forcing the brain to think through each new repetition both in preparation of and after performance of the skill. Have the student first hear the target sound in his or her head prior to initiating the sound will help slow down time in between repetitions.

Passive guidance refers to the teacher manipulating the movements of the performer. An example of passive guidance is the teacher placing a hand on the shoulders of the singer to help minimize shoulder elevation during inhalation. This risk of passive guidance is that the student will become too reliant on these tactile, hands-on cues and cannot accurately produce the desired vocal output without them. Additionally, it can prevent the natural desired errors from occurring early on in learning enhancing performance but reducing learning. As with other types of feedback and cueing, once the target movement is approximated, passive guidance should be eliminated focusing more on intrinsic feedback. Similarly, too much vocal modeling also can limit learning. Therefore, vocal modeling should be used primarily during the early stages of acquisition of a specific skill, and then faded as the student becomes more experienced with that skill.

How often a teacher gives feedback to the student can also impact learning. Frequent feedback (after every one or two trials) will increase performance but also promote learner dependency. Infrequent feedback (every 50 to 100 attempts) will certainly not result in learner dependence, but it also might not give enough guidance toward approximation of the skill especially in the early stages of acquisition. One study looked at frequency of feedback for hitting a baseball. Subjects were given feedback in intervals ranging from every attempt to every 15 attempts. Results indicated that subjects who received feedback after every five attempts exhibited the greatest integration of the given skill (Schmidt, Lange, & Young, 1990). Research on cueing and feedback from exercise physiology literature suggests that teachers should be thoughtful about structuring the amount of verbal and physical cueing and type of feedback to avoid learner dependency, and promote independent learning.

Directing Learners' Attention

Consider how you direct your student's focus during a lesson. Mental imagery is a method used by some to help provide the singer with a focus (e.g., imagine the breath is a wave and the voice rides the wave across the room). Others use anatomic imagery such as instructing a student to imagine a smile in the back of the throat to facilitate elevating the soft palate. There are two primary ways to categorize how we direct a learner's attention: internal focus and external focus.

Internal focus refers to directing the student toward movements within their body. For example, having them focus on maintaining a lowered jaw while approaching a high note. This type of focus might provide some utility during early stages of skill acquisition when the learner is still getting the sense for the physical movement and cueing and feedback are heightened; however, focusing too much on internal movements can create "paralysis by analysis," resulting in impeded learning (Prinz, 1997). As singers and teachers, we have all likely experienced this phenomenon, which can be very counterproductive. In fact, the harder we attempt to fix the internal movement, often the worse it gets.

In contrast with internal focus, exercise physiology literature supports an emphasis on external focus to enhance motor learning (Wulf, McNevin, Fuchs, Ritter, & Toole, 2000; Wulf & Prinz, 2001). In singing, this could be translated as guiding the singer to focus on the outcome of the motor skill rather than the physiologic mechanics of it. For example, asking the student to provide feedback on the feel or sound of the voice task keeps the focus external and may reduce the "locking up" that can happen from overanalyzing physical movements. The teacher should have a sense of how a student is responding to instruction and modify teaching to the focus point as needed.

Chapter Summary

Motor performance does not necessarily provide information about actual acquisition of a given skill, and the teacher must learn to discern between motor learning and motor performance in order to determine how the student is truly progressing.

Knowledge of the stages of motor learning will not only help determine appropriate training goals, but will also inform the type of cueing and feedback to give a student. Consistent voice lessons and independent practice can be structured to further maximize learning and reduce learner dependence on teacher feedback. These factors, along with how we focus learner's attention, can either impede or facilitate motor learning. An added component, for CCM performers, is that the vocal athlete often performs multiple tasks (physical and vocal) simultaneously adding a layer of complexity to internalizing vocal movement patterns learned in a studio context, to the actual performance context.

References

Bilodeau, E., Bilodeau, I., & Shumsky, D. (1959). Some effects of introducing and withdrawing results early and late in practice. *Journal of Experimental Psychology, 58*, 142–144.

Catalano, J., & Kleiner, B. (1984). Distant transfer in coincident timing as a function of variability of practice. *Perceptual and Motor Skills, 58*, 851–856.

Kleber, B., Veit, R., Birbaumer, N., Gruzelier, J., & Lotze, M. (2010). The brain of opera singers: Experience-dependent changes in functional activation. *Cereb Cortex, 20*(5), 1144–1152.

Lee, T., Magill, R., & Weeks, D. (1985). Influence of practice schedule on testing schema theory predictions in adults. *Journal of Motor Behavior, 17*, 282–299.

Prinz, W. (1997). Perception and action planning. *European Journal of Cognitive Psychology, 9*, 129–154.

Schmidt, R., & Bjork, R. (1992). New conceptualizations of practice: Common principals in three paradigms suggest new concepts for training. *Psychological Science, 3*(4), 207–217.

Schmidt, R., Lange, C., & Young, D. (1990). Optimizing summary knowledge of results for skill learning. *Human Movement Science, 9*, 325–348.

Schmidt, R., & Lee, T. (2010). *Motor control and learning: A behavioral emphasis* (5th ed.). Champaign, IL: Human Kinetics.

Schmidt, R., & Wrisbreg, C. (2008). *Motor learning and performance: A situation-based learning approach* (4th ed.). Champaign, IL: Human Kinetics.

Shea, J., & Morgan, R. (1979). Contextual interference effects on the acquisition, retention, and transfer of a motor skill. *Journal of Experimental Psychology, 5*, 179–187.

Swinnen, S., Schmidt, R., Nicholson, D., & Shapiro, D. (1990). Information feedback for skill acquisition: Instantaneous knowledge of results degrades learning. *Journal of Experimental Psychology. Learning, Memory, and Cognition, 16*, 706–716.

Wulf, G., McNevin, N., Fuchs, T., Ritter, F., & Toole, T. (2000). Attentional focus in complex skill learning. *Research Quarterly for Exercise and Sport, 71*(3), 229–239.

Wulf, G., & Prinz, W. (2001). Directing attention to movement effects enhances learning: A review. *Psychonomic Bulletin and Review, 8*(4).

Wulf, G., & Schmidt, R. (1988). Variability in practice: Facilitation in retention and transfer through schema formation or context effects? *Journal of Motor Behavior, 20*, 133–149.

Wulf, G., & Weigelt, C. (1997). Instructions about physical principals in learning a complex motor skill: To tell or not to tell. *Research Quarterly for Exercise and Sport, 68*, 4.

Yiu, E., Verdolini, K., & Chow, L. (2005). Electromyographic study of motor learning for a voice production task. *Journal of Speech, Language, and Hearing Research, 48*, 1254–1268.

17

The Art of Perfection: What Every Singer and Voice Teacher Should Know About Audio Technology

MATTHEW EDWARDS

Introduction

Whenever you listen to a recording, you are not only listening to the artistry of the performer, but also the skillfulness and artistic choices of the sound engineer. From the earliest days of audio recording, sound engineers have sought to manipulate the vocal artist and recording equipment in order to capture what the engineer believed to be the best performance (Horning, 2004). Many singers attempt to replicate the electronically altered and enhanced sounds they hear through their stereo solely with their natural acoustic voice. If a recording has been heavily processed, replicating the perceived vocal qualities on the recording with the acoustic voice alone is likely impossible. Therefore, anyone who sings or trains singers in a commercial music style should first understand the basic equipment that is available to performers and how to integrate the equipment into their performance. This chapter covers an overview of the history of sound recording, historically how and why it was important, and the current use of amplification and recording in today's commercial singing world.

Audio Engineers and the Art of Perfection

Consider for a moment your own experience of sitting in various locations of the same concert hall. Many audience members find their own favorite seat in any given hall because of the perceived sound quality and experience in that specific location. For instance, audience members listening to a concert in the front half of the orchestra section may experience a brighter timbre than those persons listening in the third row of the first balcony. Neither seating section is necessarily better than the other in quantifiable terms, but subjectively arguments can be made for both in terms of aesthetic preference of the listener. When an engineer records a performance, he or she is bringing their own personal seating preferences to the final product through microphone placement, equipment selection, and choices in the final mixing of the performance. In essence, they are manipulating the input sound of the performance in order to take you to their favorite seat in the concert hall through alteration and manipulation of the recorded sound (Buskin, 2008).

Recording in the Early 20th Century

To capture famous voices in the early 20th century, recording engineers had only one system available to them—the acoustic horn (Figure 17-1). Acoustic horn recorders utilized a long metal horn to capture acoustic vibrations for preservation. The horn sent the vibrations down a cone-shaped tube to a small metal needle. The needle vibrated with the pulsations of the

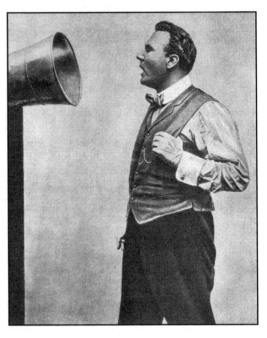

Figure 17–1. Russian bass, Feodor Chaliapin singing into a recording horn, 1913.

horn and cut small grooves into a wax cylinder to capture those vibrations. When played back, those grooves would vibrate the needle, and the horn would amplify those small vibrations into the room. It is important for singers and voice teachers to know that these early recordings did not accurately capture the entire spectrum of sound that the human ear is capable of hearing. In fact, they only captured frequencies from around 100 to 2500 Hz (Library of Congress, 2013), which fall below the typical singer's formant ("ring" in the voice) and below the upper resonance peaks of the female voice.

In addition to limited options for acoustic horn recordings, engineers had only one choice to make on increased or decreased vocal intensity: distance between the various instruments and singers from the acoustic horn. If a singer desired to make a crescendo or decrescendo, the engineer placed them on a wheel cart and moved them forward and/or backward from the horn. The methods were primitive, and the results were far from consistent. As electronic recording equipment evolved, more options became available, and engineers quickly learned to exploit the equipment's possibilities (Horning, 2004).

Modern Recording Methods

Today, sound engineers have a wide array of equipment options available at their disposal, from hundreds of microphones with varying responses, to complex soundboards, to limitless speaker choices. Many singers and teachers are unaware that this equipment is not exclusive to the recording studio, but also pervades live performances, radio, and television broadcasts as well. Audio engineering affects the way we perceive

> Terminology Defined
> - Vocoder—A voice encoder used to synthesize the human voice.
> - Spectral morphing—Uses the spectral components of multiple voices and/or instruments and blends the spectrums together to mold into a new sound.
> - Granular synthesis—Breaking a sound down into small parts and rearranging them to form a new sound.
> - Remastering—To recreate (typically through enhancement) a previous audio recording.

sound in nearly every performance venue outside of an opera house or concert hall. Here are a few real-life examples to help you form a better understanding of the use and consequence of audio enhancement.

During Paul McCartney's 2011 world tour, front-of-house engineer Paul Boothroyd customized the sound system with a unique goal in mind: to recreate the vocal tone qualities from the various eras of Paul's career. Boothroyd utilized a digital mixing board for this tour, which allowed him to preset unique combinations of vocal effects for each song in McCartney's concert. Through careful manipulation of the equalization, reverb, delays, and pitch-shift delay, Boothroyd was able to achieve this goal for the entire 4-hour concert of more than 50 songs (Benzuly, 2011).

For the 'NSync track "Pop," engineer Brian Transeau pushed the limits of his system and digital editing as a whole. Using a digital sound design environment called Kyma, Transeau wrote numerous pages of programming code so that he could run 40 different vocal treatments on the track including spectral morphing, phase vocoding, granular synthesis, and traditional vocoding, which are various forms of separating, manipulating, and combining various bandwidths of the audio spectrum. He estimated that there were over a thousand vocal edits on the final cut of the song (Buskin, 2001).

Live Performance

It may seem to many singing teachers that making extreme alterations to the acoustic voice in the recording studio would limit the ability of the artist to perform a song live. However, that is actually no longer true because sound engineering has evolved, resulting in affordable and portable equipment allowing consistent replication of the studio recording during live performance. Bands regularly use backing tracks (prerecorded audio files from the original recording session that are digitally synced with the live performers) to reproduce their recorded performance live. The development and utilization of reliable in-ear monitors has resulted in this practice becoming quite common. Essentially how this works in a live performance is that the band sets a tempo for each song during the recording session and a metronome click track is then laid down in the background with an adjustable volume level so that the drummer can clearly hear the beat. The prerecorded audio files are then played through the in-ear monitor of each band member, and the musicians add their live instruments and vocals. Through the use of the mixing board, the final "live" performance becomes a hybrid of what was recorded in the studio with some additional live input.

Broadway shows have yet to embrace and utilize the full range of vocal effects noted above during live performances, but they do employ sound systems and sound boards that rival those in use by rock bands. Andrew Lloyd Webber recorded the cast album of *Jesus Christ Superstar* in a studio, before it was performed on stage, and audiences arrived at the theatre expecting to hear the music in its "ideal" form that they had heard on the mastered recording (Grant, 2004; Wollman, 2006). Once producers began incorporating modern sound engineering techniques into the cast recordings, they had no choice but to adapt the live experience to meet audience expectations. For instance, the Broadway production of *Billy Elliot* utilizes 96 microphones under the stage floor to amplify the sounds of the tap dancers on stage (Alter, 2009). In prerecording days, the tap dancing would

not have been amplified, and the producers would have relied on the acoustic power of the dance itself to generate audience excitement. In today's marketplace, the audience expects the acoustic intensity of the tap dancing to be the same as when they listened to it in their headphones or in their car at full volume.

There is also a strange paradox that has begun to happen in some musical revivals; complex audio designs have been incorporated to make the singers appear unamplified. For the 2008 production/revival of *South Pacific* at Lincoln Center, engineer Scott Lehrer used modern technology to make the show sound reminiscent of the preamplification days (*Original South Pacific*, 1949). To achieve this effect, Lehrer used both up-close and distant microphone placement of the orchestra to combine bright and dark timbres through the system. The actors used standard head-mounted microphones with the exception of the actor playing Emile (Paulo Szot). Szot, an operatic baritone, was miked with both a head mounted unit and a chest mounted lavaliere to "warm up" his sound with some of his "natural resonance." Lehrer then tapped into the Lincoln Center's artificial reverb system and utilized 85 of the 100 speakers to run two different surround sound programs. By using a computerized system, Lehrer was able to make the actors voices appear to be coming from wherever they were standing on the stage (Alter, 2009). One may think that this is much more complicated than just returning to the days of performing acoustically, the way the show was originally performed. You would be correct. However, as pointed out earlier, modern audiences expect, and often demand, a certain sound quality in the theatre (Grant, 2004; Wollman, 2006). In order to achieve the audience desired sound night after night without damaging the singers' voices, extensive audio technology must be employed.

Opera

Even though some may wish to believe that opera has remained pure, that is unfortunately no longer true. Although artists at the Metropolitan Opera still perform acoustically in live performances, their voices are enhanced on the live broadcasts and subsequent commercial releases of those recordings. Engineer Jay David Saks uses a variety of microphone positions, which helps him combine bright and dark vocal colors in the hall. He also uses reverb, compression, and equalization to achieve what he believes to be an ideal sound. For commercial releases of performances, Saks is able to cut and paste passages from the rehearsals that may have been better than what was sung in the actual performance (Eskow, 2008). This process is comparable with autotuning and ensures that the performances we admire at home are as flawless as the marketing images that entice us to watch and listen in the first place.

Remasterings of Historic Recordings

Remasterings of historic opera recordings can also vary drastically between record labels as shown in research by Morange, Dubois, and Fontaine (2010). These researchers analyzed 11 remasterings of the same Enrico Caruso recording of Pagliacci. They found numerous digital artifacts in acoustic analysis that suggested the recordings were edited for noise reduction, removing pulse defects, and removing frequencies below 120 Hz. There were also markers suggesting equalization had been used to balance the resonance effect of the original acoustic horn. In addition, a few of the recordings had artifacts that suggested digital reverb had been added to the recording. Distinct differences in the amplitude of the singer's formant range were also visible in the spectrograms, suggesting the "ring" in the voice may have been affected by equalization (Morange, Dubois, & Fontaine, 2010).

Listening Levels

Another issue that has not gained a lot of research interest, but is nonetheless worth considering, is the difference between iPod listening levels and the actual volume levels at which singers perform. A study at Kennesaw State University found that on average, students were listening to music through their headphones at 94.8 dB. On the extreme end of the population, the students were listening to music at 110.7 dB (Alarcon & Jones, 2009). Studies examining actual vocal intensity in live performance of professional country singers found these performers produce voice between 85 and 100 dB, and researchers measuring professional belters found mean SPL ranging between 62 and 94 dB (Björkner, 2008). Both sets of measurements suggest that CCM singing styles do not necessarily require extreme volume levels. Yet voice teachers are aware that many aspiring students come into the studio attempting to sing at 100 to 110 dB to replicate the sound they have been listening to via headphones. It is this author's belief that this phenomenon is partly because of the fact that young singers are experiencing music in their headphones at average volume levels of 94.8 dB to as high as 110.7 dB (Jones & Alarcon,

2009). In most instances, attempting to replicate the perceived recorded volume level with the acoustic voice is a near impossible vocal task. Continual endeavors to reach those volume levels in the absence of amplification may result in increased collision forces and sheering stress leading to increased potential of vocal injury.

Understanding Modern Recording Technology

In order for the voice teacher to effectively train singers performing commercial music, it is imperative to have a basic understanding of the performance environments and vocal demands placed upon these artists. Additionally, the teacher should have a knowledge base of the tools available for maximizing vocal production. The next sections provide readers with the basic elements of sound systems that singers and voice specialists should be familiar with and considerations on how voice teachers can use this equipment in their work with clients to improve and enhance vocal performance.

The Signal Chain

In order to record or reinforce an audio signal, we must first capture acoustic energy and then convert it into electrical energy. Transformation of the acoustic vibrations into electrical pulses allows for transmission of that signal through a series of electrical components, which can then undergo conditioning, modification, and enhancement. The modified signal is then transmitted to a magnetic speaker where the electric pulses are turned back into

acoustic energy, and the modified signal is received by the listener.

The path described above is called the "signal chain." The complexities of the circuits, components, and infinite variations of settings within the signal chain are beyond the scope of this chapter. For more in-depth information regarding the complexities of the signal chain, the reader is referred to *Voice Processing* by Gordon E. Pelton (1993) and *Voice Science and Recording* by David M. Howard and Damian T. Murphy (2008). The focus of the following sections is on the components that vocalists and voice teachers will most likely encounter.

Microphones

Singers and those who teach singers should minimally be familiar with the following characteristics of a microphone: pickup pattern, frequency response, sensitivity, and diaphragm type. Most microphones come with a specification sheet that details these elements so that a singer can make an informed choice when making a purchase. Below you will find simple explanations of microphone traits along with implications for singers and voice teachers. Figure 17–2 provides a visual representation of how three types of microphones work (omnidirectional, unidirectional, and bidirectional).

Pickup Pattern

"Pickup pattern" is a term used to describe how a microphone's diaphragm responds to acoustic vibrations and thus "picks them up" for transmission to the audio system. Pickup patterns (also sometimes called polar patterns or directivity patterns) are visualized on a circular diagram for omni-

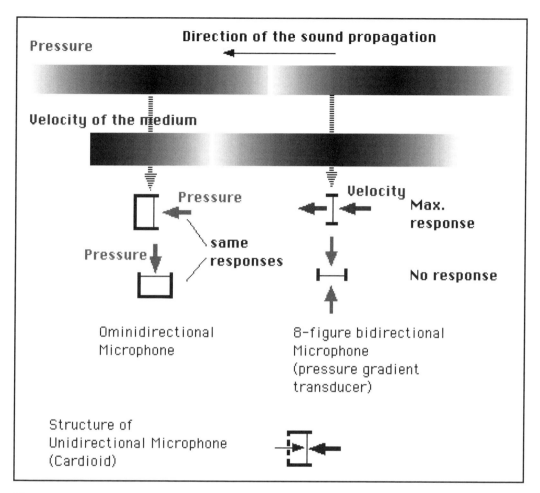

Figure 17–2. Principles of omni-uni-and 8-figure- microphones.

directional and cardioid (Figure 17-3 and Figure 17-4). The circles of the diagram indicate decreases in the sensitivity of the microphone's diaphragm. The outermost circle indicates that there is no impact on the signal approaching the diaphragm from that angle, while the inner circles each represent a -5 dB cut. While the diagram is drawn two-dimensionally, it actually represents a three-dimensional phenomenon.

To visualize this, imagine a round apple placed in front of your mouth with a long stem. Imagine that the stem is the handle of the microphone, and the opposite end of the core is the center of the microphone's diaphragm. The end of the apple in front of your lips would be labeled 0° on a pickup pattern diagram, and would be called "on-axis." The stem side of the apple would be labeled 180° on a pickup pattern, and would be called "off-axis." Now imagine two planes cutting through the apple and intersecting in the center, one horizontal and one vertical. The outer edge of the apple, where the horizontal plane breaks the skin, would be labeled as 90° on the right and 270° on the

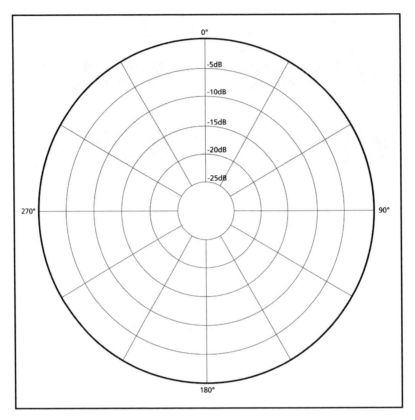

Figure 17–3. Polar pattern of omnidirectional characteristic.

left. Now imagine that you could draw a 45° angle from the center of the apple to any point of the outer skin. Now draw a circle completely around the apple at that angle. The 45° angle can now be seen from every side of the apple and represents the microphone's ability to pick up sound at that angle, regardless of which side of the microphone is facing the sound source.

Return to the two-dimensional diagram. If you draw a straight line away from the 180° label, you will see the shape of the apple as used in the example above. Within the diagram, you will see a bold black circle that indicates changes in the sensitivity of the microphone at various angles. If the bold circle touches the outermost edge of the diagram, the manufacturer is indicating that there is no amplitude loss at that angle. However, if the bold circle cuts inward at a specific angle and crosses an inner circle of the diagram, the manufacturer is indicating a decrease in amplitude response at that specific angle.

When working with this equipment, one must experiment with it to truly understand how microphones function and respond to sound source input. To gain a better understanding, go to a music store, recording studio, or other location with sound equipment and choose several microphones to attempt the following tasks:

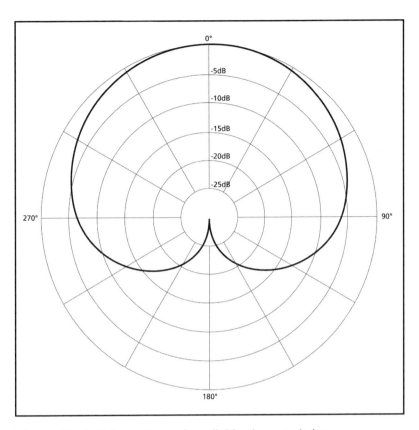

Figure 17–4. Polar pattern of cardioids characteristics.

1. Sing dead center into each microphone and note the volume level.
2. Angle each microphone so that you are singing at a 45° angle in relation to the diaphragm. Now turn the microphone 360° in your hand and sing around the entire surface of the mic at 45°. Take note of what you hear in the recording or output amplifier.
3. Repeat exercise #2, but with the microphone positioned at 90°. Take note of what you hear.

You should find that the volume level will change as you maneuver the microphone to different angles, but there will be no change when you rotate the microphone at the same angle.

Frequency Response

Frequency response is a term used to define how accurately a microphone transfers the original acoustic spectrum to the soundboard. Variations in size and materials can affect the way a microphone responds to sound. Some microphones respond very well to lower frequencies, but not high frequencies and vice versa. Variability between microphones is accounted for in frequency response curves. Take a look at the following example (Figure 17-5).

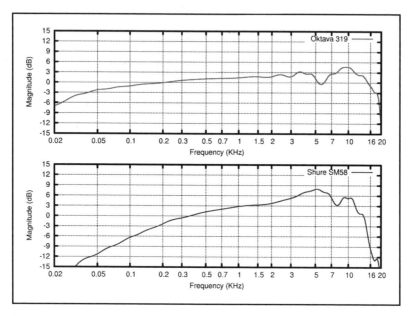

Figure 17–5. A graph comparing the frequency magnitude response of an Oktava 319 microphone versus a Shure SM 58 microphone.

The graph in Figure 17-5 represents amplitude changes on the *y*-axis and frequencies on the *x*-axis. The center line of the *y*-axis represents 0 dB, meaning that there is no cut or boost to the frequencies that intersect at that point on the graph. The Oktava 319, depicted on the upper graph, stays relatively close to the 0-dB line compared with the Shure SM 58 pictured below. The Shure SM 58 drastically cuts the frequencies below 300 Hz, by as much as –6 dB at 100 Hz and –12 dB at 50 Hz. In comparison, the Oktava 319 only cuts the amplitude of 100 Hz by about –1 to 2 dB and 50 Hz by around –2 to 3 dB. This is a significant difference and will result in quite different products. If you were to record a bass singer performing "O Isis und Osiris" from *Die Zauberflöte* or "Folsom Prison Blues" by Johnny Cash using the SM 58, you may experience a significant change in the tone quality of the lower pitches since the

SM 58 cuts the frequencies below 100 Hz by –6 dB. Choosing the Oktava 319 may be a better option in this example because the microphone only reduces the amplitude at 100 Hz by –1 to –2 dB and would therefore more accurately capture the performance.

Sensitivity

The detailed technical descriptions necessary to fully explain sensitivity are beyond the scope of this chapter. For the purposes of this chapter, a basic explanation is provided that will suffice for the needs of most readers.

Sensitivity is measured in a lab by recording the output voltage of the microphone's diaphragm in response to a 1 kHz signal with amplitude of 94 dB. The pressure of the signal used to test the microphone (1 kHz at 94 dB) is equal to one pascal. When the diaphragm moves in response to the pressure generated by the test tone, it generates an electrical signal that is sent through the microphone cable to the soundboard. The power of this signal is measured in millivolts. A microphone's sensitivity is defined as millivolts/pascal or mV/PA. The lower the mV number listed in the specification sheet, the less sensitive the microphone is and vice versa (Howard & Murphy, 2008).

Microphones with various sensitivities have different advantages. A microphone with a high sensitivity rating can be extremely useful when recording a weak-voiced singer. A high sensitivity microphone could also be useful when recording a live performance from a distance. However, microphones with high sensitivity can be problematic in a recording studio with a loud singer. Singers with significant acoustic vocal intensity can easily overblow a microphone, with high sensitivity resulting in signal distortion. In those situations, it is better to use a microphone with a lower sensitivity rating. This allows the singer to perform with their full voice and gives the audio engineer greater control at the soundboard.

Microphone Diaphragm Types

The diaphragm is the part of the microphone that receives acoustic vibrations and converts them into electrical pulses. The three most common microphone diaphragm types that a singer will encounter are dynamic, condenser, and ribbon.

Dynamic

Dynamic microphones (Figure 17–6) use a Mylar diaphragm, moving within a magnetic field, to turn vibrations into an electrical signal that can be amplified. These microphones are popular in live performance because of their low sensitivity, which minimizes feedback. However, this feature is largely because of the fact that their ability

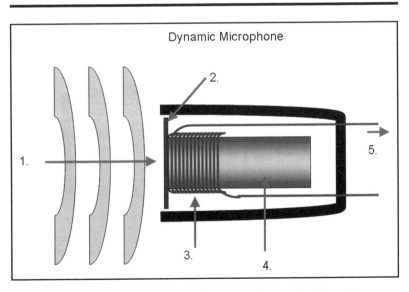

Figure 17–6. Profile of dynamic microphone. **1.** Sound waves. **2.** Diaphragm. **3.** Coil. **4.** Permanent magnet. **5.** Audio signal.

to amplify sound quickly dissipates with an increase in distance from the mouth to the microphone. Therefore, singers with decreased vocal intensity (i.e., crooners) will often sing with their lips almost touching the microphone's windscreen. Singers with increased vocal intensity will need to create some distance between themselves and the microphone; otherwise, they can overpower the diaphragm and the sound will become distorted.

Condenser

Condenser microphones (Figure 17–7) use two thin metal plates, one positive and one negative, separated by a layer of insulation. As sound hits the first thin metal plate, it vibrates and the distance between the positive and negative plates fluctuates. As the distance between the two plates changes, the microphone produces an electric signal that is then sent through the microphone cable to the amplifier.

Condenser microphones are the microphones of choice in the recording studio because of their high degree of sensitivity. They are also frequently used in headset microphones such as those found on the Broadway stage. Using a condenser microphone, performers can sing at nearly inaudible levels that when mixed in the studio will result in a final tone that is perceived as intimate and earthy. The downside of this high level of sensitivity is that these microphones are prone to feedback.

When using a condenser microphone, be aware that the magnetic plates within the diaphragm require a special power source called "phantom power" in order to operate. Phantom power sends a 48-volt power supply from the soundboard, through the microphone cable to the diaphragm. The soundboard usually has a button that can

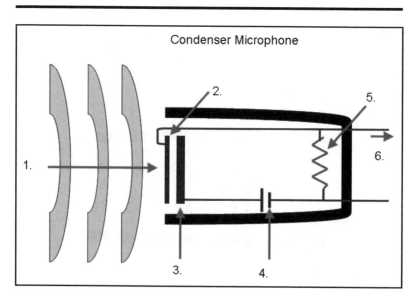

Figure 17–7. Profile of a condenser microphone. **1.** Sound waves. **2.** Diaphragm. **3.** Back plate. **4.** Battery. **5.** Resistance. **6.** Audio signal.

be used to turn phantom power on and off labeled "+48V." If you are planning on using a condenser microphone, be sure that your sound system supplies phantom power. Without a power source, these microphones will not work.

Ribbon

Ribbon microphones (Figure 17–8) use a thin metal ribbon placed between two magnets in order to capture acoustic vibrations. When the ribbon is set into motion by the sound source, the magnetic field is altered, creating an electric signal. Ribbon microphones of the past were easily broken and failed to gain the same popularity as condenser and dynamic microphones. However, recent advances in technology have enabled manufacturers to develop more durable products, and ribbon microphones are seeing a small resurgence in popularity. Be aware that phantom power can destroy

the diaphragm in a ribbon microphone. You must also be careful not to drop the microphone as a single incident can permanently damage the unit.

Making a Purchase

When purchasing a microphone, you will want to examine the "spec sheet," which details the pick-up pattern, diaphragm type, sensitivity, and frequency response for each unit. Less expensive pricing may be found online, but microphones are best purchased where you can examine the specification sheet in person, test the unit, and purchase the exact microphone that meets the needs of the singer. Microphones made by the same manufacturer may be exactly the same in design, but subtle variability between units may be noticeable to a performer. Purchasing in-store will guarantee you get exactly what you want.

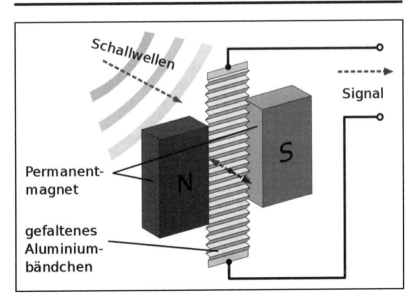

Figure 17–8. Profile of ribbon microphone.

Signal Processing

The previous discussion on the basics of the microphone provides a basis of discussion for the most common signal processing units typically encountered, what they do, and why they are important to singers.

Equalization (EQ)

If a classical singer wishes to adjust timbre, shifts and adjustments are made within their resonators to affect the perceived output. Singers spend considerable time and vocal training learning to physiologically alter the vocal tract in order to make adjustments to their timbre. However, when a singer is performing with audio technology, the audio engineer can make a few simple adjustments using an equalizer to accomplish a similar effect. Equalizers come in three main types: graphic, parametric, and shelf. Parametric and shelf equalizers enable the engineer to alter wide frequencies bands while graphic equalizers enable engineers to select specific frequencies for adjustment.

Opinions on the usage of equalization vary amongst engineers. Some would argue that equalization should only be used to remove or reduce frequencies that were not part of the original signal; others only use EQ when adjustments in microphone placement have failed to yield acceptable results. Engineers seeking a processed sound quality may choose to use equalization liberally. Equalization may also be used to compensate for a difficult acoustic setting in live performance. For instance, cutting frequencies in the 31 to 125 Hz range can reduce unwanted ambient room noise and audible breathing noise. Also, if the singer's voice sounds dull within a given space, the engineer could add "ring" or "presence" to the voice by boosting the equalizer in the 2 k to 10 kHz range. This adjustment can also be made to increase text intelligibility.

Using equalization, a singer can easily brighten or darken their voice as needed in the studio or live performance without significant resonance manipulation. While this may not be desirable for all artists or all genres, it can be very beneficial in some situations such as commercial music. It is especially important to consider that the equalization settings used in the recording studio may create a representation of the voice that is not achievable in live performance without processing.

Compression

CCM singers often use a wide variety of timbral colors and intensity levels in their performance. Drastic changes between colors and intensity levels can prove problematic for the sound team. Compression is utilized to allow the engineers to limit the output of a sound source by a specified ratio. The user sets a maximum acceptable level for the output called the threshold. Then a ratio to reduce the output once it surpasses the threshold is set. The typical ratio for a singer is between 3:1 and 5:1. A 3:1 ratio indicates that for every 3 dB beyond the threshold level, the output will only increase by 1 dB. For example, if the singer went 21 dB beyond the threshold with a 3:1 ratio, the output would only be 7 dB beyond the threshold setting.

Moving the microphone toward the mouth with decreased vocal intensity or away from the mouth with increased intensity can provide some of the same results that you can achieve with compression and is preferable for the experienced artist. However, compression provides consistency and freedom, allowing the singer to focus on artistic presentation. This additional freedom is ideal for musical theatre performers, singers using head mounted microphones, singers performing with choreography, and those new to performing with a microphone. Compression can also be helpful for classical singers whose dynamic abilities can be impressive live, but are often difficult to record.

In situations where a standard compressor alters the overall tone quality in an unacceptable manner, engineers can turn to a multiband compressor. Multiband compressors allow the engineer to isolate a specific frequency range within the audio signal and set an individual compression setting within that frequency range. For instance, if a given tenor's resonance creates a dramatic boost in the 4 kHz range every time that he sings above an A4, a multiband compressor can be used to limit the signal only in that part of the voice. By setting a 3:1 ratio in the 4 kHz area at a threshold that corresponds to the amplitude peaks that appear when the performer sings above A4, the engineer can reduce the forward placement from the sound on only those notes that are aesthetically offensive while leaving the rest of the signal untouched. These units are available in both live and studio settings and can be a great alternative to compressing the entire signal.

and recording studios are designed to inhibit natural reverb. Without at least a little reverb, even the best singer can sound harsh and even amateurish.

In the mid-20th century, engineered reverb was created using a metal spring. As sound was transmitted through the spring, the strength of the signal caused the spring to vibrate. On the other end of the spring, the sound was transferred back into the system, but with the addition of frequency variations from the vibrating spring. When combined with the original audio signal, the engineers were able to create reverb. While some engineers still use spring reverb to obtain a specific effect, most now use digital units. Digital reverb units usually have settings for wet/dry, delay time (from milliseconds to seconds), and bright/dark. The wet/dry control adjusts the amount of direct signal (dry) and the amount of reverberated signal (wet). Delay time adjusts the amount of time between when the dry signal and wet signal reach the ear. The bright/dark control helps simulate the effects of various surfaces within a natural space. For instance, harder surfaces such as marble create a brighter tone quality while softer surfaces, such as wood, create a darker tone quality. By adjusting the various settings, engineers can transform almost any room into a cathedral, concert hall, or an outdoor stadium.

Reverberation

Reverberation (known as reverb in the audio industry) is one of the easier effects for singers to identify. Natural reverb occurs when the audience hears the direct signal from the sound source and then milliseconds later, they hear the sound source again as it is reflected off the sidewalls of the performance hall. Many CCM venues

Auto-Tune

Auto-Tune was first used in studios as a useful way to eliminate minor pitch imperfections in otherwise perfect performances. However, it has now turned into an industry standard that most singers use to some extent (Tyrangiel, 2009; WENN.com, 2012). Whether or not an artist agrees with Auto-Tune, it is a reality in today's market.

The two primary developers of Auto-Tune technology are Antares and Melodyne. Auto-Tune comes in two main types: "auto" and "graphical." "Auto" Auto-Tune allows the engineer to set specific parameters for pitch correction that are then completely computer controlled. "Graphical" Auto-Tune traces the pitch of the vocal track in a recording and plots the fundamental frequency on a linear graph. The engineer can then select specific notes for pitch correction. Engineers can also drag selected pitches to a different frequency, add or reduce vibrato, and change formant frequencies with a click of the mouse.

The Basics of Live Sound Systems

Live sound systems come in a variety of sizes accommodating singers looking for an in-studio practice unit to top-of-the-line stadium setups. The majority of singers require only a basic knowledge of the components commonly found on systems with one to eight inputs. Units beyond eight inputs frequently require an independent sound engineer to operate the system during live performance and are beyond the scope of this chapter.

Following the microphone, the next element in the signal chain is usually the mixer. The mixer provides controls for equalization, volume level, and auxiliary (which controls the volume level of external effects units such as reverb). Newer units provide options for controlling on-board digital effects (e.g., reverb, compression, etc.), which can save money, time, and space as opposed to buying separate units for each effect.

Mixers

Mixers are available as powered and unpowered units. Powered mixers combine an amplifier with a basic mixer, providing a compact solution for those who do not need a complex system. Unpowered mixers do not provide amplification and require the purchase of a separate amplifier to power these systems. The amplifier or powered mixer then connects to the speaker cabinets. Sound system speaker cabinets usually contain a "woofer" and a "tweeter." The "woofer" is a large round speaker that handles the bass frequencies while the "tweeter" is a small round or horn-shaped speaker that handles the treble frequencies. Frequencies are separated and sent to the appropriate speaker (woofer or tweeter) by a device called a crossover. Speakers come in two forms: active and passive. Passive speakers require a powered mixer or an amplifier in order to operate. Active speakers have an amplifier built into the cabinet and can be used to eliminate the need for a stand-alone amplifier.

Monitors

Perhaps the most important element of the live sound system for a singer is the monitor. A monitor is a speaker that faces the singer, usually positioned on the floor, which allows the performer to hear their voice in real-time through the system as they perform. On-stage volume levels can vary considerably, depending on venue, instrumentation, and genre performed. Live percussion often produces sound levels as high as 120 dB, resulting in an inability of the singer to monitor their own voice without amplification. Performance venues that do not offer sufficient vocal monitoring for the singer may place the singer in an undesirable position of performing without hearing themselves. Natural compensation for not being aware of one's own voice can lead to hyperfunction and increased phonotrauma with potential negative vocal consequences. Understanding the proper utilization of vocal monitors for CCM singers is essential for minimizing vocal overuse, regardless of genre. In-ear monitors are another option for performers. However, research has shown that there is little to no noise reduction in the preferred listening level of performers, and therefore, they offer little to no benefit in regards to hearing safety (Federman & Ricketts, 2008). There are pros and cons to both floor and in-ear monitors, but regardless of monitor type, all CCM singers should consider utilization of vocal monitoring.

Buying a Sound System for Your Studio

For most voice teachers, a basic system is more than enough to meet the needs of the client base. Companies such as Peavey, Fender, Behringer, Phonic, Powerpod, Harbinger, Yamaha, JBL, and Bose manufacture small units that will fit in most studios and will offer more than enough power for teaching applications. When shopping for a system, look for a mixer board with one to four inputs. Smaller systems usually consist of a powered mixer and two separate speaker cabinets. In order to get the best sound from the microphone, ensure the mixer has XLR inputs with separate gain, volume, treble, mid, and bass controls. If possible, look for a system that supplies phantom power so that you may use a condenser microphone if needed. Some units will have built-in reverb, but this is not necessary if using a digital voice processor.

Digital Voice Processors

Digital voice processors are still relatively new to the market and have yet to gain widespread usage among avocational and semi-professional singers. However, they are perfect for the needs of singers in those populations as well as voice teachers, as they provide settings for compression, reverb, and auto-tune in one small, portable, easy-to-use metal box. Some manufacturers also include extra effects such as equalization, voice doublers, and harmony generators.

Several brands of digital voice processors are available on the market, but the industry leader as of this printing is a company called TC-Helicon. TC-Helicon manufactures several different units that span from consumer to professional grade. The TC-Helicon VoiceLive Play offers the perfect balance of professional level voice processing with an easy to navigate user interface at a competitive price point. One downfall of the VoiceLive Play is that it offers very little control of the individual settings for each effect. Instead, the unit relies on professionally developed presets with very basic adjustments. Most singers and teachers would rather spend their time singing instead of making adjustments to each component, which is another reason why this unit is commonly a great fit for these populations.

Teaching with Audio Equipment

Voice teachers working with CCM clients must use their knowledge of sound reinforcement and enhancement to assist with optimizing performance, reducing vocal load, and achieving vocal goals. Combining knowledge of vocal function and considering the impact of the various elements of the signal chain, the singing teacher can resolve many issues with CCM singers.

Start with the Microphone

Taking the time to choose the best microphone for each performer can reduce the need for excessive equalization and compression. The best way to choose a microphone is to set up all possible options in a straight line. Have the performer go down the line and sing into each microphone. Write down what you notice in terms of sensitivity and the overall tone quality as they perform. Engage the singer in this process and help them become aware of the differences in tone quality amongst the various microphones. Is the microphone more or less sensitive than the others? Brighter or darker? Edgier or warmer? This process is called a "mic shoot-out"; it is worth spending as much time as needed on this step since the right microphone will minimize time spent in future steps. If the singer is working in a recording studio, it is perfectly acceptable to use a different microphone for each song. If the singer is performing live, they are usually better off selecting one microphone that works best for the majority of their songs and then making soundboard adjustments for additional desired effects.

If the recording engineer is attempting to capture the sound source as accurately as possible, they will ideally try to keep equalization adjustments at a minimum. However, if you are working with a singer who is accustomed to relying on the sound equipment for additional support, you can achieve a lot with skillful manipulation of the equalizer. Consider for a moment what we know about vocal acoustics. Research has shown that classical singers have a boost in the 3 to 5 kHz range, whereas CCM singers often have a boost all the way up to 10 kHz (American Academy of Teachers of Singing, 2008). A classical singer who is overblowing the microphone and has exhausted all microphone choices will need to adjust the equalizer. Access to a spectral analyzer will be useful as you attempt to identify the frequencies that match or surpass the amplitude of the fundamental, and may be contributing to overblowing the microphone. Using the graphic equalizer, select the frequency range identified and begin reducing frequencies in that range by a few decibels at a time until the desired sound is reached.

When working with rock singers who are struggling to get "edge" in their sound, appropriate use of equalizers may help minimize vocal trauma by boosting the frequencies within the 5 kHz to 10 kHz range. Boosting the signal in this frequency range can assist in creating an "edgy" quality. Experiment with varying levels of gain until a sound that works for the artist is identified. Take note of the settings for future reference.

Working with the Beginner

Beginning pop/rock singers may have sung along with the radio and perhaps performed at karaoke night or with a small band before they embark upon singing voice lessons. However, they are generally not accustomed to performing vocal exercises and are often hesitant to experiment with strange new sounds. Having a microphone, soundboard, and amplifier in the studio may make it easier to engage a beginning level pop/rock singer to commit to vocalise and vocal training. By improving their understanding of the utility of the exercises within the context of the genre they choose to sing, the teacher can often overcome emotional barriers to making vocal progress.

Modern technology and internet resources provide limitless options and educational tools for working with this population. One exercise that can be extremely useful is to create a video playlist that shows multiple performers singing live, singing without a microphone, and singing on a studio recording. As you watch the videos together, guide the client's listening using your knowledge of sound enhancement. Educate them on equalization, compression, reverb, and microphone sensitivity. Then review the videos and point out elements in the performances that may be beneficial or detrimental to the vocal health of the performer. By using established professionals as vocal models, the teacher will often have more success in convincing the beginner to commit to technical work.

The next step in training includes vocalizing the client off-microphone with the goal of creating a sound that is free and easy, even if it does not match what they perceive to be their ideal performance sound. Once vocal improvement is noted by the teacher in the singer's raw vocal production, place them on a microphone and ask them to perform the same exercises again. A significant difference in the tone quality when singing through the microphone should be noted by the singer and teacher. Discuss with the student how the system is interacting with their instrument and dialogue about the sound quality they would ultimately like to create. Teacher unfamiliarity with a given genre may be best

addressed by listening with the student to recordings of artists that the student perceives as vocal models. As you listen, help identify, with a critical ear, the digital effects being used on the recording. Make adjustments to the microphone system in your teaching studio to begin creating the tone quality of their desired aesthetic. For instance, if the client's raw voice is airy and lacks forward placement, boost the treble frequencies from 5 to 10 kHz and turn on a preset for voice tripling on your TC-Helicon VoiceLive Play. Add compression, reverb, and delay until the client begins to hear a sound they like. This process can help the students achieve success early in the training process, which can significantly improve student retention. The sound engineering modifications are not meant to disregard the importance of continued vocal training toward optimal technique, but rather to provide the singer-in-training with options to publically present their desired vocal output as they continue to train their instrument for optimal vocal function.

It has been the experience of this author that as clients begin to perceive changes in vocal effort that result in sounds (through the audio system) which match their aesthetic preferences, they begin to readily trust the instruction they are being given. Trust between teacher and client is the first step in any teaching relationship to facilitate training, so they can produce marketable sounds without heavy processing. The premise is to provide almost immediate reduction in vocal effort with excellent perceptual output as they continue learning vocal technique for their long-term health.

Although most singers will be fascinated by the technological side of modern singing, many will also be disappointed that their favorite singers do not perform as well as they once thought. This is an ideal time to play performances by singers who do sing well acoustically. Hopefully, the client will express an interest in also being able to produce sounds without digital enhancement. When they do, begin discussing with them the value of developing multiple facets within their own voice. The awareness of the potential in their instrument will usually result in a strong commitment to the training regimen you have prescribed.

Working with Professionals

Generalization of vocal training, aesthetic quality, technique, and experience in professional pop/rock singers is variable. Some singers sound great on and off-mic but seek help because of vocal difficulty, vocal pathology, or a desire to acquire new tone qualities. Others have recorded an album in a studio that used heavy processing, and they realize they are not able to reproduce the same sounds they made in the studio on the live stage. These seem to be the two most common situations, and below is a quick look at each scenario.

"Over-Singers"

Artists complaining of vocal fatigue or vocal pathology often "over-sing" and are not using the microphone in a way that minimizes vocal load with maximal output. In these situations, it is valuable to have the client sing several songs both on and off-mic. Ask them to sing their favorite song, their loudest song, their softest song, their most upbeat song, and a ballad. One verse and chorus of each will generally suffice; feel free to stop them whenever you are sure of what you are hearing. The purpose of listening to multiple song styles is to explore their

ability to utilize a variety of vocal colors. Additionally, dynamic range and body position in relation to the microphone should be assessed during the active performance.

Many artists who concurrently play guitar lean forward into the microphone, mainly from their neck throwing the vocal instrument out of alignment. Compensation for the lack of laryngeal freedom results in constriction and pushing. Help the client make adjustments to their microphone stand and discuss the type of microphone they are currently using. If they are constantly touching their lips to the windscreen of the microphone in order to be heard, perhaps they should consider a microphone with a higher sensitivity level. If the client is consistently over-singing, use YouTube to introduce them to artists that use the microphone as an extension of their instrument to achieve vocal power (for example, Axl Rose). Discuss how a singer can achieve a variety of vocal colors that ultimately become part of the texture of the song and guide them in exploring their own possibilities. Many rock singers never consider how lyrics, timbre, and intensity can intertwine to tell a story. Exploration of new vocal possibilities typically results in decreased vocal intensity and reduction in overall vocal load during performances.

Micro Versus Macro Listening

CCM singers often only listen to the macro-level of a song. They hear percussion, guitar, bass, and vocals at near maximum volume through their headphones or a stereo system, and assume that everyone on stage is performing loudly. This can lead to over-singing as the performer attempts to reach the extreme dynamic levels that they perceive. Teaching clients to listen at the microlevel can be helpful when attempting to reduce the urge to over-sing. To demonstrate the wide variety of color and intensity choices capable in even the most extreme genres, try beginning your listening with heavy metal. Two examples worth exploring are "Nothing Else Matters" and "The Unforgiven" on Metallica's "Black" album. These two songs are perfect examples of vocal nuance in a style that is known for being excessive at the macro level.

After listening to several examples, demonstrate a few options of how you can use the microphone to assist in producing a variety of timbres and intensity combinations and work through the singer's repertoire exploring the possibilities. Biofeedback tools, such as a sound level meter, may also be useful when attempting to explore a variety of dB levels for their singing. Free downloadable decibel meter applications are readily available on smartphones, or you can purchase a handheld sound level meter at most audio and electronic stores. To reinforce the singer's trust that they are singing with adequate vocal intensity, place them on the microphone and as they sing, randomly mute and unmute the microphone (or turn the volume up and down). Encourage them to sing at a consistent intensity regardless of whether the microphone is on or off. This process can be useful in teaching them the power boosting capabilities of a sound system and getting them to relax and let the equipment do the work. Increased comfort with microphone capabilities and response will assist the singer in performing with a decreased vocal load.

The Studio Singer

Singers who have recorded a studio album and then realize that their live performance does not meet audience expectations often struggle with technical and performance anxiety issues. With these singers, an in-depth knowledge of professional sound engineering can prove very useful in solving "vocal" problems quickly.

Sit down with the client and analyze each song on the album. Ask them how they recorded each track and listen to see if you can identify what effects were used on each piece. Following song analysis, attempt to determine whether or not the singer can realistically produce the recorded sound qualities raw, or if the singer will need to rely on digital processing during live performances to replicate the recorded sound. In either case, it is likely that digital processing, at least in the short term, may be warranted.

In these instances, it is advantageous for the singer to purchase their own TC-Helicon unit. For performers who have sizable set lists, the TC-Helicon VoiceLive 2 is the best choice as it offers the ability to program multiple songs with unique settings for each section of each song. Although the upfront programming time may be cumbersome, the long-term results of reduced vocal load and consistent performance are worth the effort. It can also be valuable to have the singer watch other professionals on YouTube who also use digital enhancement (e.g., "Pumped Up Kicks" by Foster the People). In today's market, using these tools is nothing to be ashamed of; for many genres, enhancement is assumed. As singers become comfortable with their set list using the digital processing equipment, it will be helpful to pursue technical voice training that moves them away from relying solely on electronic enhancement. Although these performers may continue to use enhancement equipment even with professional training, the next time they return to the recording studio, it will hopefully be by choice and not necessity.

Dealing with Pitch Issues in the Recording Studio

Pitch inaccuracy issues in the recording studio often have more to do with adjusting to using a click track (the studio name for a metronome) and listening to oneself through headphones than actual pitch problems. If you have a singer preparing to work in a studio setting, it can be advantageous to work with both a metronome and headphones within the voice lesson. From a macro viewpoint, the vocal line in an epic ballad such as "Come Sail Away" by Styx could easily be considered "big and flowing." But careful observation at the micro-level, reveals the singer's rhythm to be very crisp. In order for a studio singer to avoid auto-tune, they need to be precise. Practicing ahead of time with a metronome will improve rhythmic accuracy before the singer is put on the spot in front of the studio microphone.

To prepare the singer for singing with headphones, ask them to bring an instrumental or karaoke track to their lesson. Plug a set of headphones into the sound system in your studio and have the student sing along with the prerecorded track (you can also listen to what they are hearing through the system by purchasing a headphone splitter at your local electronics store). As they are singing, make adjustments to the volume level of their voice and the volume level of the track. Pay close attention to when they begin singing off-pitch. Help the singer identify what seems to throw them off and help them come up with coping strategies. If nothing else, having the confidence to ask the sound engineer for more vocals in the headphones can save hours of wasted studio time.

Pitch Issues in Live Performance

Pitch issues in live performance are typically the result of poor monitor feedback. Adequate vocal monitors when performing live are essential. The TC-Helicon units have two output jacks on the back. If a client performs in venues that do not supply monitors, they can purchase their own active monitor and attach it to one of the TC-Helicon output jacks. Most monitoring systems allow the sound engineer to adjust the volume of individual instruments as well as the overall volume level of the bands, as bass guitars can sound very muddy up close. It is usually best to reduce the volume of the bass guitar in the monitor mix. The rhythm guitar and/or keyboards generally supply the tonal structure of the song. If the singer is unable to hear either instrument underneath the vocals, the singer will frequently struggle to stay on pitch. When setting up at the performance venue, sound checks should include the loudest and softest songs. Encourage the singer to talk with the sound engineer and adjust the levels of vocals and guitar/piano until they are at a comfortable level.

During private lessons, assist your clients by simulating a live situation where they cannot hear themselves. The TC-Helicon units all offer a headphone jack on the back. Plug your client's instrument into the sound system but do not turn the volume up on their microphone. Have them sing and play while you listen to their voice through the headphones. Take notes on where they are having difficulties, and then assist them with coping strategies to overcome the lack of vocal feedback. Then experiment with turning the volume up and down on the live system so that they have the experience of singing with varying levels of auditory feedback. By working on this issue during a lesson, the singer will be prepared in case a similar situation happens in live performance.

Chapter Summary

As an undergraduate conservatory student, this author experienced some older colleagues and professors dismissing singers who relied on audio technology, such as musical theatre performers and pop singers. They talked about historically great singers and the absence of such singers on the stage presently. Perhaps singers and teachers of elder generations have always lamented the loss of the great singers, while criticizing the new generation of rising vocal stars. In the 19th century, Giovanni Lamperti defined what he believed to be the "Golden Age of Song," the period when Bellini, Donizetti, and Rossini were still composing (Lamperti, 1973). In 1937, voice teacher Marcia Davenport praised great singers such as Emma Eames and Geraldine Farrar of the early 20th century who were "polished, mature, seasoned" and unlike young singers of the 1930s, which she believed were "coddled" and were "wasting their time" (Davenport, 1937). Voice teachers of the 1930s also criticized popular crooners of their era. Teachers considered crooners to be a "perversion of the natural production of the singing voice," and accused the artists of singing in a style that was "injurious to the voice" with "words and sounds of the gutter" (McCracken, 1999). By 1958 Frank Sinatra, one of the original crooners, was testifying in front of Congress about "the most brutal, ugly, desperate, vicious form of expression it has been my misfortune to hear," referring to Rock 'n' Roll (Szatmary,

1996). It seems these debates have existed for many decades, possibly even centuries.

Whether teachers of singing approve of it or not, audio enhancement of the voice is here to stay. Just as prior generations have adapted and evolved with the aesthetics of the artistic market place, this generation will morph as well. Because of internet access and abundant opportunities for consumers/producers to gain mass media attention, the public now plays a greater role than ever before in determining the artists who succeed and those who do not. Increased knowledge of available modern technologies allows for improvement in dialogue with those on the other side of the operating board who continually strive to capture performances that truthfully represent the talents of the singer.

References

Alarcon, R., & Jones, S. (2009). Measurement of decibel exposure in college students from personal music devices. *International Journal of Academic Research, 1*(2), 99–107.

Alter, G. (2009). *Four shows, four dramatically different designs.* MixOnline.com. Retrieved from http://mixonline.com/live /applications/broadway-sound-1009/.

American Academy of Teachers of Singing. (2008). NATS visits AATS. *The Journal of Singing, 65*(1), 7–10.

Benzuly, S. (2011). *Sir Paul McCartney tour profile.* MixOnline.com. Retrieved from http://mixonline.com/live/tourprofiles /sir_paul_mccartney_tour/.

Björkner, E. (2008). Musical theater and opera singing—Why so different? A study of subglottal pressure, voice source, and formant frequency characteristics. *Journal of Voice, 22*(5), 533–40. doi:10.1016/j. jvoice.2006.12.007.

Buskin, R. (2001, December). Brian transeau: Emotional experience. *Sound on Sound,* pp. 1–5. Retrieved from http://www .soundonsound.com/sos/dec01/articles /briantranseau.asp.

Buskin, R. (2008, May). Luciano Pavarotti "Nessun Dorma"—Classic tracks. *Sound on Sound.* Retrieved from http://www .soundonsound.com/sos/may08/articles /classictracks_0508.htm.

Davenport, M. (1937, December 11). "What makes a singer?" *The Saturday Evening Post,* pp. 20–21, 83–88.

Eskow, G. (2008, April). *New York's Met in HD.* Retrieved from http://mixonline.com /post/features/audio_new_yorks_met/.

Federman, J., & Ricketts, T. (2008). Preferred and minimum acceptable listening levels for musicians while using floor and in-ear monitors. *Journal of Speech, Language, and Hearing Research, 51*(February), 147–159.

Grant, M. N. (2004). *The rise and fall of the Broadway musical.* Boston, MA: Northeastern University Press.

Horning, S. S. (2004). Engineering the performance: Recording engineers, tacit knowledge and the art of controlling sound. *Social Studies of Science, 34*(5), 703–731. doi:10.1177/0306312704047536.

Howard, D. M., & Murphy, D. T. (2008). *Voice science, acoustics and recording.* San Diego, CA: Plural Publishing.

Jones, S. & Alarcon, R. (2009). Measurement of decibel exposure in college students from personal music devices. *International Journal of Academic Research, 1*(2), 99–106.

Lamperti, G. B. (1973). *Vocal wisdom; Maxims of Giovanni Battista Lamperti.* New York, NY: Crescendo Publishing.

Library of Congress. (2013). *Acoustical recording.* Retrieved from http://www.loc .gov/jukebox/about/acoustical-recording.

McCracken, A. (1999). "God's gift to us girls: Crooning, gender, and the re-creation of American popular song, 1928–1933." *American Music, 17*(4), 831.

Morange, S., Dubois, D., & Fontaine, J. M. (2010). Perception of recorded singing voice quality and expertise: Cognitive linguistics and acoustic approaches. *Journal of Voice, 24*(4), 450–7. doi:10.1016/j.jvoice .2008.08.006.

Pelton, G. E. (1993). *Voice processing.* Whitby, ON: McGraw-Hill Ryerson.

Szatmary, D. P. (1996). *A time to rock: A social history of rock and roll.* New York, NY: Schirmer Books.

Tyrangiel, J. (2009, February). Auto-tune: Why pop music sounds perfect. *Time,* pp. 1–4. Retrieved from http://www.time.com/time /printout/0,8816,1877372,00.html.

WENN.com. (2012, July 4). Bieber admits studio vocal help. *Toronto Sun.* Retrieved from http://www.torontosun.com/2012/07/04 /bieber-admits-studio-vocal-help.

Wollman, E. L. (2006). *The theater will rock: A history of the rock musical: From Hair to Hedwig.* Ann Arbor, MI: University of Michigan Press.

Index

Note: Page numbers in **bold** reference non-text material.